ON THE STUDY AND PRACTICE OF INTRAVENOUS ANAESTHESIA

ON THE STUDY AND PRACTICE OF INTRAVENOUS ANAESTHESIA

Edited by

Jaap Vuyk

Leiden University Medical Center, Leiden, The Netherlands

Frank Engbers

Leiden University Medical Center, Leiden, The Netherlands

and

Sandra Groen-Mulder

Leyenburg Hospital, The Hague, The Netherlands

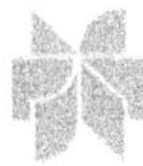

Springer-Science+Business Media, B.V.

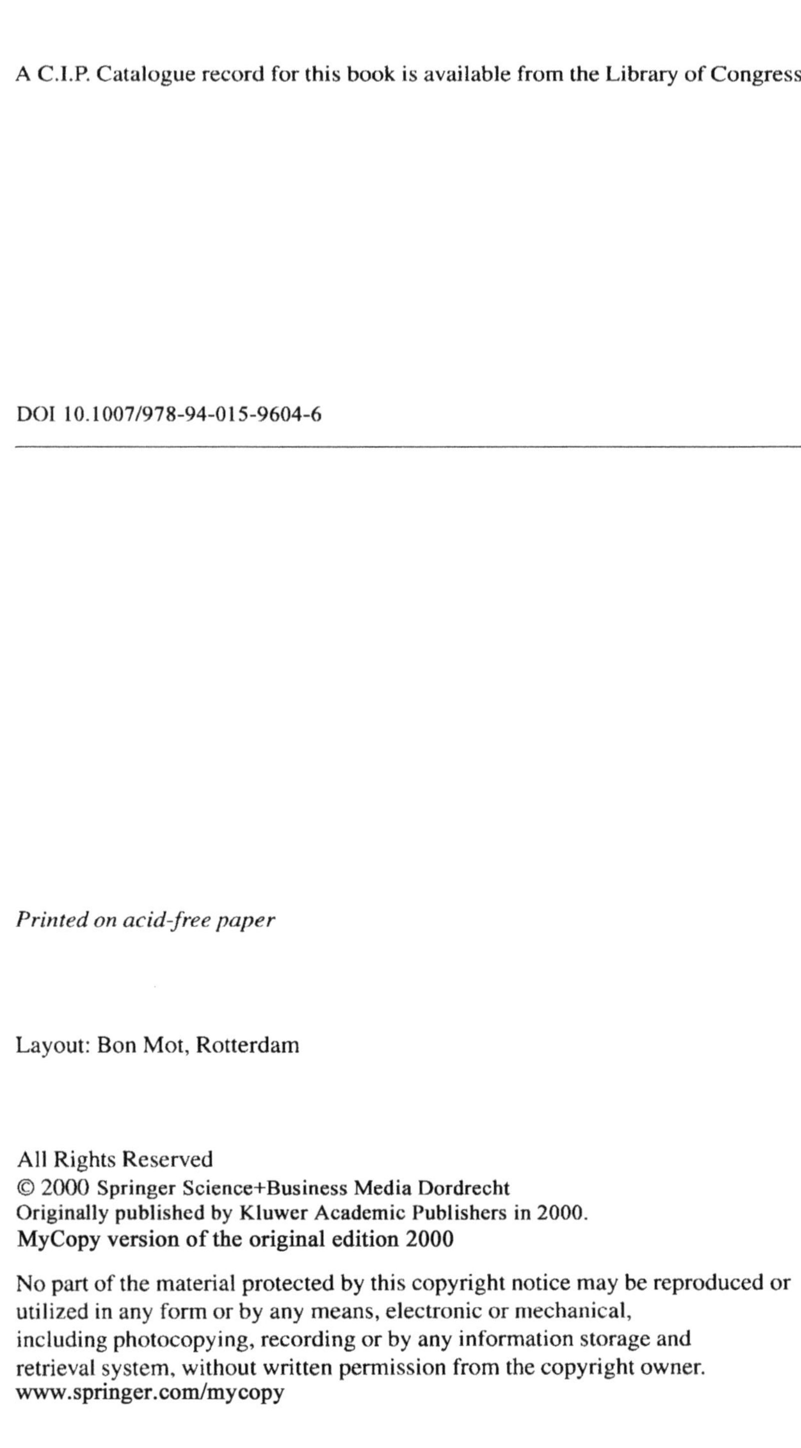

A C.I.P. Catalogue record for this book is available from the Library of Congress.

DOI 10.1007/978-94-015-9604-6

Printed on acid-free paper

Layout: Bon Mot, Rotterdam

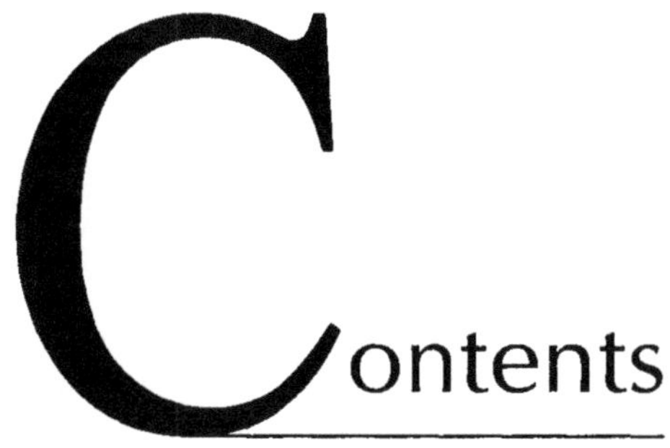

THE PERIOPERATIVE USE OF HYPNOTIC AGENTS

STATE OF THE ART ON NEUROMUSCULAR BLOCKADE

OPIOIDS FOR PERIOPERATIVE PAIN RELIEF

List of contributors

A. Absalom
University Department of Anaesthesia
Glasgow Royal Infirmary
10 Alexandra Parade, Glasgow G31 2ER, UK

D. Amutike
HCI International Medical Centre
Bearmore Street
Clydebank, Glasgow G81 4HX, UK

L. Barvais
Department of Anesthesiology
Erasme University Hospital
808 route de Lennik, B-1070 Brussels, Belgium

B. Bennett
Departments of Anesthesiology and Pharmacology, University of Colorado
Health Sciences Center, Denver, Colorado 80262
And Institute for Behavioral Genetics, University of Colorado, Boulder,
Colorado 80309, USA

V. Billard
Department of Anaesthesiology
Institut Gustave Roussy; 94805 Villejuif, France

Y. Blednov
Departments of Anesthesiology and Pharmacology, University of Colorado
Health Sciences Center, Denver, Colorado 80262
And Institute for Behavioral Genetics, University of Colorado, Boulder,
Colorado 80309, USA

A. Borgeat
Orthopedic University Clinic, Balgrist / Zurich
Forchstrasse 340, CH - 8008 Zurich, Switzerland

J. G. Bovill
Leiden University Medical Center
Albinusdreef 2, 2300 RC, Leiden, The Netherlands

E. Coussaert
Department of Anesthesiology
Erasme University Hospital
808 route de Lennik, B-1070 Brussels, Belgium

A. Craig
University of Plymouth/Derriford Hospital Plymouth
Derriford Road, Plymouth, PL6 8DH, UK

A. Dahan
Leiden University Medical Center
Albinusdreef 2, 2300 RC, Leiden, The Netherlands

C. Diefenbach
Dept. of Anesthesiology & Intensive Care
University Hospital Cologne
D-50924 Köln, Germany

F. Donati
Département d'anesthésie - réanimation de l'université de Montréal
Campus Hôtel Dieu
3840 rue Saint-Urbain
Montréal, Québec, Canada H2W 1T8

F.H.M. Engbers
Leiden University Medical Center
Albinusdreef 2, 2300 RC, Leiden, The Netherlands

S.M. Groen-Mulder
Leyenburgh Hospital
The Hague, The Netherlands

K. Ikeda
Surgical Center, University Hospital of Hamamatsu
3600 Handa, Hamamatsu 431-3192, Japan

T. Johnson
Departments of Anesthesiology and Pharmacology, University of Colorado
Health Sciences Center, Denver, Colorado 80262
And Institute for Behavioral Genetics, University of Colorado, Boulder,
Colorado 80309, USA

T. Kazama
Surgical Center, University Hospital of Hamamatsu
3600 Handa, Hamamatsu 431-3192, Japan

G.N.C. Kenny
University Department of Anaesthesia
Glasgow Royal Infirmary
10 Alexandra Parade, Glasgow G31 2ER, UK

K.S. Khünl-Brady
Department of Anaesthesia and Intensive Care Medicine
The Leopold-Franzens-University of Innsbruck, Anichstrasse 35
A-6020 Innsbruck, Austria

P. Mavoungou
Department of Anaesthesiology
Clinique Mutualiste, Nantes, France.

H. Mellinghoff
Dept. of Anesthesiology & Intensive Care
University Hospital Cologne
D-50924 Köln, Germany

K. Morita
Surgical Center, University Hospital of Hamamatsu
3600 Handa, Hamamatsu 431-3192, Japan

C. Moiny
Department of Anesthesiology
Erasme University Hospital
808 route de Lennik, B-1070 Brussels, Belgium

E. Mortier
Department of Anaesthesia
University Hospital of Gent
De Pintelaan 185, 9000 Gent, Belgium

M. van den Nieuwenhuyzen
Leiden University Medical Center
Albinusdreef 2, 2300 RC, Leiden, The Netherlands

B. Plaud
Département d'anesthésie – réanimation
Institut Gustave Roussy
39 rue Camille Desmoulins
94800 Villejuif, France

J.C. Ræder,
Department of Anaesthesia
Ullevaal University Hospital
N-0407 Oslo, Norway

B. Rikke
Departments of Anesthesiology and Pharmacology, University of Colorado
Health Sciences Center, Denver, Colorado 80262
And Institute for Behavioral Genetics, University of Colorado, Boulder,
Colorado 80309, USA

E. Sarton
Leiden University Medical Center
Albinusdreef 2, 2300 RC, Leiden, The Netherlands

S. Sato
Surgical Center, University Hospital of Hamamatsu
3600 Handa, Hamamatsu 431-3192, Japan

S. Schraag
Department of Anaesthesiology
University of Ulm
Steinhoevelstrasse 9, D-89075 Ulm, Germany

F. Servin
Département d'Anesthésie et de Réanimation Chirurgicale
C.H.U. Bichat-Claude Bernard
46, rue Henri Huchard, 75877, Paris Cedex 18, France

E. Shen
Departments of Anesthesiology and Pharmacology, University of Colorado
Health Sciences Center, Denver, Colorado 80262
And Institute for Behavioral Genetics, University of Colorado, Boulder,
Colorado 80309,USA

V. J. Simpson
Departments of Anesthesiology and Pharmacology, University of Colorado
Health Sciences Center, Denver, Colorado 80262
and Institute for Behavioral Genetics, University of Colorado, Boulder,
Colorado 80309, USA

J.R. Sneyd
University of Plymouth/Derriford Hospital Plymouth
Derriford Road, Plymouth, PL6 8DH, UK

M. Struys
Department of Anaesthesia
University Hospital of Gent
De Pintelaan 185, 9000 Gent, Belgium

N. Sutcliffe
Department of Anaesthesiology
Healthcare International
Glasgow, UK

L. Versichelen
Department of Anaesthesia
University Hospital of Gent
De Pintelaan 185, 9000 Gent, Belgium

J. Vuyk
Leiden University Medical Center
Albinusdreef 2, 2300 RC, Leiden, The Netherlands

M.Weiss
Section of Pharmacokinetics, Department of Pharmacology
Martin Luther University Halle-Wittenberg, D-06097 Halle, Germany

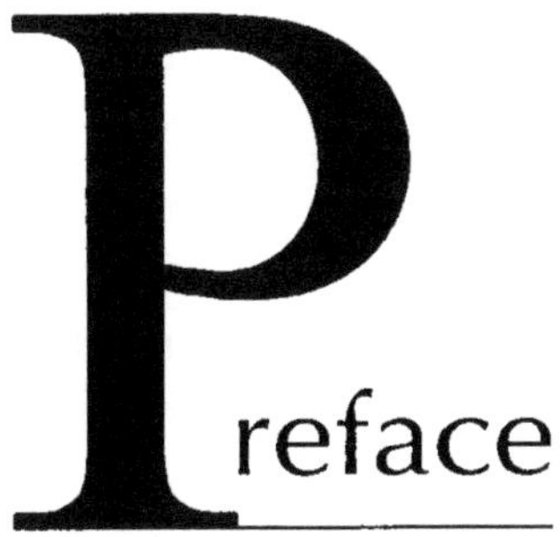

Preface

In recent years the study and practice of intravenous anaesthesia has gained increasing interest, both among the scientifically and more clinically oriented anaesthesiologists. The high standard of intravenous anaesthesia today has been achieved due to advances in technology, the development of shorter acting agents with less side effects and an increasing understanding of anaesthetic agent pharmacology and human (patho)physiology.

Modern anaesthesia has its roots in the early years of the 19th century and started on the basis of inhalational anaesthesia with ether, chloroform and nitrous oxide. Later on, also intravenous agents were used to produce the state of anaesthesia, initially with chloral hydrate, followed in the early decades of this century by barbiturates, benzodiazepines, synthetic opioids, propofol and remifentanil as the latest branches on the intravenous tree.

In contrast to the rapid developments during the first decades of this century in the inhalational anaesthetic field, resulting in sophisticated delivery and monitoring systems like vaporisers and the online measurement of the end-tidal inhalational agent concentration, most intravenous anaesthetics were, up until recently, administered in the form of droplets on a dose per kg body weight basis, a situation which resembles the administration of inhalational agents by the Schimmelbusch mask as was common practice in the period 1920-1940. This is, however, all rapidly changing now. Over the past two decades the knowledge on the pharmacokinetics and pharmacodynamics of intravenous anaesthetic agents has rapidly been growing. This has resulted in a better understanding of the drug dose - blood concentrations - biophase concentration - effect relationship. This body of knowledge has not been secluded within the close circle of anaesthetic scientists but, with the help of computer technology, has greatly influenced the practice of the modern clinical anaesthesiologist. The efforts of anaesthesiologists, pharmaceutical companies, and the development of the internet has lead to a situation that now almost every anaesthesiologist can be in close contact to anaesthetic pharmacology computer simulation programs and target controlled infusion devices. These two tools allow us to increase our understanding and improve the controllability of anaesthetic drug administration, on site, in the operating theatre. In Europe the growing enthusiasm regarding the study and practice of intravenous anaesthesia has lead to an increased output of manuscripts on this subject, the initiation of workshops on the pharmacology of anaesthetic agents and the formation of a society that embodies this spirit; the European Society for Intravenous Anaesthesia, the EuroSIVA.

EuroSIVA

The concept of EuroSIVA has been to provide a forum to co-ordinate, facilitate and promote high quality presentations in the area of intravenous drug administration. The first two meetings held in 1988 in Barcelona and 1999 in Amsterdam achieved these aims. During the Barcelona and Amsterdam meetings presenters of over 10 countries shared their knowledge with 250 and 400 participants, respectively. In addition to the EuroSIVA meetings the international board aims to promote education for those involved with intravenous anaesthesia. A central part of the educational activity has been the introduction of practical workshops that allow participants to have a hands on experience with a computer simulation program on intravenous anaesthetic agents and opioids, in small groups guided by experienced workshop trainers. These workshops have proven popular with both experienced and less experienced users, and have served to enhance the understanding for those administering drugs intravenously. The annual EuroSIVA meetings take place immediately before the meetings of the European Society of Anaesthesiology.

On the study and practice of intravenous anaesthesia

This book is the result of the efforts of the speakers and chairmen of the past two EuroSIVA meetings held in Barcelona and Amsterdam in 1998 and 1999, respectively. The manuscripts, brought together in this book, give an overview of the presentations at these meetings and thereby offer you an insight into the state of the art on intravenous anaesthesia science and the application of scientific data into clinical practice. The book is divided into 4 sections with subjects on the modelling of anaesthetic action with special interest in the effect site, the perioperative use of intravenous hypnotic agents, the state of the art of neuromuscular blockade, and lastly, on opioids as used for perioperative pain relief. We hope that this book breathes the same atmosphere of scientific forward movement and sharing of interest in intravenous anaesthetic drug pharmacology as experienced in the Barcelona and Amsterdam meetings. Furthermore we are sure that it will be of educational value to all of us who are involved in the science and clinical application of anaesthesia.

The Barcelona and Amsterdam EuroSIVA meetings would not have been possible without the strong support of AstraZeneca, GlaxoWellcome and Organon. Furthermore, we would like to acknowledge the generous financial support by GlaxoWellcome that made the publication of this book possible.

Jaap Vuyk
Frank Engbers
Sandra Groen-Mulder
Gavin Kenny

Leiden, The Hague and Glasgow, August 1999

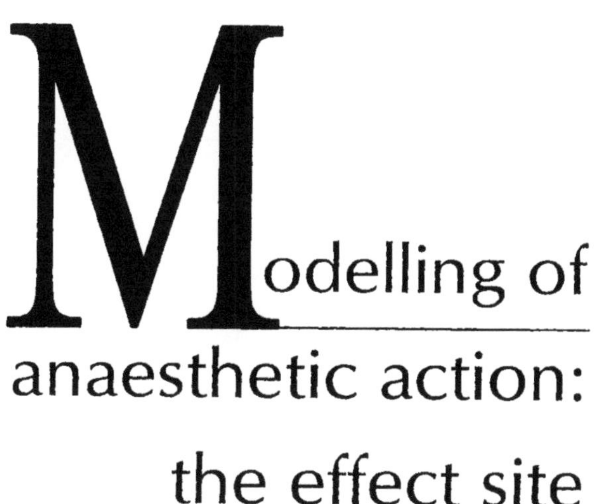

Modelling of anaesthetic action: the effect site

PHYSIOLOGICAL MODELLING AND THE EFFECT SITE

Michael Weiss

Halle-Wittenberg, Germany

Introduction

Traditional pharmacokinetic/pharmacodynamic (PK/PD) modelling is based on a concept introduced by Segre[1] more than thirty years ago: the concentration in the plasma compartment, $C(t)$, of a mammillary compartmental model is linked to the time course of the pharmacological effect, $E(t)$, via a simple first order delay (time constant $\tau = 1/k_{eo}$) determining a hypothetical concentration-time curve at the effect site [biophase level, $C_B(t)$] and a static, nonlinear $C_B(t)$ - effect relationship (figure 1).

Recently, a more general approach based on system analysis has been proposed,[2,3] to describe the behaviour of the system without making detailed structural assumptions. However, since such empirical or black-box models are based on multiexponential disposition curves they have the same limitations as compartmental models. Firstly, they do not describe the initial distribution from the injection to the effect site after bolus injection which is of importance for the onset of action when drugs have a very short effect site equilibration time, τ. Secondly, these models do not account for the influence of changes in haemodynamics on the PK profile, in contrast to the fact that convective transport by blood flow is the fundamental transport process in the body. Third, the traditional approaches fail if active metabolites are formed which contribute to the observed $E(t)$ profile. Although physiological pharmacokinetic models represent a possible alternative in these cases, questions of model selection and

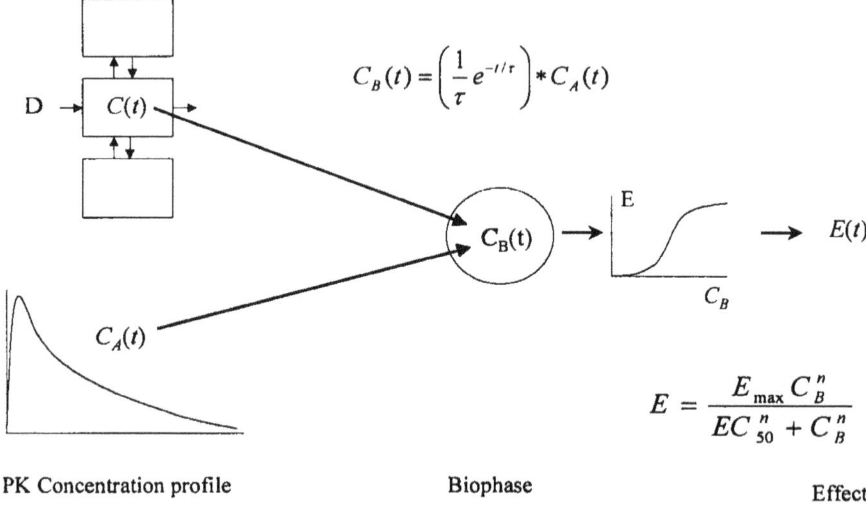

Figure 1
Structure of the PK/PD model (*denotes convolution).

experimental design are key issues since the validity of a model is always defined in terms of the modelling objectives. In this paper we will discuss these problems for short acting drugs like neuromuscular blockers and intravenous anaesthetics and drugs which form active metabolites, like morphine.

Limitations of compartmental and behavioural models

In conventional PK models distribution is assumed to take place between homogenous compartments which cannot be defined anatomically. In the present context, one main disadvantage of mammillary compartmental models is the assumption of a well-mixed plasma (sampling) compartment which is in contrast to noninstantaneous circulatory mixing, i.e. the fact that the concentration-time curve after bolus iv injection (drug disposition curve) is not monotonically decreasing.[4] This is demonstrated in figure 2 where data, simulated using a physiologic circulatory model (described below), are fitted by a two-compartmental model, i.e. a biexponential drug disposition function. The compartmental model fitted the data very well for a 5 min infusion (figure 2A1), but then failed to describe the arterial PK profile simulated by the physiological model

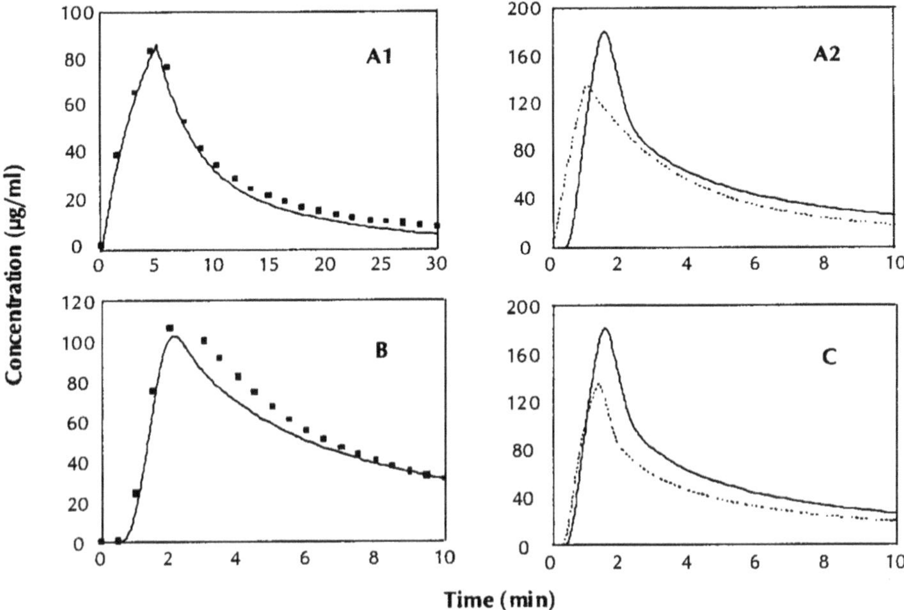

Figure 2
Recirculatory model simulations for sorbitol, a highly cleared extracellular marker[5] (see text).

for a 1 min infusion (figure 2A2, dashed line). Furthermore, a homogenous sampling compartment does not account for the transient differences between arterial and peripheral venous $C(t)$-profiles, which can be pronounced in the first minutes after injection. Thus, the use of venous instead of arterial concentration in PK/PD modelling may lead to an underestimation of the effect site equilibration time constant τ (which may become even negative).[6,7] This is illustrated in figure 2B, where for a hypothetical drug which distributes only into the extracellular space, the equilibration time constant between arterial concentration (C_A) and effect (E) is dramatically underestimated (τ = 0.2 min) when venous blood samples are used to fit the biophase $C_B(t)$ data simulated using the arterial $C_A(t)$ input and an equilibration time of τ = 1 min.

Model selection

Selection among alternative models should be based on at least three validity criteria: theoretical, empirical and heuristic validity,[8] which means that the model must be in accordance with the accepted theories and laws (e.g., conservation of matter) as well as the available experimental data, and should have explanatory power. Behavioural or black-box models may be very useful in certain cases, e.g. to control infusion pumps, but they do not have heuristic validity. To explain the behaviour of a system we need a structural model. Although the compartmental models belong to this class, their heuristic validity is low. For example, they cannot explain the effect of haemodynamics on the distribution kinetics of drugs. The explanatory power increases with increasing isomorphicity, whereby the degree of structural complexity depends on the application intended. As discussed above, compartmental models also lack empirical validity regarding the early distribution phase and this also holds for any other approach where the impulse response function of the PK system is described by a multiexponential curve.[2,3] Both model selection and experimental design must aim on an adequate characterisation of the PK profile. Another important issue is model identifiability. Although the structure of the pharmacokinetic model is well known a priori - since it is given by the circulatory multiorgan structure of the body - this model cannot be identified on the basis of plasma concentration-time data. In simplifying the model, one must avoid model misspecification since this would lead to biased parameter estimates.

Multiorgan models

As a first approximation whole body physiological models are based on organ models in its simplest form, namely well-mixed compartments, however, the latter assumption implies that the distribution kinetics within the organs is flow limited, which is a crude oversimplification for most drugs. An improvement is a two-compartment organ model where the vascular and tissue space are still well mixed but separated by a permeability barrier. Each organ and subsystem of the whole body model is then characterised by five parameters: blood flow (Q), vascular or plasma volume (V_P), permeability-surface product or distribution clearance (CL_{PT}), tissue volume (V_T), and tissue-plasma partition coefficient (K). Assuming that the physiological/anatomical parameters for the species under consideration are known, the only drug related parameter for the one-compartment organ model is the steady-state parameter, K. Any more general model can only be identified by kinetic experiments and destructive sampling,

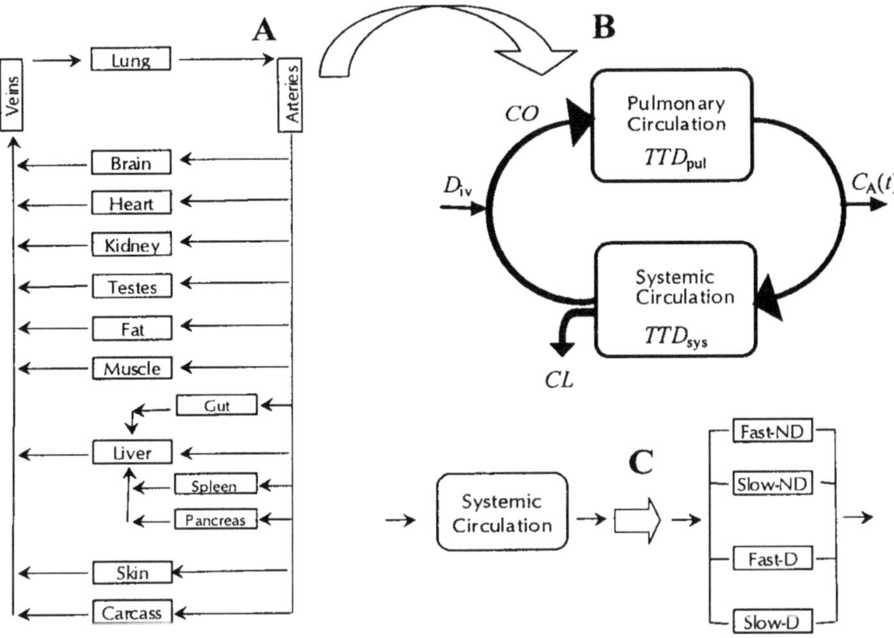

Figure 3
Physiological multi-organ model (A), recirculatory model (B) and hybrid model (C).

which means that one animal provides one point to the tissue concentration-time profiles which have to be measured for all organs in the physiological model to estimate the intrinsic distribution clearances, CL_{PT}. The fundamental work in this field has been published by the Stanford group for fentanyl, alfentanil and thiopental.[9,10] After identification of a relatively complex 12 organ model (figure 3A) by destructive sampling in rats and upscaling to humans (assuming that the organ partition coefficients and distribution clearances remained unchanged) the model well described the disposition curves of these drugs. Computer simulations then provide insight into the physiological determinants of the PK profile, as shown for the effect of cardiac output, obesity, gender and age for thiopental.[11]

Thus, physiological whole body models may be very useful to explain the sources of PK variability as also demonstrated for alfentanil and fentanyl.[12] However, such multiorgan models have two disadvantages. Firstly, they cannot be identified on the basis of clinical pharmacokinetic data (the model mentioned above contains more than 100 parameters). Secondly, they are of limited value describing the early mixing phase after bolus injection (mainly because a well-mixed vascular space is assumed for the central circulation). Thus, besides complexity reduction, the use of a concept which is not based on well-mixed spaces (also at the organ level) is an important issue.

Organ transit time distribution

To ensure the identifiability of physiological models two strategies can be applied: (i) model decomposition into subsystems which can be identified separately, and (ii) reduction of the complexity of the model, i.e. use of a simplified structural model which still satisfies the goal of the study.

Organ models which are more complex than the above mentioned two-compartment models can be identified when the organs are studied as separate subsystems. In experiments with isolated perfused organs the single-pass outflow curve is measured after bolus injection (impulse response) and under in vivo conditions the corresponding information can be obtained from the input and output concentration-time profile of the organ. The question is then how to analyse the data without assuming well-mixed spaces, i.e. using either differential equations or multiexponential response functions. The theory of organ transit time distributions is such a general framework. The unit impulse response function of the organ (normalised outflow profile) represents the transit time density function, $f_{org}(t)$. While the mean transit time, MTT [first moment of $f_{org}(t)$] determines the extent of distribution, since the steady-state volume of distribution is the product of blood flow and MTT ($V_{ss} = Q\ MTT$), the relative dispersion of transit times, RD (variance/MTT^2, calculated using the second moment), gives information on the kinetics of distribution. To utilise the information inherent in the RD estimate one needs a physiological organ model like the stochastic two-phase model[13] which has been applied to the distribution kinetics of lidocaine, diazepam and antipyrine in the isolated perfused rat hindlimb.[14] The model determines RD in terms of intravascular convective dispersion, transcapillary permeation and tissue diffusion, whereby the information on intravascular mixing is obtained from the relative dispersion (RD_P) of an intravascular indicator which is administered and measured simultaneously. These results on the distribution kinetics of diazepam and lidocaine in the isolated hindlimb indicate that binding of drug molecules to tissue constituents slows down the rate of diffusion considerably. If instead of fitting the complete model to the data only the relative dispersion has been estimated, a lower bound of the ratio organ distribution clearance to organ blood flow can be determined[13]

$$\frac{CL_{PT}}{Q} \geq \frac{2v^2}{(1+v)^2} \frac{1}{RD - RD_P}$$

where $v = (V_{ss}\text{-}V_P)/V_P$ and the vascular volume, V_P, is obtained from the *MTT* of the vascular marker, $V_P = Q\ MTT_P$. (Equality holds in the Equation when the process of intratissue diffusion is fast compared to plasma-tissue permeation.). To estimate the parameters *MTT* and *RD* the curve moments can be calculated by numerical integration or by fitting an empirical parametric function to the data.

Boer et al.[15] measured concentration-time profiles in the pulmonal artery and the aorta of pigs after a bolus dose of alfentanil and indocyanine green (ICG) as vascular marker. The estimated distribution volumes of 486 and 313 ml together with the relative dispersions of 0.42 and 0.12 for alfentanil and ICG, respectively, can be used to predict the CL_{PT}/Q ratio for alfentanil in the lungs: from the above Equation we obtain an estimate of 0.84 (Q = 2190 ml/min) which indicates permeability limited distribution (the approximation of flow limited distribution would hold for $CL_{PT}/Q >> 1$.). The role of the cardiopulmonary system as first-pass organ after the bolus injection, i.e. the fact that in the first three minutes after bolus injection the $C_A(t)$ profile is mainly determined by the transit time density of the drug through the lungs, explains the importance of more detailed organ models in intravenous anaesthesia. Physiological organ models like the stochastic two-phase model with parameters estimated in experiments with isolated perfused organs have also been used as subsystems in whole body multiorgan models to reveal the effect of intravascular mixing and slow tissue diffusion on the disposition of fentanyl, alfentanil and thiopental.[16]

Recirculatory minimal models

The organ transit time density functions determine the residence time distribution of the drug in the body,[17] as shown by recirculatory modelling more than 20 years ago.[18,19] Complexity reduction is the idea behind the introduction of so-called minimal models; although all physiological models are recirculatory models this term is mostly used for a model consisting of only two subsystems (figure 3B) which can be used to analyse clinical pharmacokinetic data.

For iv injection and arterial sampling the subsystems are the pulmonary and the systemic circulation. This model has been used to analyse the disposition of sorbitol in humans after bolus injection.[5] Assuming an empirical transit time density function (inverse Gaussian density) for both subsystems, six parameters have to be estimated: cardiac output (*CO*), systemic clearance (*CL*), the steady-state distribution volumes (V_{pul}, V_{sys}) and relative transit time dispersions (RD_{pul}, RD_{sys}) of the pulmonary and systemic circulation, respectively. One advantage of this minimal recirculatory model is the noncompartmental assessment of distribution kinetics utilising the information given by the relative dispersion of circulation times. The latter determines the whole body distribution clearance which can be presented in terms of the intercompartmental distribution clearances of mammillary compartmental models.[20] For sorbitol it could be shown that the distribution clearance correlates with cardiac output, in agreement with the results obtained by Henthorn et al.[21] for alfentanil using a compartmental model. A recirculatory model also well accounts for the effects of a change in haemodynamics induced by an infusion of the β-adrenoceptor agonist orciprenaline on sorbitol kinetics in healthy volunteers.[22] Orciprenaline increased cardiac output (*CO*) by 60 % which led to a decrease in peak concentration as demonstrated in figure 2C for a 1 min infusion (solid line, control; dashed line, orciprenaline). This effect which may be important for short acting intravenous anaesthetics follows from the fact that the area under the concentration peak, AUC_1 (i.e. the first-pass outflow curve of the pulmonary circulation neglecting recirculation) is given by $AUC_1 = D_{iv}/CO$. While the inverse Gaussian density function containing only two adjustable parameters *V* and *RD* has been found suitable for sorbitol and other extracellular indicators, it is not flexible enough to describe the long-tailed systemic transit time distribution of tissue bound drugs. For fentanyl and alfentanil a three-exponential function is sufficient if the drugs are administered as short-term infusions (unpublished results). This is in accordance with the results of Wada and Ward.[23] They used the term hybrid modelling for the reduction of the systemic circulation to four well-mixed compartments arranged in parallel (cf. figure 3C). Since this model corresponds to a four-exponential systemic transit time density function the underlying modelling philosophy is the same, namely to find a function which describes the systemic circulation time density of a drug. Simulating alfentanil data with the recirculatory model these authors already demonstrated the limitations of the compartmental (or multiexponential) approach as PK model for the control of infusion pumps (similarly as shown in figure 1A for sorbitol). The most advanced approach is the recirculatory model identified by the multiple indicator method used by Krejcie et al.[24] in dog experiments. Their model of the systemic circulation shown in figure 3C consists of fast and slow nondistributive (ND) and distributive (D) subsystems, respectively. While the D-systems are well-mixed compartments, the ND-systems are described by Erlang density functions and account for intravascular mixing (a similar transit time model was used for the lungs). The kinetics of ICG, inulin and antipyrine as markers of blood, extracellular space and total body water were analysed simultaneously using frequent arterial blood sampling after bolus injection of the markers. The model provided an excellent description of the concentration during the early distribution phase and the effect of halothane.[25] The results well reflected the increase in the areas under the first-pass $C_A(t)$ profiles (AUC_1) for ICG, inulin and antipyrine as expected from the decrease in cardiac output for increasing doses of halothane. The significant (more than 2-fold) increase in the initial *AUC* of antipyrine may be of importance for the maximum effect of intravenous anaesthetic drugs which are characterised by similar early disposition phase. Recently, this approach has been applied to study the influence of cardiac output on the initial mixing kinetics of alfentanil in pigs.[26]

While frequent early blood sampling is essential to observe the early concentration peak after rapid injection, less frequent sampling and a simpler recirculatory model may be sufficient for short term infusions (10 seconds and more), especially if an independent estimate of cardiac output is available.[5,27] Thus, from a practical point of view, two systemic compartments in parallel may be sufficient as proposed for propofol by Upton and Ludbrook.[28] A most interesting aspect of their approach is the inclusion of the brain (as effect-site organ) in the physiological recirculatory model. The concentration in brain tissue is not only linked to the anaesthetic effect but also used to model the feedback reduction of cerebral blood flow to account for the fact that propofol affects its own distribution kinetics to the effect site. One should note, however, that this is only possible if relevant a priori information on the kinetics in the effect-site organ is available since the distribution kinetics to the brain in general does not affect the whole body disposition curve, i.e. the PK profile does not react sensitive enough to changes in the parameters of brain kinetics. Thus, effect-site organ models (identified by separate experiments) in physiological models are a promising approach to improve the PK/PD model for drugs which influence the blood flow to the effect site.[29,30] It should be emphasised that the recirculatory models are not only necessary to describe the initial mixing phase and first-pass transit through the lungs in the case of short acting drugs, but are very useful to explain the effects of changes in haemodynamics on pharmacokinetics. The latter is of importance, for example, to improve our understanding of haemodynamic drug interactions with respect to distribution kinetics, where previous results obtained by compartmental analysis[31] may be of limited value.

Semiphysiological models

For drugs with a relatively long effect site equilibration time, when the onset of drug effect is slow even after rapid intravenous injection, multiexponential drug disposition curves may be sufficient as PK models. For oral administration, however, a minimal representation of the PK model is a decomposition of the system in two subsystems describing the absorption and disposition process, respectively. The crucial point is the selection of an empirical absorption time distribution which is flexible enough to describe also the input profile of slow release formulations.[32] As in bioavailability studies the model can be identified when the drug disposition curve (iv administration) is studied separately. This model can be extended to account for the formation of an active metabolite. For oral administration the model consists of three subsystems: the input system, which describes absorption into the portal vein, first-pass extraction (drug) and formation (metabolite) in the liver (including the effect of hepatic transit time), and the disposition systems of the drug and the (preformed) metabolite, respectively, which must be analysed separately.[33] The model describes the PK profiles of the parent drug, $C(t)$, and the generated active metabolite, $C_M(t)$, which both contribute to the observed time course of effect $E(t)$. Note that not only $C(t)$ and $C_M(t)$ are different but also the corresponding equilibration time constants, τ and τ_M , since in general metabolites are more hydrophilic with a lower capillary permeability (especially in the brain). Since this structural model still retains physiological information we call it semiphysiological. This approach has been used to model the pharmacokinetics of morphine and its metabolite morphine-6-glucuronide (M6G) in humans after intravenous and oral administration.[34,35] The different C-E equilibration time constants of morphine (τ = 17 min) and M6G (τ_M = 20 h) together with the high first-pass formation of M6G (71 %) make this modelling approach particularly interesting. A simulation study suggested that the effect site concentration of M6G formed from morphine after multiple dosing is approximately two times higher than that of morphine. Thus, the semiphysiological model may serve as a basis to explain a possible contribution of M6G to the analgesic effects of morphine.

Future

Having highlighted the advantages and chances of physiological pharmacokinetic modelling in relation to the effect site, the model linking arterial concentration and effect remained empirical, i.e. a simple behavioural model (figure 1). Such an empirical link model can be extended to include the effects of tolerance development and sensitisation.[36,37] A more challenging problem is the development of more realistic physiological models of the processes of drug distribution to the effect site and drug receptor interaction. Such models should include blood flow, permeation across the capillary wall, intratissue diffusion as well as nonspecific (tissue) and specific (receptor) binding kinetics. The fact that in the conventional link model only one parameter (τ) accounts for all these processes indicates that more detailed information is lacking in available PK/PD data. Furthermore, the reliability of estimation of the parameters of the static C_B-E model (figure1) on the basis of clinical data has been challenged.[38] Novel experimental designs and methods as, for example, kinetics in isolated organs, dynamic positron emission tomography and - if the distribution process is sufficiently slow - also microdialysis can be useful to identify more complex link models. Regarding drug receptor interaction the time course of the effect may depend on the rates of association and dissociation of a ligand-receptor complex as well as the density of available binding sites. The latter was recently demonstrated by Zhu et al.[39] for doxacurium. Finally, so-called indirect response models are necessary to explain the PK/PD relationship when the effect is not caused "directly" by drug-receptor interaction.[40]

References

1. Segre G: Kinetics of interaction between drugs and biological systems. Il Farmaco 1968; 23:907-18
2. Modi NB, Veng-Pedersen P: Validation of a variable direction hysteresis minimization pharmacodynamic approach: Cardiovascular effects of alfentanil. Pharm Res 1994; 11: 128-35
3. Schwilden H, Schüttler J: Model-based adaptive control of volatile anesthetics by quantitative EEG, Control and Automation in Anaesthesia. Edited by H Schwilden, H Stoeckel. Berlin Heidelberg , Springer, 1995, pp 163-74
4. Ducharme J, Varin F, Bevan DR, Donati F: Importance of early blood sampling on vecuronium pharmacokinetic and pharmacodynamic parameters. Clin Pharmacokinet 1993; 24:507-18
5. Weiss M, Hübner GH, Hübner GI, Teichmann W: Effects of cardiac output on disposition kinetics of sorbitol: recirculatory modelling. Br J Clin Pharmacol 1996; 41:261-8
6. Stanski DR, Hudson RJ, Homer TD, Saidman LJ, Meathe E: Pharmacodynamic modeling of thiopental anesthesia. J Pharmacokin Biopharm 1984; 12:223-40
7. Tuk B, Danhof M, Mandema JW: The impact of arteriovenous concentration differences on pharmacodynamic parameter estimates. J Pharmacokin Biopharm 1997; 25:39-62
8. Cobelli C, Carson ER, Finkelstein L, Leaning MS: Validation of simple and complex models in physiology and medicine. Am J Physiol 1984; 246:R259-R66
9. Björkman S, Wada DR, Stanski DR, Ebling WF: Comparative physiological pharmacokinetics of fentanyl and alfentanil in rats and humans based on parametric single-tissue models. J Pharmacokin Biopharm 1994; 22:381-410
10. Ebling WF, Wada DR, Stanski DR: From piecewise to full physiologic pharmacokinetic modeling: Applied to thiopental disposition in the rat. J Pharmacokin Biopharm 1994; 22:259-92
11. Wada DR, Björkman S, Ebling WF, Harashima H, Harapat SR, Stanski DR: Computer simulation of the effects of alterations in blood flows and body composition on thiopental pharmacokinetics in humans. Anesthesiology 1997; 87:884-99
12. Björkman S, Wada DR, Stanski DR: Application of physiologic models to predict the influence of changes in body composition and blood flows on the pharmacokinetics of fentanyl and alfentanil in patients. Anesthesiology 1998; 88:657-67
13. Weiss M, Roberts MS: Tissue distribution kinetics as determinant of transit time dispersion of drugs in organs: application of a stochastic model to the rat hindlimb. J. Pharmacokin. Biopharm. 1996; 24:173-96

14. Weiss M, Koester A, Wu Z.-Y, Roberts MS: Distribution kinetics of diazepam, lidocaine and antipyrine in the isolated perfused rat hindlimb. Pharm Res 1997a; 14:1640-3
15. Boer F, Hoeft A, Scholz M, Bovill JG, Burm AGL, Hak A:. Pulmonary distribution of alfentanil and sufentanil studied with system dynamics analysis. J Pharmacokin Biopharm 1996; 24:197-218
16. Weiss M, Geschke D: Estimation and model selection in pharmacokinetics: the effect of model misspecification, Modelling and Control in Biomedical Systems. Edited by DA Linkens, E Carson, Elsevier, 1997, pp 123-27
17. Weiss M: The relevance of residence time theory to pharmacokinetics. Eur J Clin Pharmacol 1992; 43:571-9
18. Weiss M, Förster W: Pharmacokinetic model based on circulatory transport. Eur J Clin Pharmacol 1979; 16:287-93
19. Cutler DJ: A linear recirculation model for drug disposition. J Pharmacokin Biopharm 1979; 7:101-16
20. Weiss M, Ring A: Interpretation of general measures of distribution kinetics in terms of a mammillary compartmental model. J Pharm Sci 1997; 86: 1491-93
21. Henthorn TK, Krejcie TC, Avram MJ: The relationship between alfentanil distribution kinetics and cardiac output. Clin Pharmacol Ther 1992; 52:190-6
22. Weiss M, Sziegoleit W, Hübner GI: Effects of hemodynamics in the pharmacokinetics of sorbitol in healthy volunteers: Recirculatory vs. compartmental modeling. Eur J Pharm Sci 1999; 8:A149
23. Wada DR, Ward DS: The hybrid model: A new pharmacokinetic model for computer-controlled infusion pumps. IEEE Trans Biomed Eng 1994; 41:134-42
24. Krejcie TC, Henthorn TK, Niemann CU, Klein C, Gupta DK, Gentry WB, Shanks CA, Avram MJ: Recirculatory pharmacokinetic models of markers of blood, extracellular fluid and total body water administered concomitantly. J Pharmacol Exp Ther 1996; 278:1050-57
25. Avram MJ, Krejcie TC, Niemann CU, Klein C, Gentry WB, Shanks CA, Henthorn TK. The effect of halothane on the recirculatory pharmacokinetics of physiologic markers. Anesthesiology 1997; 87:1381-93
26. Kuipers JA, Boer F, Olofson E, Olieman W, Vletter AA, Burm AGL, Bovill JG: Recirculatory and compartmental pharmacokinetic modeling of alfentanil in pigs. Anesthesiology 1999; 90:1146-57
27. Weiss M: Errors in clearance estimation after bolus injection and arterial sampling: nonexistence of a central compartment. J Pharmacokin Biopharm 1997; 25: 255-60
28. Upton RN, Ludbrook GL: A physiological model of induction of anaesthesia with propofol in sheep. 1. Structure and estimation of variables. Br J Anaesthesia 1997; 79:497-504
29. Upton RN, Ludbrook GL, Grant C, Gray EC: In vivo relationships between the cerebral pharmacokinetics and pharmacodynamics of thiopentone in sheep after short-term administration. J Pharmacokin Biopharm 1996; 24:1-18
30. Wada DR, Harashima H, Ebling WF, Osaki EW, Stanski DR: Effects of thiopental on regional blood flows in the rat. Anesthesiology 1996; 84:596-604
31. Wood M: Pharmacokinetic drug interactions in anaesthetic practice. Clin Pharmacokinet 1991; 21:285-307
32. Weiss M: A novel input function for the assessment of drug absorption in bioavailability studies. Pharm Res 1996; 13:1545-51
33. Weiss M: Analysis of metabolite formation pharmacokinetics after intravenous and oral administration of the parent drug using inverse Laplace transformation. Drug Metab Disp 1998; 26:562-65

34. Loetsch J, Weiss M, Kobal G, Geisslinger G: Pharmacokinetics of morphine-6-glucoronide and its formation from morphine after intravenous administration. Clin Pharmacol Ther 1998; 63:629-39
35. Lötsch J, Weiss M, Ahne G, Kobal G, Geisslinger G: Pharmacokinetic modeling of M6G formation after oral administration of morphine in healthy volunteers. Anesthesiology 1999; 90:1026-38
36. Ouellet DM-C, Pollack GM: A pharmacokinetic-pharmacodynamic model of tolerance to morphine analgesia during infusion in rats. J Pharmacokin Biopharm 1995; 23:531-49
37. Mandema JW, Wada DR: Pharmacodynamic model for acute tolerance development to the electroencephalographic effects of alfentanil in the rat. J Pharmacol Exp Ther 1995; 275:1185-94
38. Dutta S, Matsumoto Y, Ebling WF: Is it possible to estimate the parameters of the sigmoid E_{max} model with truncated data typical of clinical studies? J Pharm Sci 1996; 85:232-39
39. Zhu Y, Audibert G, Donati F, Varin F: Pharmacokinetic-pharmacodynamic modeling of doxacurium: effect of input rate. J Pharmacokin Biopharm 1997: 25:23-37
40. Jusko WJ, Ko HC: Physiologic response models characterize diverse types of pharmacodynamic effects. Clin Pharmacol Ther 1994; 56:406-19

TARGETING THE EFFECT SITE

James G. Bovill

Leiden, The Netherlands

Introduction

The availability of commercial devices (Diprifusor™) that provide computerised control of the plasma concentrations of propofol has focused attention on Target Controlled Infusion (TCI) techniques in anaesthesia. TCI devices can rapidly achieve and maintain any desired target concentration of a drug, and allow the target concentration to be changed when required by the clinical situation. While they cannot deliver an ideal concentration profile such as that shown in figure 1a, they can come quite close (figure 1b). Figure 1b shows a simulated plasma propofol concentration profile obtained using the STANPUMP program written by Dr Steven Shafer, Department of Anesthesiology, Stanford University, California, USA.*

While plasma concentrations can be increased very rapidly to a higher level, the fall in concentration when the target is lowered depends on the pharmacokinetic parameters of the drug being infused and the previous infusion history. The decrease follows a multiexponential process. This is the major difference between the two profiles shown in figure 1.

The ability to achieve a plasma concentration profile such as that in figure 1b, and thus to be able to respond to changing patient requirements during surgery is often claimed to be one of the major advantages of TCI. This appar-

* This program is freely available and can be downloaded from the World Wide Web site, http://pk-pd.icon.palo-alto.med.va.gov/

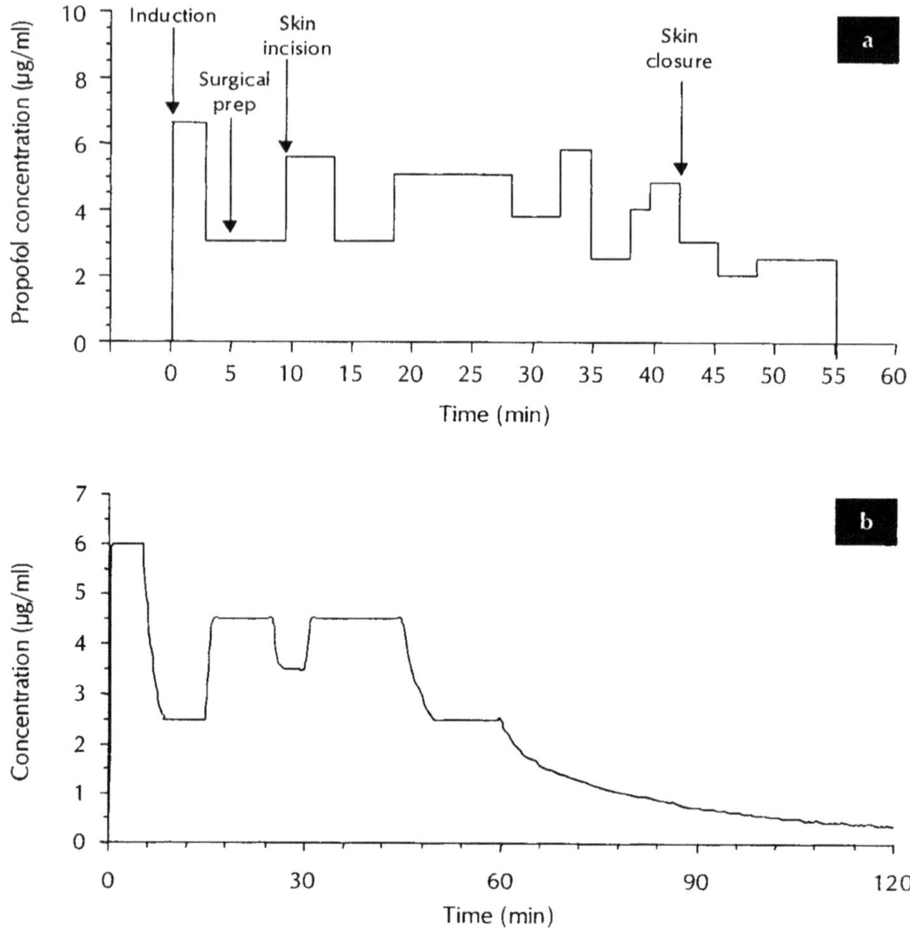

Figure 1
(a) Ideal intraoperative propofol concentration profile, (b) the propofol concentration profile for a real TCI device simulated using STANPUMP.

ent ability to control the depth of anaesthesia is, however, an illusion since the plasma is not the site of action of anaesthetic drugs. These act either within the central nervous system or, in the case of neuromuscular blocking drugs, at the motor end plate of somatic muscles.

While we cannot sample drug concentration directly in these sites, it is possible, using the concept of a theoretical effect site (sometimes referred to as the biophase) and pharmacokinetic-pharmacodynamic modelling techniques, to obtain an estimate of the apparent effect site concentration for any form of drug input. An extension of this has been the development of software allowing the effect site to be targeted with TCI technology. This manuscript describes the place of the effect site in modern anaesthesia and the development of effect site targeted target controlled infusion.

The effect site

Because most drugs act at sites remote from the blood stream, there will be a temporal delay between changes in plasma drug concentration and measured effect. This delay is a consequence of the finite time needed for drug molecules to equilibrate with the effect site. Equilibration between plasma and effect site is rapid for thiopentone[1], propofol[2], alfentanil[2,3], and remifentanil[4], and intermediate for fentanyl and sufentanil[5] and the nondepolarizing muscle relaxants[6,7]. A consequence of a delay in equilibration is that a plot of pharmacodynamic response (effect) against plasma concentration measured during and after a short intravenous infusion will show an anticlockwise hysteresis loop. By manipulation of this hysteresis loop so that the loop collapses it is possible to obtain an estimate of the underlying effect site concentration and the blood-effect site delay. This is the principle of pharmacokinetic-pharmacodynamic modelling, in which the drug concentration in the hypothetical effect or biophase compartment is derived by simultaneous consideration of the plasma concentration and the measured effect.

The effect site is modelled as an additional compartment linked to the central compartment of a conventional 2- or 3-compartment pharmacokinetic model by a single first-order process (Fig 2). This approach was first proposed by Segre[8] and used by Hull et al.[9] to model the effect of pancuronium. Hull introduced the term 'biophase'. The biophase or effect site compartment is assumed to be negligibly small (typically taken as 1/10 000 of the volume of the central compartment). In figure 2 the first-order rate constant connecting the effect compartment to the central compartment is k_{1e}. Since V_e is negligible, k_{1e} can be assumed to be negligible also since $k_{1e} = V_e \cdot k_{e1} / V_1$. This ensures that the transfer of drug to the effect compartment is negligible, so that the effect-site processes do not influence the pharmacokinetics in the rest of the body, in particular the plasma disposition. The rate constant for drug removal

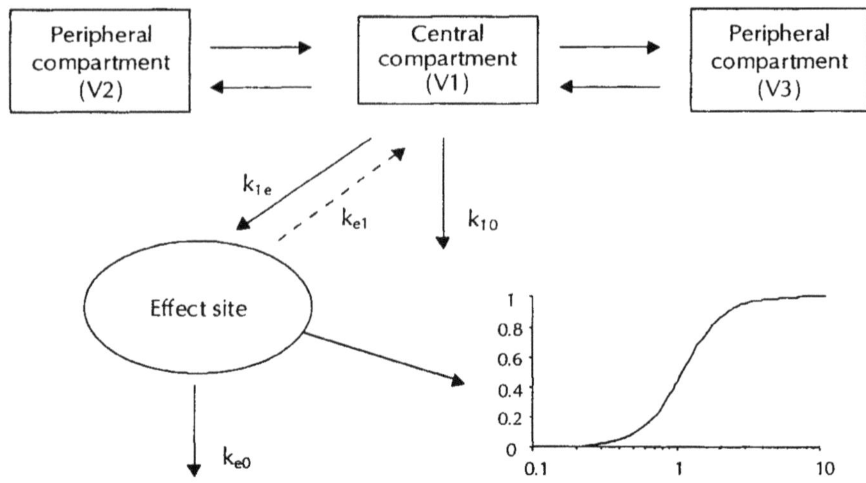

Figure 2
Three-compartment pharmacokinetic model with the effect compartment linked to the central compartment.

from the effect compartment is k_{e1}. However, because negligible mass of drug transfers to the effect compartment, the subsequent loss of this negligible mass is, by convention, taken to be to the outside rather than back into the central compartment[6], and the rate constant k_{e0} is used instead of k_{e1}. As with other rate constants, k_{e0} can be converted into a half-life using the formula

$$T_{1/2}k_{e0} = \frac{\ln 2}{k_{e0}} = \frac{0.693}{k_{e0}}$$

$T_{1/2}k_{e0}$ is the time for the effect site concentration to reach 50% of the plasma concentration when the plasma concentration is maintained constant. For drugs with a short $T_{1/2}k_{e0}$ (high k_{e0}) equilibration between plasma and the effect compartment will be rapid (e.g. thiopentone or alfentanil) while equilibration will be slow for those with a long $T_{1/2}k_{e0}$ (low k_{e0}) such as morphine. The converse may not always be true since the decline in the effect compartment concentration will also depend on the concentration gradient between the biophase and plasma, and the latter is determined by the pharmacokinetics of a drug.

This important pharmacodynamic parameter, k_{e0}, can be determined from plots of simultaneously measured plasma concentrations against an effect, producing the previously mentioned hysteresis loop. By successive approximations of k_{e0}, a value can be found which collapses the hysteresis loop to give the true value of k_{e0}. Hull et al.[9] were the first to use this approach, using pancuronium and muscle twitch tension as the measured effect. They used only two points on the hysteresis loop, one during drug input when the pancuronium concentration was rising and one when the concentration was falling, when pancuronium produced 70% of maximum block. K_{e0} was estimated as the value producing identical concentrations of drug in the biophase at these two times. This approach was subsequently extended by Sheiner et al.[6] who used the "negligible biophase" concept of Hull to derive a full-range model for tubocurarine in which all data points in the hysteresis plot were used. The Sheiner model has been extensively used to characterise the pharmacodynamics of a variety of drugs, including intravenous anaesthetics and opioids. In most of these a parameter derived from the EEG, such as the spectral edge frequency or median frequency, has been used as a surrogate measure of pharmacological effect. When derived in this way k_{e0} can be considered as a composite rate constant reflecting access to the biophase receptor from the plasma, the kinetics of drug interaction with the receptor, and elimination of drug from the effect compartment[10].

Modelling the effect site

The amount of drug in the effect compartment at time t is the convolution of the input from the central compartment with the first-order exponential function e^{-ke0t} describing the loss of drug from the effect site. Mathematically this is described as

$$A_e(t) = k_{1e} \int_0^t e^{-k_{e0}(t-\tau)} A_1(\tau)\, d\tau$$

where A_e and A_1 are the amounts of drug in the effect and central compartments, respectively. In non-mathematical terms convolution can be considered as a slurring or spreading out of the plasma concentration profile by the effect compartment disposition function e^{-ke0t}. This is illustrated in figure 3, which shows the disposition of the effect site concentration resulting from the plasma propofol concentration profile of figure 1b. The precise control of plasma su-

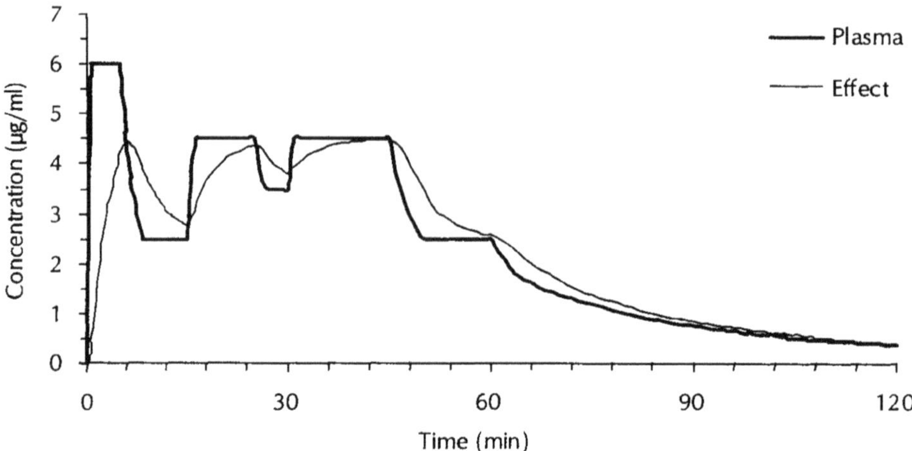

Figure 3
Simulated effect site propofol concentration resulting from the plasma concentration profile in figure 1b.

fentanil concentration has been transformed into a slurred rise and fall of drug concentration at the effect site, and the illusion of precise control of anaesthetic depth has been shattered. Obviously more precise control of effect would be obtained by using a TCI system that targeted the effect site rather than the plasma. This is, however, more difficult to achieve.

Exact solutions of the equations giving the infusion rates needed to control target plasma concentrations have been described[11-14]. These are based on modifications of the BET ("Bolus, Elimination, Transfer") infusion scheme[15], which is only applicable to the maintenance of a single target concentration. Unfortunately there are no exact solutions that will allow the calculation of infusion rates needed to precisely achieve, maintain and change drug concentrations at the effect site, and numerical solutions are required. Algorithms for targeting the effect site using TCI have been published[16,17], and several other algorithms are also routinely used, including the one used by the author developed by Dr. Frank Engbers of the Leiden University Medical Center.

One cannot administer a drug directly into the effect compartment, it must be delivered via the blood stream. Drug entry to the effect site then depends on a concentration gradient between the plasma and the effect site. Conse-

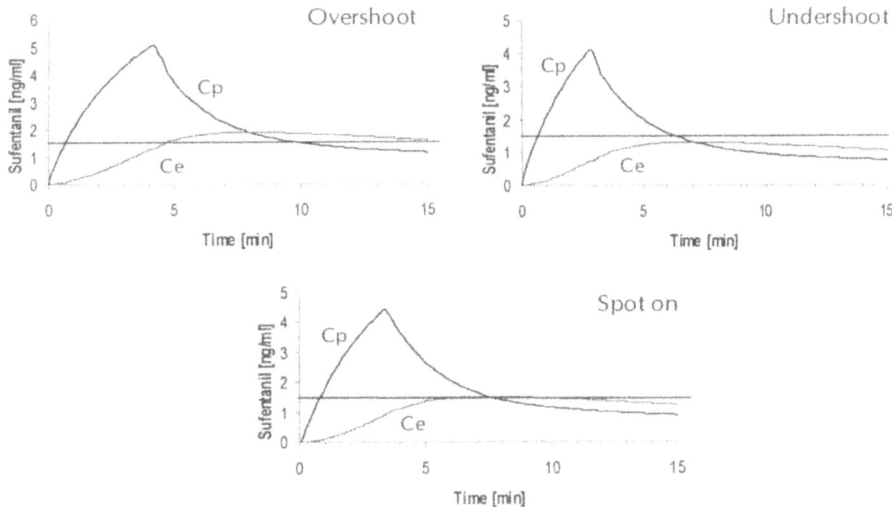

Figure 4
The approach to targeting the effect site concentration without overshoot using plasma concentration "overpressure".

quently effect site TCI systems rely on the principle of 'overpressure'. In essence, the infusion pump is instructed to deliver drug at a high infusion rate, which may often be the maximum rate available (e.g. 1200 ml/h). The computer must calculate the time at which the infusion must be stopped so that the resultant effect site concentration peaks at the desired target concentration without overshoot (figure 4). Once the peak has been reached, the effect and plasma concentrations are in equilibrium. The target effect concentration can then be maintained by continuing to maintain the plasma concentrations at this level using a conventional plasma-targeted TCI algorithm. This approach is used in the STANPUMP system; other systems use more complex algorithms.

The necessity for the above approach has several important clinical implications. The iterative approach in effect-compartment control algorithms is computationally much more intensive compared to plasma concentrations control algorithms. This is not a real problem with modern high-speed and powerful computers. Indeed, in their effect-site control algorithm Shafer and Gregg[16] were able to perform the real time calculations with an iteration interval of 1 sec using a 4.77 MHz 8088 microprocessor without benefit of a

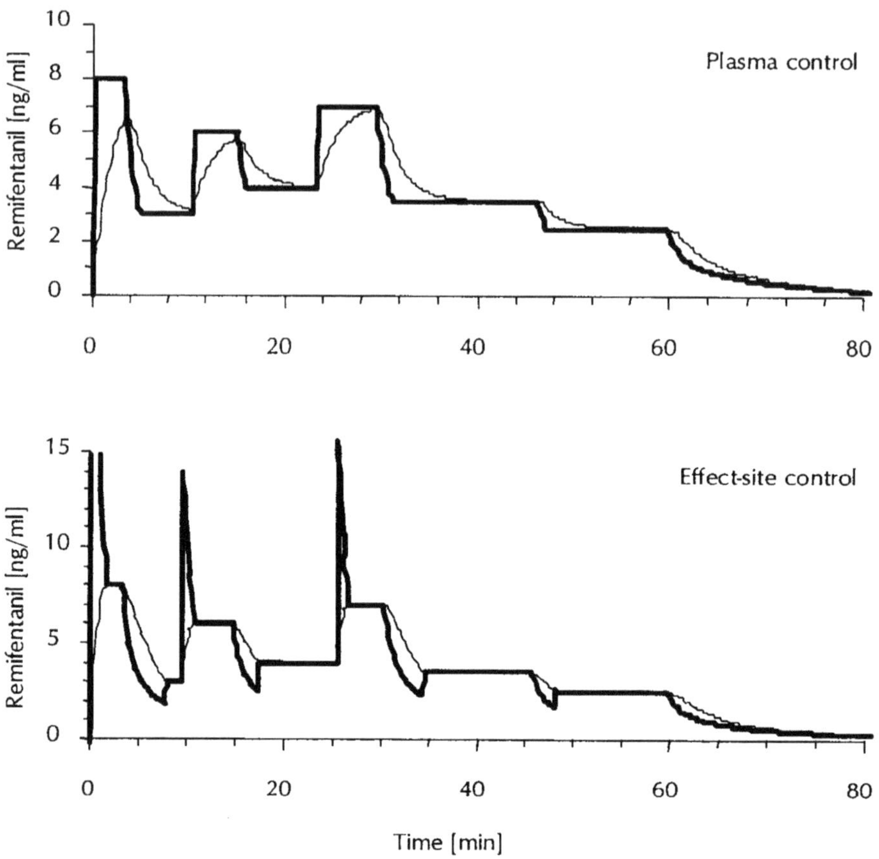

Figure 5
Simulated target plasma and effect site concentrations of remifentanil during TCI. The dark line is the target plasma concentration, the light line the target effect site concentration.

floating point coprocessor. Today's processors are up to 100 times faster and more powerful by several orders of magnitude.

Secondly, since the effect site cannot respond as quickly as the plasma, control of the effect site concentration will never be as fast as with central compartment control. This is simply a consequence of the finite delay in drug transportation into the effect compartment. The rapidity of the effect site response is obviously dependent on the value of k_{e0} (or $T_{½}k_{e0}$). More precise control will be achieved by using a drug with more rapid equilibration between the plasma and the effect site, i.e. one with a shorter $T_{½}k_{e0}$. Figure 5 compares the plasma and effect site concentrations of remifentanil during TCI when targeting the plasma and the effect site. Even for remifentanil, which has a rapid effect site equilibration (k_{e0} = 0.525 min^{-1}, $T_{½}k_{e0}$ = 1.32 min) there is a small, but appreciable, benefit from targeting the effect site.

A potential disadvantage of targeting the effect site is the inevitable overshoot in the plasma concentration when the target is increased. This will be particularly marked at the beginning of a case when no drug is present in the body and relatively high effect site targets are set for induction of anaesthesia. The smaller the value of k_{e0} (longer $T_{½}k_{e0}$) the greater will be the degree of plasma concentration overshoot. This could result in an increased risk of adverse effects, particularly of those side effects, that will be more closely related to the plasma concentration. This could result, for example, in potentially greater haemodynamic disturbances than might be seen with control of the plasma concentration. There is, however, little evidence that targeting the effect site results in a greater incidence of adverse effects compared to plasma control, and that the observed advantages outweigh the theoretical disadvantages[18]. Another potential problem with effect site control could be the use of parameters derived from the EEG as surrogate pharmacological end points for determining k_{e0}. Again, however, clinical experience suggests that this is not a real problem. For thiopentone, the values of k_{e0} derived using clinical (loss of muscle power) and EEG (burst suppression) end points were identical[1].

Conclusion

In conclusion, there are good theoretical reasons for using TCI systems targeting the effect site rather than the plasma or blood. Despite the potential disadvantages of this approach, e.g. increased risk of haemodynamic side effects, clinical experience in several hundred patients suggests that the potential advantages outweigh the disadvantages. This has never been tested, however, in well-controlled clinical trials comparing these two methods of TCI. There is a need for such a study. It is to be hoped that future versions of commercial TCI systems will offer effect site control as an alternative to the conventional central compartment control now available.

References

1. Shanks CA, Avram MJ, Krejcie TC, Henthorn TK, Gentry WB. A pharmacokinetic-pharmacodynamic model for quantal responses with thiopental. J Pharmacokinet Biopharm 1993;21:309-321.
2. Billard V, Gambus PL, Chamoun N, Stanski DR, Shafer SL. A comparison of spectral edge, delta power, an bispectral index as EEG measures of alfentanil, propofol and midazolam drug effect. Clin Pharmacol Ther 1997;61:45-58
3. Scott JC, Ponganis KV, Stanski DR. EEG quantitation of narcotic effect: The comparative pharmacodynamics of fentanyl and alfentanil. Anesthesiology 1985;62: 234-241.
4. Egan T D, Minto CF, Hermann DJ, Barr J, Muir KT, Shafer SL. Remifentanil versus alfentanil: comparative pharmacokinetics and pharmacodynamics in healthy adult male volunteers. .Anesthesiology 1996;84 :821-833.
5. Scott JC, Cooke JE, Stanski DR. Electroencephalographic quantitation of opioid effect : Comparative pharmacodynamics of fentanyl and sufentanil. Anesthesiology 1991;74:34-42.
6. Sheiner LB, Stanski DR, Vozeh S, Miller RD, Ham J. Simultaneous modelling of pharmacokinetics and pharmacodynamics: Applications to d-tubocurarine. Clin Pharmacol Ther 1979;25:358-371.
7. Fisher DM, Szenohradszky J, Wright PM, Lau M, Brown R, Sharma M. Pharmacodynamic modeling of vecuronium-induced twitch depression. Rapid plasma-effect site equilibration explains faster onset at resistant laryngeal muscles than at the adductor pollicis. Anesthesiology. 1997 ; 86: 558-566.
8. Segre G. Kinetics of interaction between drugs and biological systems. Il Farmaco 1968;23:907-918.
9. Hull CJ, Van Beem HBH, McLeod K, Sibbald A, Watson MJ. A pharmacodynamic model for pancuronium. Br J Anaesth 1978;50:1113-1123.
10. Nony P, Cucherat M, Boissel J-P. Revisiting the effect compartment through timing errors in drug administration. Trends Pharmacol Sci 1998;19:49-54.
11. Shafer SL, Siegel LC, Cooke JE, Scott JC. Testing computer-controlled infusion pumps by simulation. Anesthesiology 1988;68:261-266.
12. Jacobs JR. Analytical solution to the three-compartment pharmacokinetic model. IEEE Trans Biomed Eng 1988;35:763-765.
13. Jacobs JR. Algorithm for optimal linear model based control with application to pharmacokinetic model-driven drug delivery. IEEE Trans Biomed Eng 1990;37:107-109.
14. Bailey J, Shafer SL. A simple analytical solution to the three-compartment pharmacokinetic model suitable for computer-controlled infusion pumps. IEEE Trans Biomed Eng 1991;38:522-525.
15. Schwilden H. A general method for calculating the dosage scheme in linear pharmacokinetics. Eur J Clin Pharmacol 1981;20:379-383.
16. Shafer SL, Gregg KM. Algorithms to rapidly achieve and maintain stable drug concentrations at the site of drug effect with a computer-controlled infusion pump. J Pharmacokinet Biopharm 1992;20:147-169.
17. Jacobs JR, Williams EA. Algorithm to control "effect compartment" drug concentrations in pharmacokinetic model-driven drug delivery. IEEE Trans Biomed Eng 1993;40:993-999.
18. Jacobs JR. Infusion rate control algorithms for pharmacokinetic model-driven drug infusion schemes. Int Anesthesiol Clin 1995;33:65-82.

EFFECT SITES OF INTRAVENOUS ANAESTHETIC AGENTS

Koji Morita, Tomiei Kazama, Shigehito Sato and Kazuyuki Ikeda

Hamamatsu, Japan

Pharmacokinetics

A drug that is administered by bolus into the blood, flows in the form of a cluster to the peripheral tissues through the heart and pulmonary veins, to return to the heart and lung again. This circulation is repeated and the cluster of drug that is carried by the blood perfusion gradually is distributed into the whole blood compartment after several circulations. During the distribution process the drug is transferred from the blood into the vessel- rich and vessel-poor compartments, and vice-versa, following the principle of equilibration. The metabolism and/or excretion has started simultaneously as the distribution. The time course of the concentration after a bolus administration of a drug, follows an exponentially decaying curve. The gradient of the curve can be expected to agree with the number of the compartments the model is thought to have. In the above notation, the number is three; blood in the vessels, the vessel-rich tissue, and the vessel-poor tissue. The mathematical model that can satisfy these natures had been well described by Gibaldi and Perrier[1], and is shown in figure 1. The system of first-order differential equations governs mass transfer between the compartments and to the outside of the body. This can be described as

$$\begin{bmatrix} dX_1/dt = -E_1X_1 + E_2X_2 + E_3X_3 + R \\ dX_2/dt = -K_{12}X_1 - E_2X_2 \\ dX_3/dt = -E_{13}X_1 - E_3X_3 \end{bmatrix} \cdots\cdots \text{(Eq.1)}$$

Herein

$E_1 = K_{12} + K_{13} + K_{10}$

$E_2 = K_{21}$

$E_3 = K_{31}$

X_i : Mass in i – th compartment, $X_i = V_i C_i$

V_i : Volume in i – th compartment, C_i : Concentration in i – th compartment

K_{ij}: Rate constant from compartment$_i$ to compartment$_j$

R : Infusion rate

Solving these equations will predict the time course of drug concentration.

Pharmacodynamics

The plasma or blood concentration can be predicted by solving the model shown above. The target concentration that the anaesthesiologist desires is based on the pharmacodynamic data of the drug. The time course of the analgesic and sedative effects of fentanyl, sufentanil[2], alfentanil[3] and propofol[4] were determined on the basis of surrogate effects as e.g. taken from the procession of the electroencephalogram (EEG). The median power frequency, power in the delta region and the spectral edge frequency were used in this context. Recently the bispectral index (BIS) had been developed[5] to quantify the sedative level of propofol[6] and inhalation anaesthetics.[7] These effect parameters are related to the concentration in the blood or plasma by a simple model. Suppose an agent-D and its receptor-R are bound to each other, get in equilibrium, and after they had completed their equilibration, the following relation can be derived.

$DR \leftrightarrow D + R$, where $K = [D][R]/[DR]$ - - - -(Eq.2 - 1)

K : Equilibration coefficient

$[X]$: Concentration or density of X, X denotes D, R and DR(conjunct of D and R)

There are receptors of which some are conjugated with agent-D and others that are not occupied yet after equilibration. Hence the total concentration of receptors [Rt] can be shown as:

$$[R_t] = [R] + [DR]$$

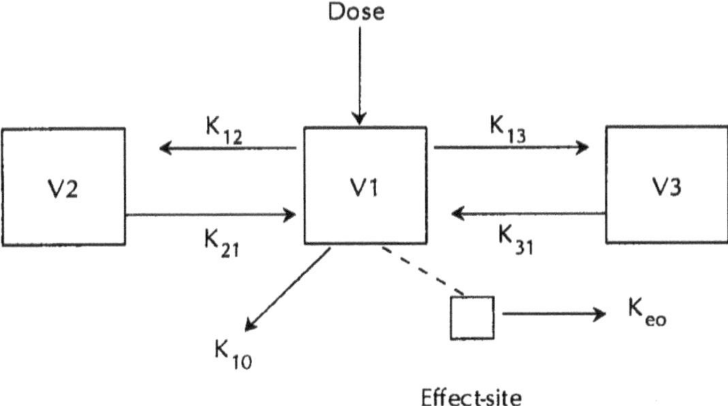

Figure 1
The 3-compartment model connected to an effect site compartment. V1, V2 and V3 are volume of the central, shallow and deep compartments, respectively. Rate constant Kij denotes proportional constant to time derivative of mass transfer rate from. the i-th compartment to the j-th compartment. After drug is administered into the central compartment, drug begins to be distributed to peripheral compartments and excreted. The effect site is a hypothetical compartment in which the concentration has a time delay from that in the central compartment.

The pharmacological effect F shall be:

$$F = [DR]/[R_t]$$

Hence *F/(1-F)* can be derived as:

$$\begin{aligned} F/(1-F) &= [DR]/([R_t]-[DR]) \\ &= [DR]/[R] \\ &= [D]/K \quad \text{----(Eq. 2-2)} \end{aligned}$$

Suppose $[D_{50}]$ denotes concentration of *D* at the condition of *F=1/2*, then following relation can be derived from Eq.2-2.

$$[D_{50}]/K = 1 \text{ and } K = [D_{50}] \quad \text{----(Eq. 2-3)}$$

From Eq.2-3 and Eq.2-2, we can find

$$F/(1-F) = [D]/[D_{50}] \text{ or } F = 1/(1+[D_{50}]/[D]) \quad \text{-----(Eq. 2-4)}$$

Table 1
Pharmacodynamic parameters of propofol. Propofol has several sets of pharmacodynamic parameters. They are dependant on the background fentanyl concentration (ng/ml, mean ± SD) and the type of stimulus tested. D_{50} (mean and confidence limits) denotes the concentration that causes 50% of depression of the control response. γ is a steepness factor.

Fentanyl concentration (ng/ml)		Group 1 (0)	Group 2 (1.2±0.3)	Group 3 (2.6±0.5)	Group 4 (4.1±0.7)	Group 5 (5.5±0.8)
Stimulation						
Verbal Command	D50 (μg/ml)	4.4 (3.8-5.0)	4 (3.5-4.5)	3.6 (3.1-4.0)	3.5 (3.1-4.0)	3.2 (2.8-3.6)
	γ	5.143	5.131	5.118	5.009	5.100
Tetanus	D50 (μg/ml)	9.3 (8.3-10.4)	7.8 (6.8-8.7)	5.1 (.4.5-5.8)	4.2 (3.6-4.7)	3.7 (3.2-4.3)
	γ	4.152	4.248	4.132	4.323	4.167
Laryngoscopy	D50 (μg/ml)	9.8 (8.9-10.8)	10.1 (9.2-11.1)	6.3 (5.6-7.0)	5.6 (5.0-6.2)	4.6 (4.0-5.1)
	γ	5.787	5.592	5.874	5.931	6.193
Intubation	D50 (μg/ml)	17.4 (15.1-20.1)	16.4 (14.2-18.8)	10.6 (9.1-12.3)	9.8 (8.3-11.6)	7.9 (6.6-9.3)
	γ	4.248	4.286	4.248	4.248	4.287
Skin incision	Cp50 (μg/ml)	10 (8.1-12.2)	9.8 (7.7-12.2)	5.7 (4.3-7.4)	5 (3.7-6.5)	4.2 (3.0-5.5)
	γ	5.157	5.129	5.147	5.209	5.199

Applying this equation to the experimental result of pharmacodynamic equilibration, a correction coefficient γ is added and finally the pharmacodynamic equation becomes

$$F = 1/\left(1 - \left([D_{50}]/[D]\right)^{\gamma}\right) \text{----(Eq. 2-5)}$$

This equation is well known as Hill equation. The constants in equation 2-5 for propofol in fentanyl background are shown in table 1[8].

The effect site

In clinical practice anaesthesiologists experience a dissociation between the time of administration of a drug and its effect as predicted by equation 2-5. The

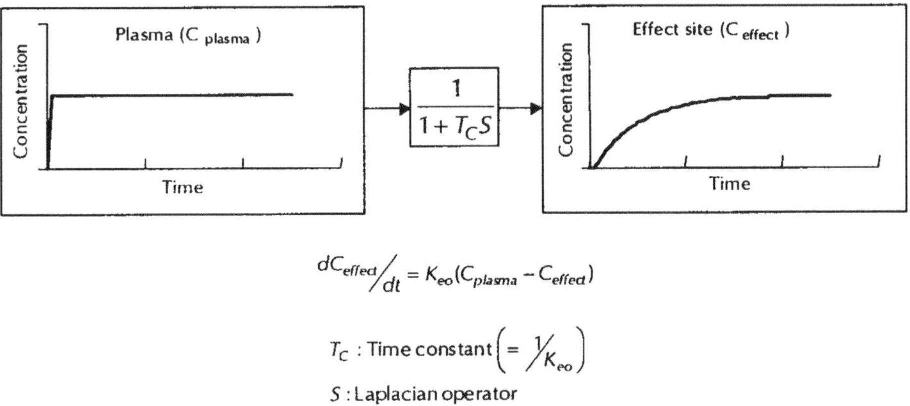

$$dC_{effect}/dt = K_{eo}(C_{plasma} - C_{effect})$$

T_C : Time constant $\left(= 1/K_{eo}\right)$

S : Laplacian operator

Figure 2
The effect site model. The relationship between input and output functions of the effect site compartment. The output time profile of the effect site has a first-order time delay as is shown in the formula.

delay can be explained by the model shown in figure 2. The differential equation shown there is consistent with the historical equation derived by Hull[9] or Sheiner[10] under the assumption that the concentration at the effect site increases and finally becomes equivalent to the plasma concentration. The delay in the equation is characterised by the time-constant: k_{e0}, in which a larger k_{e0} leads to a faster rise in effect than with a smaller k_{e0}. This k_{e0} is the rate constant from inside to outside the effect compartment. The k_{e0} (min^{-1}) of fentanyl is 0.105 ($t_{½}k_{e0}$ = 6.6 min)[2] and that for propofol is 0.239 ($t_{½}k_{e0}$ = 2.9 min).[11] Recently, we have determined the $t_{½}k_{e0}$ by measuring the bispectral index (BIS) in 41 patients aged from 20 to 85 years. K_{e0}'s of BIS for propofol were 0.3, 0.301, 0,303, and 0.292 for patients aged 20-39, 40-59, 60-69, and 70-85 years, respectively.[11] Age thus did not affect k_{e0}. The k_{e0} of fentanyl is about half of that of propofol, which means that twice the time is required for the plasma fentanyl concentration to equilibrate with the effect site compared to propofol.

Because an anaesthetic agent has more than one effect it may also have more than one k_{e0}, each related to a specific effect. The main effect of propofol is hypnosis, an important side effect is haemodynamic depression. We have studied k_{e0} of propofol for the haemodynamic side effect by measuring the response of the systolic blood pressure (SBP) against the change of the concentration of propofol. The k_{e0} 's were 0.118, 0.117, 0.0781 and 0.0678 for patients aged 20-39, 40-59, 60-69, and 70-85 years, respectively.[12] There was a significant difference ($P < 0.05$) in between the k_{e0} 's of the patients aged 70-85 and 20-39 years. The equilibration half-life for the haemodynamic depressant effect of propofol was three times longer than that for the induction of hypnosis.

The propofol concentrations that caused half of the maximal decrease (IC_{50}) from the control systolic pressure to 80 mmHg were 4.61, 4.13, 3.96 and 2.09 μg/ml for patients aged 20-39, 40-59, 60-69 and 70-85 years, respectively.[12] The EC_{50}'s of BIS were 5.60, 6.76, 8.21 and 7.67 μg/ml for patients aged 20-39, 40-59, 60-69 and 70-85 years, respectively. There was a significant difference between the EC_{50} of systolic blood pressure decrease in the patients aged 70-85 years and that in the patients of the other groups ($p < 0.05$). These results suggest that the blood pressure in elderly patients decreases slower than in younger patients and that the magnitude of the decrease in systolic pressure is more significant in elderly than in young patients.

Predicting the time course of pharmacological effect

We have described above that the plasma concentration-time profile that can be predicted quantitatively by a pharmacokinetic model. Furthermore, we have shown that the effect can be modelled by adding an effect compartment. Although the pharmacological effect can be determined on the basis of either the plasma or the effect site concentration, derivation by plasma will be associated with a time lag (first-order delay) but derivation by the effect site will not be accompanied with such a time lag. Hence, the prediction of the effect site concentration reflects pharmacological effect more directly than that of the plasma concentration.

Finding an adequate infusion rate

In the following section, we will describe a method to find an appropriate infusion rate or dose to achieve a desired concentration and associated effect in the desired time period. Solving equation 1 (Eq. 1) by Euler's principle, the following equations can be derived:

$$X_1[i+1] = X_1[i] + (-E_1X_1[i] + E_2X_2[i] + E_3X_3[i] + R[i])\Delta t \text{ -------(Eq. 5-1)}$$
$$X_2[i+1] = X_2[i] + (K_{12}X_1[i] - E_2X_2[i])\Delta t \text{ -------(Eq. 5-2)}$$
$$X_3[i+1] = X_3[i] + (K_{13}X_1[i] - E_3X_3[i])\Delta t \text{ -------(Eq. 5-3)}$$
$$C_e[i+1] = C_e[i] + K_{eo}(C_1[i] - C_e[i])\Delta t \text{ -------(Eq. 5-4)}$$

To achieve the desired concentration $C_{1\ target}$ at time period (i+1)Δt, R[i] can be derived from Eq.5-1;

$$R[i] = (V_1C_{1\,\text{target}} - V_1C_1[i])/\Delta t + E_1V_1C_1[i] - E_1V_2C_2[i] - E_3V_3C_3[i] \text{ -----Eq. 5-5}$$

This equation shows that when the rate R is maintained during time iΔt, the plasma concentration can attain the target concentration of $C_{1\ target}$ at the time of (i+1)Δt. Finding the rate to achieve a pre-set effect site concentration ($C_{e\ target}$), the following equation can be derived from Eq.5-4:

$$\begin{aligned} C_{e\,\text{target}} &= C_e[i+2] = C_e[i+1] + K_{eo}(C_1[i+1] - C_e[i+1])\Delta t \\ &- C_e[i+1](1 + K_{eo}\Delta t) + K_{eo}C_1[i+1] \\ &= (C_e[i] + K_{eo}(C_1[i] - C_e[i])\Delta t)(1 + K_{eo}\Delta t) + K_{eo}C_1[i+1] \text{ ----Eq. 5-6} \end{aligned}$$

The desired effect site concentration $C_{e\ target}$ can be calculated from the current C_e, C1 and C_1[i+1]. Hence, C_1[i+1] have to be controlled appropriately. Suppose this C_1[i+1] is $C_{1\ required}$, we can find the currently required infusion rate R[i] by substituting $C_{1\ target}$ in Eq.5-5 for this $C_{1\ required}$ to achieve the desired effect site concentration at the time period of (i+2)Δt. By solving the differential PK/PD equations with Euler's method, the infusion rate to achieve the desired concentration in the plasma or the effect compartment can be determined analytically. However, Euler's method uses only the first order of Taylor's approximation in estimating the next value from the current value. This may cause an error that becomes apparent in dynamic conditions e.g. when the infusion rate is changed frequently over a great range. The Runge-Kutta's method uses the first to fourth order of Taylor's expansion series, and can decrease the error to $1/10^3$ of Euler's one. However, contrasting to its high accuracy, there is a difficulty in finding analytical solutions to achieve the desired concentrations. An alternative method that can find the target numerically, an iterative "half-interval searching" method, is called "Regula-falsi". The principle of this method will be explained briefly here. At first, the infusion rate is set to the initial value of R_0 ($mg.kg^{-1}.min^{-1}$), then the plasma or the effect site concentration is calculated by solving the equation of the pharmacokinetic model under the assumption that the rate R_0 is kept for the desired time interval (iteration period). When the estimated concentration is lower than the desired target, the rate will be increased by ΔR and the rate R_1 becomes $R_1=R_0+\Delta R$. This step of iteration will be repeated for n times until the calculated concentration will pass above the target concentration, and then the appropriate rate R_{root} may be in the range between R_{n-1} and R_n, and the approximated rate R_{app} can be estimated by linear interpolation as:

$$\left|f\left(R_{app}\right)\right| \leq \varepsilon$$

If $f(R_n)f(R_{app}) < 0$, R_{root} will be on the right side of R_{app}, then the new R_{n-1} shall be substituted by R_{app}. Contrarily, if $f(R_{n-1})f(R_{app})<0$, R_{root} will be on the left side of R_{app}, then the new R_n shall be substituted by R_{app} and find the new R_{app} by Eq.5-7. This process will be repeated until

$$R_{app} = R_{n-1} + f\left(R_{n-1}\right)\left(R_n - R_{n-1}\right)/\left(f\left(R_{n-1}\right) - f\left(R_n\right)\right) \quad \text{----(Eq. 5-7)}$$

Herein $f(R) = $ (concentration kept at infusion rate of R) − (target concentration)

Herein is ε a small value like 10^{-5}. Finally we can find the R_{app} within the permitted error to the extent of less than ε. This method can be used to find an appropriate infusion rate at any period to get the desired concentration both in the plasma and the effect site.

Comparing effect site and plasma controlled TCI by simulation

We have evaluated both the performances of a TCI device controlling the plasma concentration and of a TCI device controlling the effect site concentration. To evaluate their performances we have compared the time needed to reach a specified target level. Kazama et al.[8] reported that the Cp_{50} of propofol for intubation, in the presence of a plasma fentanyl concentration of 2.6 ng/ml, was 10.6 μg/ml. We assumed we could start intubation after the effect site concentration had reached this blood propofol concentration of 10 μg/ml. We

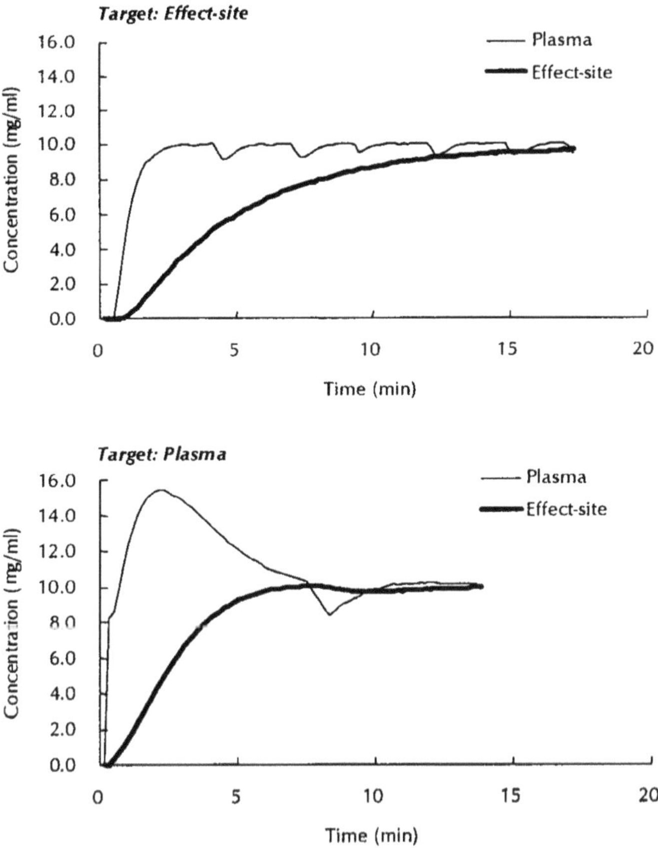

Figure 3
The concentration-time profiles of a plasma controlled and effect site controlled TCI. Simulated concentrations of plasma and effect site are shown. *Left:* During plasma controlled TCI a plasma concentration of 10 µg/ml was preset as the target of the TCI system. A 95% level of this target plasma concentration was reached at 2.17 min after the start of the infusion, but the effect site concentration was still 22% below the target. A level of 95% of the maximum effect site concentration was reached at 15 min after the start of the infusion. *Right:* During effect site controlled TCI an effect site concentration of 10 µg/ml was preset as the target of TCI. An overshoot was seen in the plasma concentration and its maximum was 15.4 µg/ml. However, the effect site concentration reached 95% of the preset target value at 5.5 min after starting the TCI.

simulated the plasma and effect site concentration-time profiles of a TCI device controlling either a plasma concentration of 10 µg/ml or an effect site concentration of 10 µg/ml. The concentration-time courses of both methods are shown in figure 3.

The required time to reach the level of 95% of the maximum effect site concentration (0-95% response-time) was 15 min versus 5.5 min in the plasma and the effect site controlled TCI, respectively. A significant overshoot of the plasma concentration was seen in the effect site controlled TCI, a maximum plasma concentration of 15.4 μg/ml was reached at 2 min from the initial start-up. The cumulative dose of propofol that had been infused to achieve 95% of the maximum effect site concentration (9.5 μg/ml) was 11.8 versus 8.09 mg/kg, respectively, in the plasma and the effect controlled TCI setting. The reason that the required dose in the effect site controlled TCI setting was smaller than that in the plasma controlled setting is supposed to be due to the difference in the length of time interval required for the concentration to reach the pre-set target level. Directly after the infusion is started, the inter-compartmental transfer of drug from the central to the peripheral compartments and the metabolic clearance from the central compartment, has its way. Thus, if a longer time is required to reach the pre-set concentration, more drug will be required to compensate for this outflow.

Comparing effect site and plasma controlled TCI in a clinical setting

When studying muscle relaxants, the pharmacological effect can be evaluated directly by measuring the muscle twitch response to electrical nerve stimulation. Hence, with muscle relaxants it is easy to compare plasma and effect site controlled TCI, clinically. The concentration of vecuronium needed to cause 95% (EC_{95}) depression of the control response, measured at the abductor pollicis, to electrical ulnar nerve stimulation is 0.2 μg/ml. To evaluate the plasma and effect site controlled TCI, the target concentration was set equal to the EC_{95} in both devices. The time courses in both cases are shown on the left and right side of figure 4, respectively. The times required to cause 95% depression in muscle response were 27.5 (estimated) and 13.8 min (measured), and 6.6 (estimated) and 3.8 min (measured) for the plasma and the effect site controlled TCI devices, respectively. The short required time for the effect site controlled TCI device (less than one third) to cause a 95% response leads us to conclude that this is the method of administration to be used preferably when

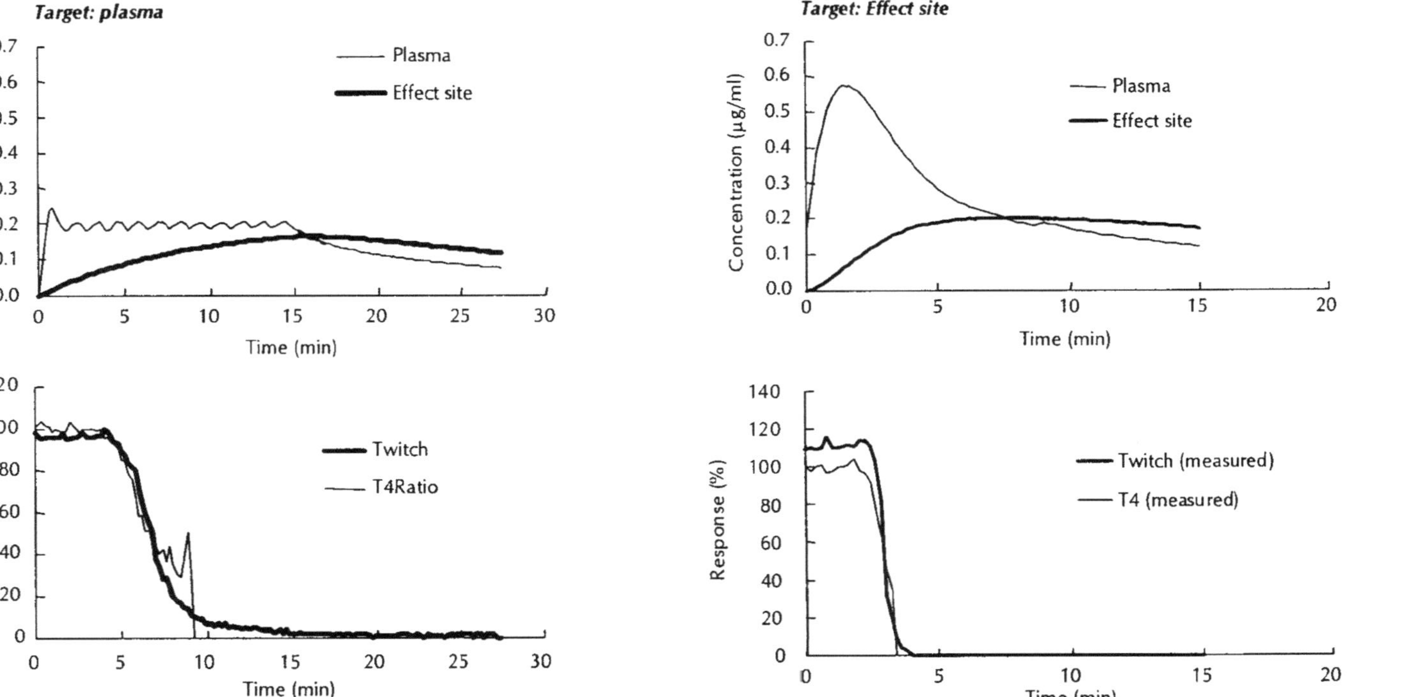

Figure 4
Muscle relaxant TCI. The muscle relaxation by vecuronium was evaluated clinically. Concentration-time-profiles were simulated numerically under the following two conditions. A target plasma concentration of 0.2 µg/ml was preset as the target (left panel). A target effect site concentration of 0.2 µg/ml was preset as the target (right panel). The muscle response was evaluated by measuring the twitch ratio with an electrical nerve stimulation. *Left panel:* In the plasma controlled TCI 95% of the preset concentration was reached 0.5 min after the start of infusion but the effect site concentration remained less than 5% of the target, and another 25 min were required to reach 95 % of the target effect site concentration. The measured twitch response decreased less than 5% of the control value at 13 min after the infusion started. *Right panel:* The effect site concentration reached 95% of the preset level at 5.2 min and the measured response decreased to 5% of the control value at 3.8 min after the TCI started.

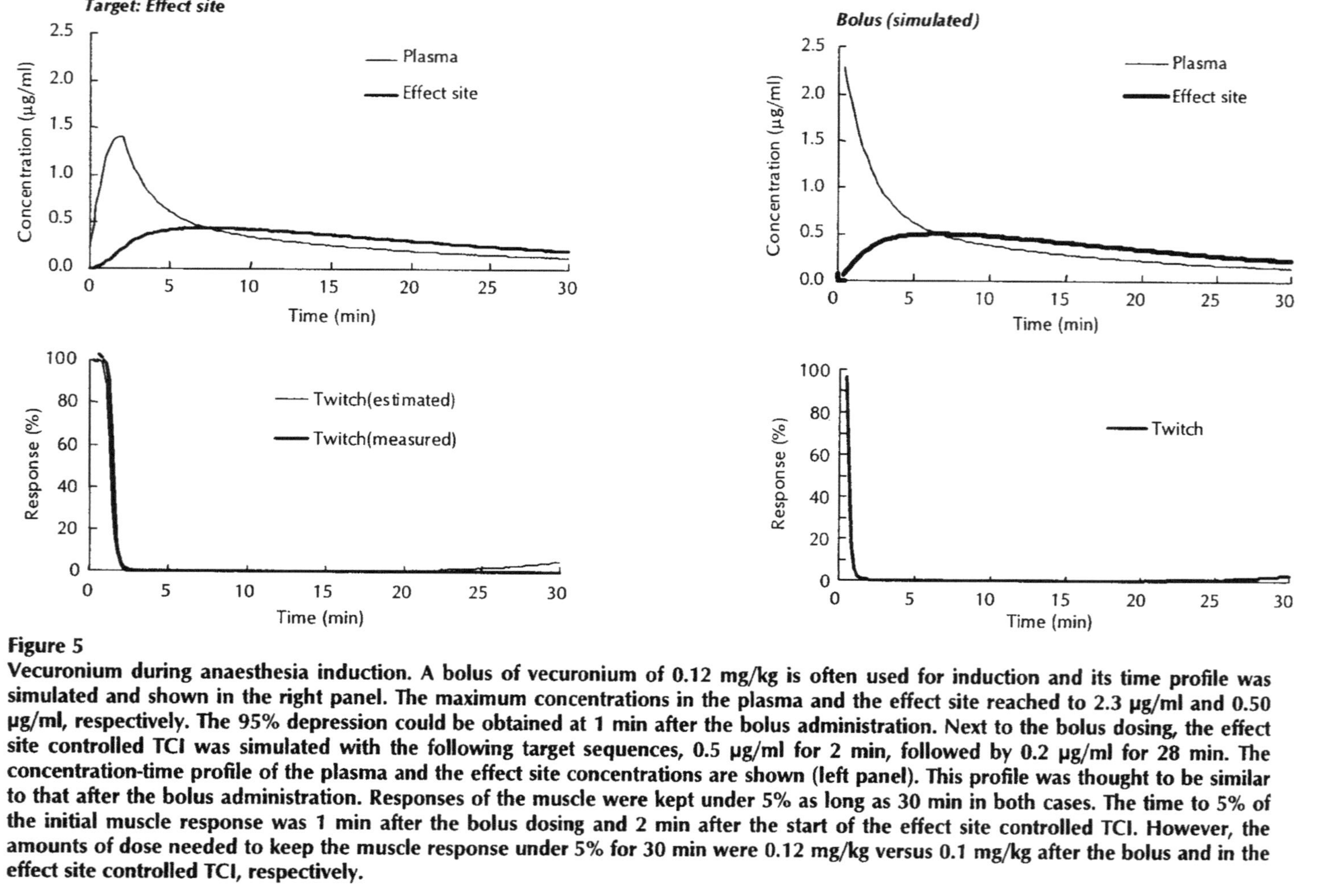

Figure 5
Vecuronium during anaesthesia induction. A bolus of vecuronium of 0.12 mg/kg is often used for induction and its time profile was simulated and shown in the right panel. The maximum concentrations in the plasma and the effect site reached to 2.3 µg/ml and 0.50 µg/ml, respectively. The 95% depression could be obtained at 1 min after the bolus administration. Next to the bolus dosing, the effect site controlled TCI was simulated with the following target sequences, 0.5 µg/ml for 2 min, followed by 0.2 µg/ml for 28 min. The concentration-time profile of the plasma and the effect site concentrations are shown (left panel). This profile was thought to be similar to that after the bolus administration. Responses of the muscle were kept under 5% as long as 30 min in both cases. The time to 5% of the initial muscle response was 1 min after the bolus dosing and 2 min after the start of the effect site controlled TCI. However, the amounts of dose needed to keep the muscle response under 5% for 30 min were 0.12 mg/kg versus 0.1 mg/kg after the bolus and in the effect site controlled TCI, respectively.

immediate control of the muscle response is required. Anaesthesia induction is such a typical application.

For intubation, a bolus of vecuronium of 0.12 mg/kg is often used. We simulated the time profile following this bolus dose as is displayed in figure 5 on the right side. The maximum concentrations in the plasma and in the effect site were 2.3 and 0.50 μg/ml, respectively. The 95% depression was obtained 1 min after the bolus administration. In our comparison we evaluated the effect site controlled TCI to the previous plasma controlled administration of vecuronium with the following sequences; the effect site target was pre-set at 0.5 μg/ml for 2 min, followed by a target effect site concentration of 0.2 μg/ml for 28 min. The estimated time courses of the plasma and effect site concentrations are shown on the left side of figure 5. Responses of the muscles were kept well under 5% the of control value for as long as 30 min after the administration started, in both cases. The required time to cause 5% of the muscle response was obtained at 1 min after the bolus dose and at 2 min in the patients receiving the effect site controlled TCI. The amounts of dose needed to keep the muscle response under 5% for 30 minutes were 0.12 versus 0.1 mg/kg for the bolus and effect site controlled TCI administration, respectively.

Accuracy

The accuracy of the prediction of the acquired concentration can be evaluated by the performance error (PE) and the median PE (MDPE) or median absolute PE (MDAPE), which are defined as:

$$PE = \frac{\text{Measured} - \text{Predicted}}{\text{Predicted}}$$
$$\text{MDPE} = \text{median}\{PE_i, i = 1 \text{ to } n\}$$
$$\text{MDAPE} = \text{median}\{|PE_i|, i = 1 \text{ to } n\}$$

The PE denotes the normalised residuals describing the difference between measured and predicted concentrations. The MDPE reflects the presence of systematic under dosing or overdosing by the TCI algorithm, while the MDAPE is not influenced by a positive or negative discrepancy between the measured and predicted values and thus represents the magnitude of the PE. Shafer et al.[13] applied their TCI algorithm to 21 patients and evaluated the accuracy of the used fentanyl pharmacokinetic parameter set. They derived various pharmacokinetic parameters from each of four previous studies[3, 14 - 16], then applied each of these sets and their own parameter set to their own observed fentanyl data set. The MDAPE's were 22, 33, 44, 59 and 21 %, respectively. Glass et al.[17] assessed the accuracy of fentanyl TCI in 24 patients using their pharmacokinetic model-driven infusion pump (CACI) based on parameters taken from McClain and Hug. Their MDAPE was 21%. Maitre et al.[18] reported a mean absolute PE (MAPE) of 22.3 % in 19 patients who were anaesthetised by alfentanil in the presence of 66% nitrous oxide. Lastly, with respect to the propofol pharmacokinetics, Schnider et al.[19] reported that the MDAPE was 23.0 %. These results suggest that the inaccuracy of TCI devices is in the order of 21 % - 59 %. Hence, the inaccuracy in the prediction of the effect site concentration will be in the same order of magnitude.

Factors of influence on pharmacokinetic parameters

These accuracy variations are partially the result of the pharmacokinetic variation that exists in between individual patients. Factors of influence are age, body weight, height and gender. Maitre et al.[20] reported that bodyweight had significant influence on the volume of the central compartment (Vc) of alfentanil, i.e. normalisation of Vc for bodyweight yielded a significant improvement of the fit. Total clearance (Cl) and K_{31} were decreased in patients aged older than 40 years, and male patients had a significant smaller Vc than female patients. The author concluded that the fit was improved from 24 to 20% after correction of the measured data by these parameters. Meanwhile, Schnider et al.[19] showed factors that influenced the propofol pharmacokinetics, in which age was a significant covariate for V_2 and for rapid peripheral clearance, and bodyweight, height and lean body mass were significant covariates for metabolic clearance. The goodness of fit was improved from 23 to 17.39% of the MDAPE after applying these corrections to the pharmacokinetic parameters.

Closed loop

In the search for the appropriate rate to infuse a drug to the patient, the TCI algorithm compares the difference between the current concentration and desired target value. Herein the concentration is not directly measured but it is estimated from the numerical model based on the population pharmacokinetics. After adjustment of covariates related to individual patient pharmacokinetics the goodness of fit was increased but still an inaccuracy of 17–20 % exists. In this context, current TCI devices have no real feedback source. Recently, the bispectral analysis of electroencephalography was introduced[5] to quantify the depth of anaesthesia. The bispectral index (BIS), which is one of the statistical scores derived from the bispectral analysis was reported to be closely related with hypnosis induced by propofol.[6,7] Hence, the BIS could be used as a feedback source of the TCI instead of the predicted pharmacological effect.

Conclusions

A time delay exists between the step change in the plasma concentration and the onset of pharmacological effect. This delay can be described by the constant k_{e0} (min^{-1}). The effect site is a hypothetical compartment in which this k_{e0} is included to denote the time-course of the effect site concentration. The concentration of the effect compartment is by definition closely related with the pharmacological effect without time delay. Controlling the pharmacological effect is the final objective of TCI and controlling the effect site concentration is the method to accomplish this. Controlling the effect site concentration can be accomplished by the following two iterative processes; A: comparison of the current predicted effect site concentration and the desired target concentration, B: determination of the appropriate infusion rate at the current step to decrease the difference between the target concentration and the future one, several steps later. Finding this infusion rate is a key point in this type of effect controlled TCI algorithm. It can be derived by either an analytical or a numerical method. If the measured pharmacological response could be used instead of the predicted concentration in the iterative process, the controlling accuracy of effect controlled TCI would markedly increase. The bispectral index may be an effective parameter to accomplish this.

References

1. Gibaldi M & Perrier D: Pharmacokinetics 2nd Edition, Section 2 (p45-111), Marcel Dekker, New York

2. Scott JC, Cooke JE, Stanski DR: Electroencephalographic quantitation of opioid effect: Comparative pharmacodynamics of fentanyl and sufentanil. Anesthesiology 1991; 74:34-42
3. Scott JC, Stanski DR: Decreased fentanyl and alfentanil dose requirements with age. A simultaneous pharmacokinetic and pharmacodynamic evaluation. Journal of pharmacology and experimental therapeutics 1987; 240:159-166
4. Forrest FC, Tooley MA, Sauders PR, Prys-Roberts C: Propofol infusion and the suppression of consciousness: the EEG and dose requirements. British Journal of Anaesthesia 1994; 72: 35-41
5. Sigl JC, Chamoun NG: An introduction to bispectral analysis for the electroencephalogram. Journal of Clinical Monitoring 1994; 10:392-404
6. Kearse LA, Manberg P, Chamoun N, deBros F, Zaslavvsky A: Bispectral analysis of the electroencephalogram correlates with patient movement to skin incision during propofol/nitrous oxide anesthesia. Anesthesiology 1994; 81;1365-1370
7. Katoh T, Suzuki A, Ikeda K: Electroencephalographic derivatives as a tool for predicting the depth of sedation and anesthesia induced by sevoflurane. Anesthesiology 1998; 88(3):642-50
8. Kazama T, Ikeda K, Morita K: The pharmacodynamic interaction between propofol and fentanyl with respect to the suppression of somatic or hemodynamic responses to skin incision, peritoneum incision, and abdominal wall retraction. Anesthesiology 1998; 89(4):894-906
9. Hull CJ, Van Beem HBH, McLeod K, Sibbald A, Watson MJ: A pharmacodynamic model for pancuronium. British Journal of Anaesthesia 1978; 50: 1113-1122
10. Sheiner LB, Stanski DR, Vozeh SV, Miller RD, Ham J: Simultaneous modeling of pharmacokinetics and pharmacodynamics: Application to d-tubocurarine. Clinical Pharmacology and Therapeutics 1979; 25:358-371
11. Schuttler J, Schwilden H, Stoeckel: Pharmacokinetic-dynamic modeling of diprivan. Anesthesiology 1986; 65: A549
12. Kazama T, Ikeda K, Morita K: Comparison of the effect-site keos of propofol for blood pressure and EEG bispectral index in elderly and younger patient. Anesthesiology 1999; June (in press)
13. Shafer SL, Varvel JR, Aziz N, Scott JC: Pharmacokinetics of fentanyl administered by computer-controlled infusion pump. Anesthesiology 1990; 73:1091-102
14. McClain DA, Hug CC: Intravenous fentanyl kinetics. Clinical Pharmacology and Therapeutics 1980; 28:106-114
15. Hudson RJ, Thomson JR, Cannon JE, Friesen RM, Meatherall RC: Pharmacokinetics of fentanyl in patients undergoing abdominal aortic surgery. Anesthesiology 1986; 64:334-338
16. Varvel JR, Shafer SL, Hwang SS, Coen PA, Stanski DR: Absorption characteristics of transdermally administered fentanyl. Anesthesiology 1989; 70:928-934
17. Glass PSA, Jacobs JR, Smith LR, Ginsberg B, Quill TJ, Bai SA, Reves JG: Pharmacokinetic model-driven infusion of fentanyl: Assessment of Accuracy. Anesthesiology 1990; 73:1082-90
18. Maitre PO, Ausem ME, Vozeh S, Stanski DR: Evaluating the accuracy of using population pharmacokinetic data to predict plasma concentrations of alfentanil. Anesthesiology 1988; 68:59-6717)
19. Schnider TW, Minto CF, Gambus PL, Andresen C, Goodale DB, Shafer SL, Youngs EJ: The influence of method of administration and covariates on the pharmacokinetics of propofol in adult volunteers. Anesthesiology 1998; 88:1170-82

20. Maitre PO, Vozeh S, Heykants J, Thomson DA, Stanski R: Population pharmacokinetics of alfentanil: The average dose-plasma concentration relationship and interindividual variability in patients. Anesthesiology 1987; 66:3 -12

EXPLORING THE PLASMA-EFFECT SITE CONCENTRATION DIFFERENCE DURING EFFECT SITE CONTROLLED INFUSION

Catherine Moiny, Edouard Coussaert and Luc Barvais

Brussels, Belgium

Introduction

Based on pharmacokinetic models, target-controlled infusion (TCI) systems have been developed to reach and maintain any desired plasma concentration of a drug during anaesthesia. These TCI systems control the plasma concentration and clinical effects are often deferred. The delay between the peak plasma concentration (Cp_{max}) and maximal clinical effect is called hysteresis. To explain this hysteresis, a new compartment has been added to the pharmacokinetic model; the effect compartment (see the chapter by Bovill). To characterise the rate of distribution elimination of intravenous anaesthetic drugs to and from the effect compartment parameters derived from the EEG such as the spectral edge and the bispectral index have been used. For a drug, if the plasma concentration is at a semi-steady state, the concentration in the effect compartment (Ce, effect site concentration) will rise following a simple increasing exponential curve. The effect site concentration is proportional to the plasma concentration: $Cp.\ (1\text{-}e^{-kt})$. The effect site concentration is characterised by the quantity of drug entering the effect compartment. The effect site concentration depends on the gradient between the plasma and the effect site concentration and by the value of the elimination rate constant of the effect compartment (k_{e0}). The k_{e0} value is different for each drug but is fixed in a specific pharmacokinetic model for one drug. For a plasma concentration at steady state, the required time needed to obtain Ce = ½ Cp is called $T_{1/2}k_{e0}$. This is dependent on the elimination rate constant from the effect site: $T_{1/2}k_{e0} = \ln 2 / k_{e0}$. The longer the $T_{1/2}k_{e0}$, the more the time delay to reach a steady state between the plasma and the effect site concentration is required. Moreover, with a long $T_{1/2}k_{e0}$, a damping in the rise and fall of the effect site concentration is observed compared to the peaks and valleys of the blood concentration.

For drugs with a very short half-life in plasma, like adenosine, the peak of the effect site concentration is obtained very quickly, no matter the k_{e0} value. Among the commonly used intravenous anaesthetic drugs, k_{e0} plays a role. Thiopental, alfentanil and remifentanil in young patients have a rapid $T_{1/2}k_{e0}$, shorter than 2 min. Propofol and remifentanil in old patients have a $T_{1/2}k_{e0}$ between 2 and 5 min. Midazolam, fentanyl and sufentanil have an intermediate $T_{1/2}k_{e0}$ of about 5 min, while morphine has a small k_{e0} and its $T_{1/2}k_{e0}$ therefore is quite long.

Wakeling et al.[1] showed that when different values of k_{e0} are taken for propofol administered as a single bolus dose, the rate of distribution from the plasma to the effect site changes. For a large k_{e0} value, $T_{1/2}k_{e0}$ is short and the effect site concentration will show a peak faster and higher than for a small k_{e0}. But the design of the curve stays similar: maximum plasma concentration is instantaneously reached and then decreases. The effect site concentration rises to reach an equilibrium (Ce = Cp). Then, the effect site concentration decreases because the drug is eliminated from the effect site.

During parametric modelling of the effect compartment, the concentration of drug in the effect compartment (Ce) varies according to the entry of drug into the effect site and its elimination. If the parameters characterising the elimination (k_{e0} and $T_{1/2}k_{e0}$) are fixed, the way out will be constant. Variations of the gradient between the plasma and the effect site concentrations will then be the most important factor that will affect the concentration in the effect site. That allows us to determine the influence of different concentration gradients between the plasma and effect site, on the time delay to reach a certain effect (Ce). For a high concentration gradient, the drug will be forced into the effect compartment to reach as fast as possible a target Ce. To limit this concentration gradient, a maximum value of Cp can be defined. Under these conditions, the target Ce will be obtained less rapidly and the pharmacodynamic effect will be

Table 1
Population pharmacokinetic parameters of remifentanil by Minto et al.[3, 4] as calculated for 3 different age groups.

Volumes (L)	
Central compartment:	5.1 - 0.0201 * (Age - 40) + 0.072 * (LBM - 55)
Rapid peripheral compartment:	9.82 - 0.0811 * (Age - 40) + 0.108 * (LBM - 55)
Slow peripheral compartment:	5.42
Clearance (L/min)	
Metabolic:	2.6 - 0.0162 * (Age - 40) + 0.0191 * (LBM - 55)
Rapid peripheral	2.05 - 0.0301 * (Age - 40)
Slow peripheral	0.076 - 0.00113 * (Age - 40)
K_{e0} (min^{-1})	0.595 - 0.007 * (Age - 40)

	20 years	50 years	80 years
keo (min^{-1})	0.735	0.525	0.315
$t_{1/2}$ keo (min)	0.943	1.32	2.2
Volume central compartment (L)	6.058	5.455	4.852
Clearance of the central compartment (L/h)	184.287	155.127	125.967

delayed. The purpose of the following simulations was to evaluate the influence of limitation of the maximum plasma concentration during effect site controlled TCI on the time that the desired Ce is reached. Remifentanil was chosen as an example because Minto et al.[3, 4] have studied a population pharmacokinetic set including the k_{e0} which identifies the effect of age and lean body mass (LBM) on the pharmacokinetic parameters of remifentanil.

Materials and methods

In collaboration with the Department of Computer Sciences of the University of Brussels, a simulation program has been developed to control the effect site concentration. In this software program, the pharmacokinetic and pharmacodynamic population models of Minto et al.[3, 4] for remifentanil are included (table 1).

The following simulations are restricted to the initial infusion of remifentanil in different patient settings according to the population pharmacokinetic model of Minto.[3, 4] A given effect site concentration is targeted and the software computes the bolus dose of remifentanil required to reach a peak plasma concen-

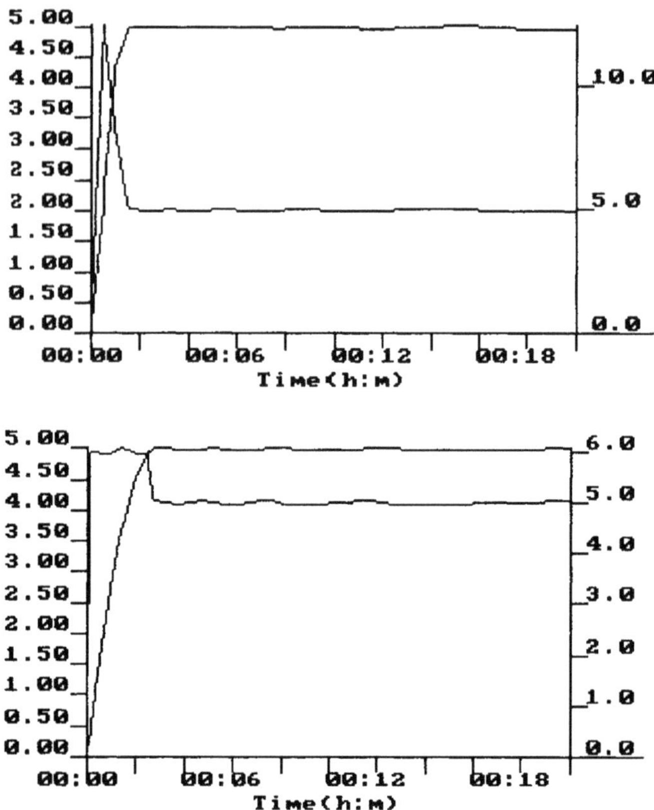

Figure 1
Graph simulation to obtain an effect-site remifentanil concentration of 5 ng/ml using the pharmacokinetic set of Minto et al.[3,4] in a 50-year old patient. In the upper part, the peak plasma concentration is limited to 12 ng/ml and in the lower part to 6 ng/ml. The left Y-axis is the effect site concentration scale and the right Y-axis is the plasma concentration scale.

tration within 30 sec. This peak of the plasma concentration is of a higher value than the target effect site concentration.

As the plasma concentration decreases, the effect site concentration rises to reach the targeted effect site concentration. Once the semi-steady state is reached, the plasma concentration and the effect site concentration are at the same value and the pump is programmed to infuse remifentanil to maintain a constant plasma concentration. This constant plasma concentration will then assure a constant effect site concentration.

The program allows the peak plasma concentration to be limited to a predetermined value. Consequently, the difference between the plasma concentration and the effect site concentration is limited. The plasma concentration will be maintained at its maximal value on a "plateau phase" as the effect site concentration rises. Then, the plasma concentration decreases to reach the value of semi-steady state with the effect site concentration. The dilution of remifentanil used for the simulation is 0.01 mg/ml (1 mg in 100 ml). All the simulations are performed using a Fresenius Pilot Anaesthesia pump. Its maximal flow rate is 1500 ml/h. The loading bolus dose is given over 30 sec.

For the first simulation set, a 50-year old male patient with a lean body mass of 62.7 (weight 80 kg, length 180 cm) is selected (tables 2 and 3, and figures 1 and 2). Those characteristics determine the pharmacokinetic and pharmacodynamic model and are kept constant throughout the simulation (k_{e0} = 0.525 min^{-1}). Then, an effect site concentration of 10 ng/ml of remifentanil is targeted. In the first situation, the peak plasma concentration is only limited by the maximal delivery rate of the pump. The required times to reach 80%, 90%, 95% and 100% of the targeted effect site concentration are measured. The same measurements for a peak plasma concentration limited to 15 ng/ml, 11 ng/ml, 10 ng/ml are also simulated. This means that the difference between the plasma concentration and the effect site concentration is limited to 50%, 10% and 0% of the target effect site concentration, respectively.

In the second simulation, the effect of age is studied. Two patients are studied. The first one is a male of 20 years old, 80 kg and 180 cm and the second one is a male patient of 80 years old, 80 kg and 180 cm. For both patients, the LBM is 62.7. As the age increases, the k_{e0} value decreases from 0,735 min^{-1} to 0,375 min^{-1}. The pharmacokinetic parameters (volume of distribution and clearance) are also adapted (table 1). The same simulations are performed in the 2 different patient settings (table 4 and figure 3). For both patients, the effect site concentration is targeted at 5 ng/ml and the time required to reach this target effect site concentration is calculated in different situations in which Cp_{max} becomes progressively limited to 5, 5.2, 5.4, 5.6, 5.8, 6, 7, 8, 9, 10, 11, 12 and 15 ng/ml. The situation where the peak plasma concentration is only limited by the pump delivery is also simulated.

Table 2
Time delay to obtain 100, 95, 90 or 80 % of the effect site remifentanil target concentration (Ce) of 10 ng/ml, when the peak plasma concentration (Cp) is limited to 17, 15, 11 or 10 ng/ml. In clinical practice, the initial loading dose is administered over a 30-sec period using the maximum pump flow rate of the selected infusion device (1500 ml/hr) and using remifentanil at a dilution of 0.01 mg/ml.

Time to attain 10 ng/ml of Ce of remifentanil if:	Peak Cp at 17 ng/ml	Peak Cp at 15 ng/ml	Peak Cp at 11 ng/ml	Peak Cp at 10 ng/ml
100 % of Ce	2:00	2:37	4:40	10:18
95 % of Ce	1:58	2:28	4:06	5:40
90 % of Ce	1:56	2:20	3:35	4:30
80 % of Ce	1:54	2:07	2:52	3:10

Table 3
Percentage of time increase to reach 100, 95, 90 or 80 % of the target effect site remifentanil concentration (Ce) of 10 ng/ml, when the peak plasma concentration (Cp) had been limited to 15, 11 or 10 ng/ml compared to when the peak plasma remifentanil concentration had not been limited (17 ng/ml). This peak plasma concentration of 17 ng/ml corresponds to the administration of the initial loading dose over a 30 sec period using the maximum pump flow rate of 1500 ml/h and using remifentanil at a dilution of 0.01 mg/ml.

	Peak Cp at 15 ng/ml	Peak Cp at 11 ng/ml	Peak Cp at 10 ng/ml
100 % of Ce	30.83	133.33	415.00
95 % of Ce	25.42	108.47	188.14
90 % of Ce	20.69	85.34	132.76
80 % of Ce	11.40	50.88	66.67

Results

Simulation 1: male patient; 50 years, 80 kg, 180 cm, target remifentanil Ce: 10 ng/ml

When the peak plasma concentration of remifentanil is not limited, only 2 min are required to obtain 100% of the target effect site concentration of remifentanil in this patient (table 2). When the peak plasma concentration of remifentanil is not limited, the effect site concentration reaches the level of the target effect site concentration rapidly. To reach 95%, 90% and 80% of the effect site concentration, only 2, 4 and 6 seconds are needed, respectively (table 2 and

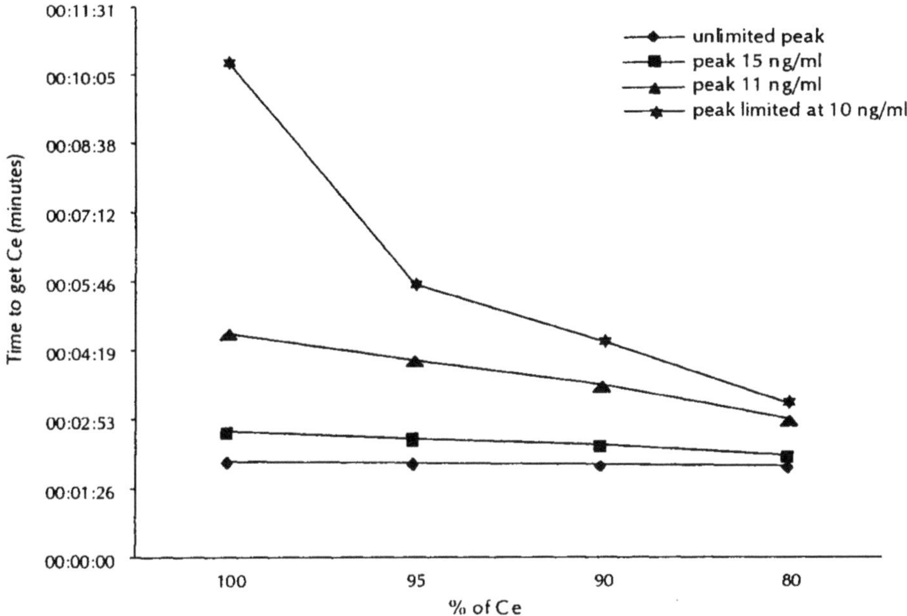

Figure 2
Influence of the peak plasma remifentanil concentration to obtain 80 %, 90 %, 95 % or 100 % of a target effect site concentration of 10 ng/ml in a 50-year-old patient if the plasma concentration is not limited (17 ng/ml) or limited to 50 % (15 ng/ml), 10 % (11 ng/ml), or 0 % (10 ng/ml) overshoot.

figure 2). In contrast, limitation of Cp_{max} influences greatly the delay to get to the required effect site concentration. For example, if the difference between the plasma concentration and the effect site concentration is restricted to 10%, this means that for a target effect site concentration of 10 ng/ml, a highest plasma concentration of only 11 ng/ml is allowed.

Nearly 5 min are required to obtain the target effect site concentration of 10 ng/ml of remifentanil. This corresponds with a supplementary time delay of 160 sec. The time delay is increased by 133 % compared with the unlimited Cp_{max} (table 3). However, when the plasma concentration is limited to only 10 % above the desired effect site concentration, 80% of the target effect site concentration is obtained after 172 sec, which only corresponds to a 50 % increase of the time delay compared with the administration of a non limited overshoot.

Table 4
Comparison of the time delay to reach a theoretical effect site target remifentanil concentration of 5 ng/ml according to the gradient between the plasma (Cp) and the effect-site (Ce) concentration using the population pharmacokinetic parameters of Minto et al.[3,4], either in young (20 years) or old (80 years) patients.

Maximal peak plasma concentration of remifentanil (ng/ml)	% difference between Cp and Ce	Time delay to get Ce of 5 ng/ml in a 20 year old patient (min:sec)	% of the time delay increase compared with non limited Cp in a 20-year-old patient	Time delay to get Ce of 5 ng/ml in a 80 year old patient (min:sec)	% of the time delay increase compared with non limited Cp in a 80-year-old patient
5		7:18		17:27	
5.2	4	4:38	219.54	10:35	320.53
5.4	8	3:40	152.87	8:30	237.75
5.6	12	3:06	113.79	7:21	192.05
5.8	16	2:57	103.45	6:35	161.59
6	20	2:42	86.21	5:42	126.49
7	40	2:03	41.38	4:26	76.16
8	60	1:46	21.84	3:41	46.36
9	80	1:37	11.49	3:15	29.14
10	100	1:32	5.75	3:00	19.21
11	120	1:29	2.30	2:51	13.25
12	140	1:27	0.00	2:41	6.62
15	200	1:27	0.00	2:31	0.00
17		1:27		2:31	

The limitation of the allowed peak plasma concentration at 50 % of the effect site concentration value does not influence the time scheme as much as a 10 % overshoot limitation. Only, 37, 30, 24 and 13 supplementary sec are required to reach 100, 95, 90 and 80 % of the targeted effect site concentration, respectively (table 2). Eighty percent of the target effect site concentration is obtained after 127 sec, which is approximately the same time duration as the minimum required period to reach 100% of the effect site concentration when the allowed plasma concentration is not limited (table 2).

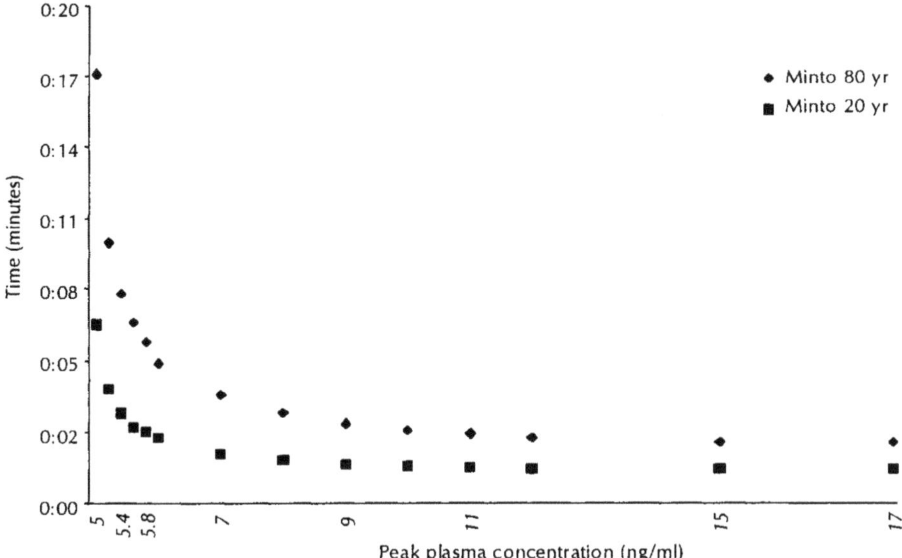

Figure 3
Time delay to reach a theoretical remifentanil effect-site concentration of 5 ng/ml, according to the peak of the plasma concentration, using the population pharmacokinetic parameters of Minto et al.[3, 4] for either a 20 yr old or a 80 yr old patient.

When remifentanil is administered by a TCI system controlling the plasma concentration, the time to a semi-steady state between the plasma and the effect site concentration is lengthened. More than 10 min are required to reach an effect site concentration plateau of 10 ng/ml (table 2). The time delay to reach 10 ng/ml is prolonged by 415 % if the maximal plasma concentration is limited at the same level (table 3). However, the time delay to reach 80 % of the target effect site concentration of 10 ng/ml is prolonged by only 66.67 %, if the plasma concentration is limited at 10 ng/ml (table 3).

Simulation 2: 20- and 80-year old males of 80 kg and 180 cm, target remifentanil Ce: 5 ng/ml

Using the population set of Minto et al.[3,4] for a 20-year-old patient, the time delay to reach an effect site concentration of 5 ng/ml is very short (87 sec) when the maximum plasma concentration peak is not limited (table 4). When the difference between the plasma and the effect site concentration is limited to 100 %, the percentage increase of the time delay to reach the target effect concentration is only 5.75 %. When this difference between the plasma and the effect site concentration is limited to less than 50 %, the time delay to get the target effect concentration starts to increase abruptly. More than 7 min are required to attain the effect site concentration when the plasma concentration is limited at the same level (table 4).

Using the population set of Minto et al.[3,4] for an 80-year-old patient, the time delay to reach an effect site concentration of 5 ng/ml is longer than in a 20-year-old (table 4). When the maximum plasma concentration is limited to 100 %, the percentage increase of time delay is 19.21 %. When the difference between the plasma and effect site concentration is limited to less than 50 % of the target effect site concentration, the time delay increases more than in young patients. Over 17 min are required to attain an effect site concentration of 5 ng/ml when the maximum plasma concentration is limited at the same level of 5 ng/ml (table 4).

Discussion

The relationship between the dose the anaesthesiologist injects and the generated blood concentration is described for all intravenous anaesthetic agents. For propofol, the pharmacokinetic parameter set described by Gepts et al.[6] and modified by Marsh et al.[7] has been demonstrated to be associated with a low bias (+ 5.7 %) and an acceptable precision (25.5 %) in healthy adult patients[8], but also in patients during coronary bypass grafting[9] and elderly patients.[10] Glass et al. have demonstrated that a TCI of fentanyl provides an acceptable accuracy within a homogeneous patient population of ASA 1-2 adult patients.[11] Other studies have demonstrated a good predictive accuracy for remifentanil, alfentanil, fentanyl and sufentanil.[3,4, 12, 13, 14]

In Europe, the Diprifusor has been commercialised thanks to the collaboration of the infusion system manufacturers and the Zeneca pharmaceutical company. The Diprifusor is a TCI system controlling the plasma concentration of propofol. It consists of a module in which infusion control algorithms are linked to a pharmacokinetic simulation program, which includes the conventional 3-compartment pharmacokinetic parameter set of Marsh.[7] The Diprifusor controls the amount of propofol delivered to achieve and maintain the calculated target blood propofol concentration in adult patients. It enables the anaesthetist to titrate the target blood propofol concentration, to assess the adequacy of hypnosis and to adjust it either upwards or downwards according to the surgical stimulation, the patient's requirements and the concomitant use of other anaesthetic drugs. The Diprifusor system also provides information on the effect site concentration of propofol. The value of the k_{e0} of 0.297 included in the Diprifusor is not derived from the same pharmacokinetic study because EEG parameters have not been measured in the initial pharmacokinetic study of Gepts et al.[6]. Unfortunately, up to now, there is no commercialised TCI system for any of the other intravenous anaesthetic drugs, except those developed as research tools.[3,4,11,14]

The ability to control the plasma concentration of the intravenous hypnotic or opioid drugs does not automatically imply instantaneous control of the level of hypnosis or analgesia. The primary site of action of the anaesthetic drugs is the central nervous system. The transfer through the blood-brain barrier and the equilibrium between the plasma and the so-called effect site or the biophase takes time. This delay is defined by the parameter k_{e0}. So, it would be more logical to control the effect site concentration rather than the blood concentration. Algorithms to control the effect site have been developed.[15,16] Pharmacokinetic simulation programs and new TCI systems developed can also target the effect compartment concentration.[15] These TCI systems act by giving a predetermined bolus of the drug in the blood. This overshoot produces a large concentration gradient between the plasma concentration and the effect site concentration, which forces the drug into the effect site. The target effect site concentration is attained very rapidly if the maximum plasma peak is not limited. If the peak plasma concentration is restricted, the time to get the target effect site concentration is delayed but still shorter compared to a standard TCI system controlling the blood concentration. The difference or the gradient between the plasma concentration and the effect site concentration is the major factor that is of influence on the delay to attain a desired effect because k_{e0} is fixed.

In the first simulation, increasing the gradient between Cp and Ce decreases the time required to reach the targeted Ce (table 2 and figure 2). When peak plasma concentration is limited, the time delay to attain Ce increases. This time augmentation is less evident if the practitioner is satisfied when 80 % to 90 % of the target Ce is reached (table 2). This practice can be justified because a chosen effect concentration might be appropriate for someone but not for another one because of the interindividual variability among people.

In the second simulation, two patients with a similar LBM but with different ages are selected. Ageing is accompanied by a decrease of the remifentanil clearance and the k_{e0} value (table 1). This simulation shows that the limitation of the gradient between the plasma and the effect site concentration increases the time delay to reach the target Ce more in the 80-year-old patient (k_{e0} = 0.315 min^{-1}) than in the 20-year-old patient (k_{e0} of 0.735 min^{-1}) (table 4 and figure 3). For example, in the old patient, the limitation of the plasma concentration by only 4% greater than the effect site concentration, increases four-times the delay compared to when Cp_{max} is not limited. The same limitation of Cp_{max} by 4% greater than the effect site concentration, increases only three-times the time delay in the young patient (table 4). The limitation of Cp_{max} at 20 % above the target effect site concentration only prolongs by 75 seconds the time delay in the young patient but more than by 3 minutes in the elderly patient (table 4). When the peak of the plasma concentration is permitted to reach a concentration twice that of the target effect site concentration, the time delay is prolonged by 20 % in the elderly patient (table 4). When k_{e0} is small, the time delay to reach the target effect site concentration is prolonged because of the distribution of the drug from plasma to peripheral compartments. In this case, peripheral compartments play a role of reservoir.

Wakeling et al.[1] have shown the importance of targeting the effect site concentration in achieving loss of consciousness. By targeting the effect site concentration instead of the plasma concentration, loss of consciousness is more rapidly induced. However, until now no clear data exist demonstrating the poor influence of the peak plasma concentration of the intravenous anaesthetic drugs on the haemodynamic stability.[1,17] Although a reduction in blood pressure has been demonstrated during induction of anaesthesia with propofol[18], Wakeling et al. could not show any heart rate or blood pressure differences when propofol was given to titrate the blood or the effect compartment in healthy young volunteers.[1] Recently, Kazama et al.[17] have demonstrated that the effect of propofol on BIS occurs more rapidly than its effects on systolic blood pressure. Different values of the $T_{1/2}k_{e0}$ for the plasma-effect-site equilibration for BIS and systolic blood pressure reductions were determined.

Moreover, in elderly patients, systolic blood pressure decreased to a greater degree but more slowly than in young patients.

Conclusions

The modern daily clinical practice of intravenous anaesthesia has changed significantly with the introduction of TCI systems such as the Diprifusor. Using a TCI system, anaesthesiologists do not need to calculate the amount of the intravenous loading dose expressed in µg/kg and to convert the maintenance infusion rate from µg/kg/min into the units of the pump syringes. They target and adapt the plasma concentration of the hypnotic or the opioid in a simple and controlled manner. If the TCI system calculates or controls the effect site concentration, the delay of the drug transfer to the site of action is taken into account and the anaesthesiologist better controls the drug action. From our simulations, limited overshoots of 20 % to 100 % of the plasma concentration above the effect site concentration seem to be appropriate to rapidly obtain 80 to 100 % of the target effect site concentration. Moreover, when k_{e0} is small, the gradient between the plasma and the effect-site concentrations has to be increased, if the desired level of the effect concentration has to be reached rapidly. More studies on the titration of the effect site concentration of intravenous anaesthetic drugs in different clinical situations are still required to validate this concept. In the next century, the future generation of TCI systems may allow the simultaneous and independent titration of the effect-site concentration of hypnotic and analgesic drugs.

References

1. Wakeling HG, Zimmerman JB, Howell S, Glass PSA (1999) Targeting effect compartment or central compartment concentration of propofol. Anesthesiology 90: 92-97
2. Schnider TW, Minto CF, Stanski DR (1994) The effect compartment concept in pharmacodynamic modelling. Anaesthetic Pharmacology Review 2: 204-213
3. Minto CF, Schnider TW, Egan TD, Youngs E, Lemmens HJ and colleages (1997) Influence of age and gender on the pharmacokinetics and pharmacodynamics of remifentanil- Model development. Anesthesiology 86: 10-23
4. Minto CF, Schnider TW, Shafer SL (1997) Pharmacokinetics and pharmacodynamics of Remifentanil-Model application. Anesthesiology 86: 24-33

5. Wakeling HG, Zimmerman JB, Howell S, Glass PSA (1999) Targeting effect compartment or central compartment concentration of propofol. Anesthesiology 90: 92-97
6. Gepts E, Camu F, Cockshott ID et al (1987) Disposition of Propofol administered as constant rate intravenous infusions in human. Anesth. Analg. 66 : 1256-1263
7. Marsh P, White M, Morton N et al (1991) Pharmacokinetic model - driven infusion of Propofol in children. Br. J. Anaesth. 67 : 41-48
8. Coetzee JF, Glen JB, Wium CA et al (1995) Pharmacokinetic model selection for target controlled infusions of Propofol. Anesthesiology 82 : 1328-1345
9. Barvais L, Rausin I, Glen JB et al (1996) Administration of Propofol by target-controlled infusion in patients undergoing coronary artery surgery. Journal of Cardiothoracic and Vascular Anesthesia 10 : 877-883
10. Swinhoe CF, Peacock JE, Glen JB et al (1998) Evaluation of the predictive performance of a Diprifusor TCI system. Anaesthesia 53 : 61-67
11. Glass PA, Jacobs JR, Smith LR et al (1990) Pharmacokinetic model-driven infusion of Fentanyl: assessment of accuracy. Anesthesiology 73 : 1082-1090
12. Raemer DB, Buschman A, Varvel JR et al (1990) The prospective use of population pharmacokinetics in a computer-driven infusion system for alfentanil. Anesthesiology 73 : 66-72
13. Shafer SL, Varvel JR, Aziz N et al (1990) Pharmacokinetics of Fentanyl administered by computer-controlled infusion pump. Anesthesiology 73 : 1091-1102
14. Pandin P, Ewalenko P, d'Hollander A et al (1997) Long-term predictive accuracy of target controlled infusion of Propofol and Sufentanil. Anesthesiology 87 : A319
15. Shafer SL, Gregg KM (1992) Algorythms to rapidly achieve and maintain stable drug concentrations at the site of drug effect with a computer-controlled infusion pump. J Pharmacokinet Biopharm 20: 147-169.
16. Jacobs JR, Williams EA (1993) Algorythm to control effect compartment drug concentrations in pharmacokinetic model-driven drug delivery. IEEE Trans Biomed Eng 40:993-999
17. Kazama T, Ikeda T, Morita K, Kikura M, Doi M , Ikeda T, Kurita T, Nakajima Y (1999) Comparison of the effect site keos of propofol for blood pressure and EEG bispectral index in elderly and younger patients. Anesthesiology 90: 1517-1527.
18. Billard V, Moulla F, Bourgain JL, Megnigbeto A, Stanski DR (1994) Hemodynamic : reponse to induction and intubation. Propofol/fentanyl interaction. Anesthesiology 81: 1384-1393.

GENETIC MODELS AND MAPPING GENES IN THE STUDY OF ANAESTHETIC ACTION

Victoria J. Simpson, Brad Rikke, Elaine Shen, Beth Bennett, Yuri Blednov and Thomas Johnson

Denver and Boulder, Colorado, USA

Introduction

The molecular action of anaesthetic agents is a problem well studied but not well understood. A novel approach to identifying molecular pathways involved in anaesthetic drug action involves isolating the genes mediating anaesthetic sensitivity in animal models. Several animal models have been derived using differential drug sensitivity as a screening phenotype. This method has produced both invertebrate (*Drosophila melanogaster, Caenorhabditis elegans, Saccharomyces cerevisiae*) and vertebrate (rodent) animal lines that differ in their central nervous system (CNS) response to anaesthetic agents. Lines can be derived from spontaneous or induced mutagenic processes, or selective breeding schemes. Inbred and recombinant lines possessing inherent differential drug sensitivities also are available. All can be used in a method of gene mapping known as quantitative trait loci (QTL) mapping. Anaesthetic sensitivity is a quantitative measure and is likely influenced by multiple genes known as QTLs where each QTL corresponds to a single gene. In this review we describe several genetic models currently used in studying anaesthetic action. We focus primarily on a mouse model which has been used to identify a QTL mediating propofol neurosensitivity in a selectively bred mouse line known as Long Sleep (LS) and Short Sleep (SS) mice.

Invertebrate models systems

Lower organisms such as *Drosophila, Caenorhabiditis elegans* and *Saccharomyces cerevisiae* provide the ability to study newly induced mutations influencing anaesthetic sensitivity. They have a rapid life cycle, are easy to maintain and large numbers of animals can be phenotyped in a very short time. The invertebrate models systems have been very good for producing mutants resistant or sensitive to the inhalational agents, but none have been isolated based on their resistance or sensitivity to any of the intravenous agents. A summary of invertebrate models discussed below is presented in table 1.

Drosophila melanogaster

Mutations have been identified that confer resistance to volatile anaesthetics.[1,2] Several mutants strains (*har38, Har56, Har63, har 85* for "halothane resistance") have been isolated which demonstrate increased resistance to halothane using the loss of motor control as screening assay. Both *har38* and *har85* mutations have been mapped to the 12E region of the X chromosome, but no candidate gene has been identified. In addition, mutations which produce increased sensitivity to halothane are likely due to ion channel mutations.[3]

The *Shaker* (*sh*) mutant demonstrates an abnormal shaking movement when exposed to diethylether.[4] They demonstrated abnormal conductance through the I_A K^+ channel. In addition, the ShakerB K^+ channel demonstrates differential sensitivity to certain volatile agents when expressed in *Xenopus* oocytes.[5]

Caenorhabditis elegans

The nematode *Caenorhabditis elegans* has been used to generate some very interesting and informative mutants to the effects of volatile agents. Analysis of the *C. elegans* mutants has been most useful in studying the volatile agents, probably because of ease of drug administration. Several possible protein targets have been identified in *C. elegans.*[6-8] Researchers using *C elegans* have developed at least two different behavioural assay end points in screening for anaesthetic resistant mutants. A reversible inhibition of movement is seen in *C elegans* upon exposure to halothane at relatively high levels of halothane and has been used to isolate halothane resistant mutants such as *unc-1* and *gas-1.*[9] Two potential protein targets have been identified which are related to the loss of movement.[6, 7] *Gas-1* is a mitochondrial protein and a homologue of a subunit

Table 1
Invertebrate animal models used in anaesthetic drug studies

Species	Drug Response/ Behavior	Proposed Protein Target	Reference
Drosophila	Volatile anaesthetics: loss of motor control	K^+ channel (Shaker mutant) Ion channels	Krishnan and Nash, 1990;Leibovitch et al, 1995; Correa, 1998
Caenorhabditis elegans	Volatile anaesthetics: immobility/ behavioral dysfunction	Mitochondrial NADH:ubiquione-oxireductase homologue Stomatin homologue Syntaxin, syntaxin - binding proteins	Kayser et al, 1999; Rajaram et al, 1998; van Swinderen et al, 1999
Saccharomyces cerevisiae	Volatile anaesthetics: Inhibition of growth	Not identified	Wolfe et al, 1998

of NADH:ubiquinone-oxireductase. *Unc-1* is a stomatin homologue and may be involved with regulating membrane ion channels. At lower levels of halothane, changes in several behavioural parameters such as inhibition of mating, slowing of pharyngeal pumping mechanisms, and decrease in rate of defecation can be observed and halothane and isoflurane resistant mutants have been isolated.[10] A mutation in the neuronal syntaxin gene is associated with volatile agent resistance. Syntaxin is a protein component of the regulatory mechanism of synaptic vesicle exocytosis.[8]

Saccharomyces cerevisiae

Mutants in yeast have been isolated which are sensitive to the effects of volatile anaesthetics. Volatile anaesthetics inhibit the growth of wild-type yeast (Zzz^+) but not anaesthetic-resistant (Zzz^-) mutants. Lipophilic volatile compounds which are not anaesthetics in mammals do not inhibit the growth of either strain.[11] These authors suggest that yeast behave in a parallel manner to mammals and are a viable model for investigation of molecular action of anaesthetics.

Table 2
Selected rodent lines used in anaesthetic drug studies.

Animal line	Drug	Behavioral Assay	Reference
Mouse			
HI/LO	Nitrous Oxide	Loss of righting reflex	Koblin et al, 1980
LS/SS	Ethanol, inhalational anaesthetics, propofol, etomidate, ketamine	Loss of righting reflex	McClearn and Kakihana, 1981, Baker et al, 1980, Simpson and Blednov, 1995, Simpson et al, 1998
DS/DR	Diazepam	Ataxia, Loss of righting reflex	Gallaher et al, 1987, McCrae et al, 1991
HAR/LAR, HA/LA	Morphine	Analgesic tests	Marek et al, 1993
Rat			
HAS/LAS	Ethanol	Loss of righting reflex	Draski et al, 1992

Rodent Model Systems

The mouse and rat models are popular models derived for assessing intravenous agent response. The ease of drug administration in a rat or mouse, the similarity of mammalian neurobiology and the highly developed genetics of rodents make them an attractive system. A few lines (both mouse and rat) derived for ethanol sensitivity also display cross-sensitivities to anaesthetic agents (see table 1). Strains used for anaesthetic drug studies are usually inbred strains or selected lines.

Inbred Mouse Strains

An inbred mouse strain is produced by at least 20 generations of brother-sister matings. This inbreeding strategy insures that strains are homozygous at all genetic loci. Any variation in drug response among inbred strains is due to differences in genes mediating the drug's actions. C57BL/6J and DBA/2J are two popular inbred strains which have been reported to have variations in morphine analgesia as assessed by the hotplate test.[12,13]

Selected Mouse Lines

Mouse lines bred for specific drug sensitivities can be used for mapping and identification of genes mediating anaesthetic drug action. A selected mouse line is produced by breeding strategies designed to produce a desired trait or phenotype such as drug sensitivity or resistance. Lines selected for differential drug sensitivity are created by screening a genetically heterogeneous population of mice. The extreme responders, either with respect to resistance or sensitivity, are selected for breeding. This selection procedure continues over many generations until there is no more response to the screening test in the offspring. All of the rodents listed in table 2 were produced by this kind of scheme. The name designations of the lines are as follows: HI/LO = high anaesthesia requirement, low anaesthesia requirement, LS = long sleep and SS =short sleep, DS = diazepam sensitivity and DR = diazepam resistant, HAR high analgesia (swim-stressed) and LAR low analgesia (swim-stressed), HA/LA high and low levorphanol analgesia.

Recombinant Inbred Mouse Strains

Recombinant inbred (RI) strains of mice are generated by mating F2 offspring generated from two existing parental inbred strains. The offspring from this mating are used for brother-sister matings for 20 generations to produce the RI strain. RI strains are useful for identifying and mapping provisional quantitative trait loci associated with drug sensitivities.

Quantitative trait loci mapping of propofol neurosensitivity genes in LS/SS mice

The LS and SS mice have been used to map genes that mediate propofol neurosensitivity. Although these mice were originally bred for their high or low sensitivity to ethanol, they have been very useful for identifying genes controlling sensitivity to other anaesthetic drugs, such as propofol. The LS and SS mice were originally bred for their sensitivity or resistance to ethanol (McClearn and Kakihana, 1981). A dose of 4.1 gm/kg ethanol induces a loss of righting reflex (LORR) of about 2 h in LS mice and of only 15 min in SS mice. Blood and brain ethanol differences are also significantly different at awakening between the lines, indicating that the differences are at the level of the central nervous system and not just due to differences in ethanol clearance. In addition to ethanol,

LS and SS mice have been found to be differentially sensitive to a number of other CNS depressants including propofol.[14, 15] A dose of 20 mg/kg given retroorbitally will produce a LORR of 3.5 min (SD = 1.01) in SS mice while the LORR for the LS mice is approximately 2.2 min longer. SS mice regain the righting reflex at about twice the brain level of the LS mice indicating that the differences are at the level of the central nervous system rather than pharmacokinetic. It is interesting that the LS and SS do not differ in their response to activation of the γ-aminobutyric $acid_A$ ($GABA_A$) chloride channel by propofol despite the fact that propofol is known as a potent activator of $GABA_A$ receptors.[14, 15]

Positional cloning is a strategy used by geneticists to identify where genes to be cloned are located on the chromosome. This is known as "gene mapping". The propofol neurosensitivity gene has been mapped using LSXSS recombinant inbred (RI) strains of mice. The RI strains were derived by crossing LS and SS mice and then intercrossing their F1 progeny. Chromosomal recombination in the F1 gametes produces chromosomes in the F2 generation that are a mix of LS and SS DNA. F2 progeny are then inbred by brother-sister matings for more than 20 generations resulting in chromosome pairs that are identical or homozygous at all gene loci. The entire genome of each RI strain was genotyped in DNA marker studies, indicating the LS or SS origin of selected chromosomal regions.[16] This information is known as strain distribution patterns. Once the strain distribution patterns for the LS, SS and RI strains are known, then phenotypic differences between the LS and SS, such as sensitivity to propofol, can be mapped by using these DNA markers to find allelic associations, or genetic linkage.

The LS and SS lines are different at the albino locus (*Tyr*) on chromosome 7 where all SS mice are albinos and all LS mice are pigmented. The 24 RI strains also exist as albino (11) or pigmented (13). A comparison of propofol sleep times show the albino RI strains have a mean LORR of 4.8 min (SEM, 0.4), while the LS have a mean LORR of 9.3 min (SEM, 0.4). This suggests a QTL for propofol neurosensitivity may be located close to the *Tyr* locus. The region around the *Tyr* locus was genetically mapped in the LSXSS RI strains using a regression approach.[17] Genotypes of seven DNA markers were determined on a 50 cM span of chromosome 7 and a significant QTL was identified at 44 cM. This QTL is known as *LORP1* (loss of righting reflex, propofol) and it explains about 80% of the genetic variance between LS and SS strains.

The region around 44 cM on chromosome 7 was further explored using the NMR deletional mutant mice. These mice carry a deletion of a small region of chromosome 7 which includes the *Tyr* locus and causes them to be albino (private communication, B.A. Rikke). Some of the mice have been engineered to carry a yeast artificial chromosome (YAC) which contains a normal *Tyr* gene and will cause the mouse to be a pigmented mouse. *LORP1* has been genetically mapped close to *Tyr* and if *LORP1* is carried on this YAC, then animals carrying the YAC should display an increased sensitivity to propofol. We tested this theory by crossing the NMR mice carrying the YAC with SS mice. F1 mice are approximately 50% albino and 50% pigmented. The albino mice do not carry the YAC while the pigmented mice do. Testing the propofol sleep times in the F1 show a statistically significant increase in propofol LORR in the pigmented mice suggesting that *LORP1* is contained within the YAC (BA Rikke, unpublished data). The YAC is approximately 250 kilobases in size and it is possible to identify genes contained within by determining its DNA sequence. Parts of the YAC have been sequenced and two candidate genes have been identified which may be *LORP1*. One of these genes is mGluR5, a metabotropic glutamate receptor gene. The other is 14-3-3 protein, a brain protein which is involved in regulating tyrosine and tryptophan hydroxylase activity. Whether either of these genes is LORP1 is yet to be determined, but they remain strong candidate genes, although others may be present on parts of the YAC which have not yet been sequenced.

Conclusion

Studies in several model systems have shown that anaesthetic action is mediated by individual genes. These studies suggest that at least in select cases, the mode of anaesthetic action is due to action at membrane protein receptors. Mapping quantitative trait loci's for anaesthetics in the mouse has identified the first locus, *LORP1*, specifying differential sensitivity for propofol, a clinically important intravenous anaesthetic. Single gene mutants in non-mammalian species such as *Drosophila melanogaster* and *Caenorhabditis elegans* have been identified which determine halothane sensitivity in these species. There is much optimism in this field that identifying genes and their products will elucidate the molecular pathways involved in mediating anaesthetic action.

References

1. Krishnan KS and Nash HA (1990). A genetic study of the anesthetic response: Mutants of Drosophila melanogaster altered in sensitivity to halothane. Proc Natl Acad Sci USA 87:8632-36
2. Nash HA, Campbell DB and Krishnan KS (1991). New mutants of Drosophila that are resistant to the anesthetic effects of halothane. Ann NY Acad Sci 625:540-44
3. Leibovitch BA, Campbell DB, Krishnan KS, Nash HA (1995). Mutations that affect ion channels change the sensitivity of Drosophila melanogaster to volatile anesthetics. J Neurogenet;10:1-13
4. Solc CK and Aldrich RW (1988). Voltage-gated potassium channels in larval CNS neurons of Drosphila. J Neurosci 8:2556-70
5. Correa AM (1998). Gating kinetics of Shaker K+ channels are differentially modified by general anesthetics Am J Physiol;275:C1009-21
6. Kayser EB, Morgan PG, Sedensky MM (1999). GAS-1: a mitochondrial protein controls sensitivity to volatile anesthetics in the nematode Caenorhabditis elegans. Anesthesiology; 90:545-54
7. Rajaram S, Sedensky MM, Morgan PG (1998). Unc-1: a stomatin homologue controls sensitivity to volatile anesthetics in Caenorhabditis elegans. Proc Natl Acad Sci USA 95: 8761-6
8. van Swinderen B, Saifee O, Shebester L, Roberson R, Nonet ML, Crowder CM (1999). A neomorphic syntaxin mutation blocks volatile-anesthetic action in Caenorhabditis elegans. Proc Natl Acad Sci USA; 96:2479-84
9. Sedensky MM, and Meneely PM (1987). Genetic analysis of halothane sensitivity in Caenorhabditis elegans. Science 236:952-954
10. Crowder CM and Schedl T (1994). Reexamination of C. elegans as a model system for the study of volatile anesthetic mechanisms. Anesthesiology 81:A898
11. Wolfe D, Hester P, Keil RL (1998). Volatile anesthetic additivity and specificity in Saccharomyces cerevisiae: implications for yeast as a model system to study mechanisms of anesthetic action. Anesthesiology; 89:174-81
12. Racagni G, Bruno F, Iuliano E, Paoletti R (1979). Differential sensitivity to morphine-induced analgesia and motor activity in two inbred strains of mice: Behavioral and biochemical correlations. J Pharmacol Exp Ther 209:11-116
13. Filibeck J, Castellano C and Oliverio A (1981). Differential effects on behavior of opiate agonists-antagonists on morphine-induced hyperexcitability and analgesia in mice. Psychopharmacology 73:134-1136
14. Simpson VJ and Blednov Y (1996). Propofol produces differences in behavior but not chloride channel function between selected lines of mice. Anesth and Analg 82:327-331
15. Simpson VJ, Rikke BA, Costello JM, Corley R, Johnson TE (1998). Identification of a genetic region in mice that specifies sensitivity to propofol. Anesthesiology 88:379-389
16. Markel PD, Bennett B, Beeson MA, Gordon L, Simpson VJ, Johnson TE (1996). Strain distribution patterns for genetic markers in the LSXSS recombinant-inbred series. Mamm Genome 7:408-12.
17. Haley CS and Knott SA. A simple regression method for mapping quantitative trait loci in line crosses using flanking markers. Heredity 1992; 69:315-24
18. McClearn GE and Kakihana R (1981). Selective breeding for ethanol sensitivity: Short-sleep and long-sleep mice. In "Development of Animal Models as Pharmacogenetic Tools" (GE McClearn, RA Deitrich and VG Erwin, eds), Research Mono-

graph No. 6, pp. 147-159. U.S. Department of Health and Human Services, Rockville, MD.

19. McCrae AF, Gallaher EJ, Winter PM, Firestone LL (1993). Volatile anesthetic requirements differ in mice selectively bred for sensitivity or resistance to diazepam: Implications for the site of Anesthesia. Anesth Analg 76:1313-1317
20. Baker R, Melchoir C and Deitrich R (1980). The effect of halothane on mice selectively bred for differential sensitivity to ethanol. Pharmacol Biochem Behav 12:691-695
21. Draski LJ, Spuhler KP, Erwin VG, Baker RC, Deitrich RA (1992). Selective breeding of rats differing in sensitivity to the effects of acute ethanol administration. Alcohol Clin Exp Res 6:48-54
22. Gallaher EJ, Hollister LE, Gionet SE (1987). Mouse lines selected for genetic differences in diazepam sensitivity. Psychopharmacology 93:25-30
23. Koblin DD, Dong DE, Deady JE, Eger EI II (1980). Selective breeding alters murine resistance to nitrous oxide without alteration in synaptic membrane lipid composition. Anesthesiology; 52:4101-4107
24. Marek P, Mogil JS, Belknap JK, Sadowski B, Liebeskin JC (1993). Levorphanol and swim stress-induced analgesia in selectively bred mice: Evidence for genetic commonalilties. Brain Res 608:353-357

The perioperative use of hypnotic agents

TOTAL INTRAVENOUS ANAESTHESIA: THE EQUIPMENT

Frank H.M. Engbers

Leiden, The Netherlands

Introduction

Only a few years ago Total Intravenous Anaesthesia (TIVA) was advocated and used by only a few enthusiasts. Reasons for prevalence of intravenous anaesthesia above inhalational anaesthesia vary. There are theoretical arguments like having control over the separate components of anaesthesia: analgesia, hypnosis and muscle relaxation, but increasingly the argument of environmental pollution is a consideration in the choice between inhalational and intravenous anaesthesia. In some hospitals pregnancy of the personnel is a reason to avoid specific environments; such as the ENT departments, where frequently tonsillectomies with inhalational anaesthesia are performed, or the recovery rooms, where avoidance of the pollution with inhalational waste products is almost impossible. Although the effects of nitrous oxide and inhalation anaesthesia on the embryonic development remain controversial, personnel in operating theatres logically tend to avoid any risk. There may be also pure practical problems that can be solved by using TIVA, e.g. the need for higher oxygen concentrations or the inability to provide inhalational anaesthesia in the presence of a difficult airway. Fiberscopic intubation, jet ventilation and lung surgery are just a few other examples, next to the necessity to provide anaesthesia outside our 'natural' environment for its use in the operating theatre with its ready to use vaporisers and scavenging systems. Many procedures are now done on radiology departments with minimal invasive techniques. Often these patients require more than just sedation. Only the anaesthesiologist, with knowledge and access to the modern intravenous anaesthetic drugs, and expertise in applying life support techniques can safely guide these patients through these procedures.

It is certainly true that the development of intravenous drugs with a desirable pharmacokinetic-pharmacodynamic profile has led to the increased interest and more widespread use of TIVA in recent years in most parts of the world. It should not be forgotten that also the development and availability of the drug delivery system; the infusion pump plays an important role. For a successful administration of intravenous anaesthesia, knowledge of the pitfalls of applying the TIVA technique per se is important. Because most of the research has focused on revealing the properties of the drug itself, little is known on the influence of the practical application on the blood or plasma concentration of the drug. For example, what is the influence of the inflation of a non-invasive blood pressure cuff on the blood concentration of a drug that is infused in the arm where the cuff is on? These factors would hardly have had influence on the 'stability' of the intravenous anaesthesia in the past because the half-lives of the pharmacokinetic processes and blood-brain equilibration of the drugs that we used back then where of such an order that a flow interruption of a few min would not cause any change in the effect. However, the more precisely we are able to titrate a drug (and stay just above the threshold of inadequate anaesthesia), the shorter acting our drugs, and the more supra-additive (see chapter by Vuyk) the interaction is, the more likely the interruption of the drug flow will be recognisable by a change in the anaesthetic state of the patient. It is the author's experience and belief that many of the problems encountered in intravenous anaesthesia are caused by the handling of the pump and infusion line and can simply be avoided once recognised. This chapter deals with some of these factors regarding intravenous anaesthesia and Target Controlled Infusion (TCI)

The infusion pump for manual controlled TIVA

For drug infusions such as used in TIVA the syringe pump is the most commonly used device in Europe. In the past these where mechanically relative simple devices that where meant to take over the function of the human hand for slowly injecting drugs. These systems had only limited functions and alarms.

Also the syringe inlay was primitive and some pumps did not withhold the backside of the syringe plunger leading to dangerous situations caused by siphoning (see there). An example of a development dedicated syringe pump for intravenous anaesthesia was the Ohmeda 9000[1] and the InfusOR (Bard).

The user interface

More and more functions have been added to the infusion pumps since the early days, leading to devices that are almost impossible to control without extensive study and thereby creating the danger of over-complexity. Now, some of the infusion pumps have the possibility of entering the body weight and drug concentration so that dosing on a concentration unit per kg per time basis is possible. Increased computer power has made it even possible to store complete drug databases inside one syringe pump. Although this seems to be an advance in technical development, it may not be an advance clinically. First of all, although we usually dose our drugs on the weight of the patient, there is very little evidence that the weight of the patient is an important factor in the pharmacokinetic differences between patients. Secondly, there is no standard in the dosing unit. Some drug dosing schemes are for example in $mg.kg^{-1}.h^{-1}$, whereas others may be dosed as $\mu g.kg.^{-1}min^{-1}$. This may vary also between departments and even between users. Every added function attenuates the complexity and the possibility of mistakes. When there is no scientifically proven advantage of this increased functionality for patient or user, it should not be implemented. Users who know the dosing schemes and how to set up these complex functions of the pumps do not need it, and people who do not know the infusion schemes should not use the drug or the pump. Unless technology is added to these pumps to protect users from making mistakes, such as an automatic drug and dilution detection, pumps should be as simple as possible. Numerical input will evoke typing errors. The same goes for semi-automatic dosing schemes that can be pre-programmed into some infusion pumps. These are useless for intravenous anaesthesia because they neglect the fact that anaesthesia is a dynamic process that requires adjustments of the drug dosing dependent on the stimulus and the sensitivity of the patient. In daily practice most of the features of the very advanced infusion pumps are seldom, if ever, used.

There are, however, some requirements for infusion devices used for intravenous anaesthesia that can be helpful.

- *Bolus*

  Immediate change of the anaesthetic status is often necessary. This should be possible with one button push giving a high flow of at least 800 ml/h, without the necessity of prior stopping the pump. The advantage of this immediate response and fall back to the pre-set infusion rate will also make sure that the pump is not forgotten to be restarted after a bolus.

  The so-called 'hands free' bolus, where a pre-programmed amount of drug is injected has the advantage that other activities can be employed during the bolus delivery, but has the danger that the bolus may not be appropriate for the drug in use.

- *Flow rate*

  Pumps for intravenous anaesthesia should have the possibility of high flow rates. It is obligatory to use the same pump for induction and maintenance. Induction with some of the anaesthetic drugs requires flow rates of at least 600 ml/h. On the other hand the pump must also be usable at low infusion rates with adjustments of 0.1 ml/h.

- *Alarms*

  Indication of correct syringe and plunger inlay is essential (see below). An adjustable pressure alarm is desirable. The pressure alarm should automatically adjust itself to the installed syringe size to prevent extreme high pressures being build up in smaller syringes.

  Other obligatory alarms are the indication of stopped infusion and the end of syringe and near end of syringe alarms. Most important is that the alarm philosophy is well evaluated. Too many false negative alarms will annoy the user and lower his alertness to respond. Lastly, some alarms have a certain pitch that makes the place of origin very difficult to locate.

- *Battery*

  One of the advantages of intravenous anaesthesia is that with only a few components it can be admitted everywhere with an appropriate battery. Unfortunately battery technology in infusion pumps is lagging severely behind compared to for example the home video equipment. Intelligent battery

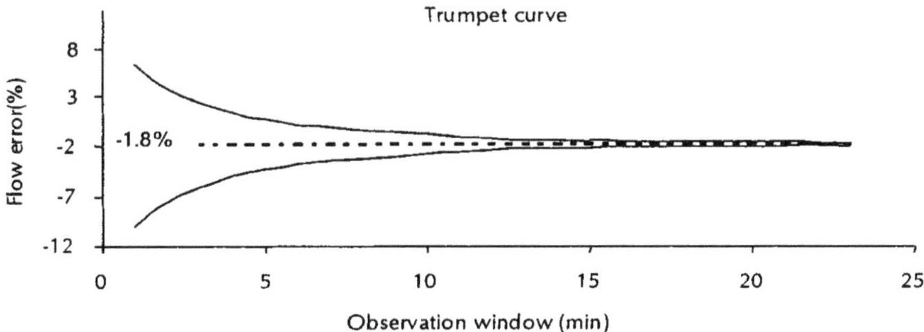

Figure 1
Accuracy of a typical infusion pump related to the observation time at a flowrate of 5 ml/hr. Nominal error: -1.8%.

loading and indication of duration of battery powered operation would be of great value.

- *Tight syringe fitting.* See below

Accuracy of the infusion pump

If an infusion pump is to be judged on the suitability for use for intravenous anaesthesia, nominal (or averaged) accuracy is probably not the most important item. Accuracy is usually represented by a so-called trumpet curve (figure 1) where at a typical flow of 5 ml/h the error is plotted against the observation time. The shape is often trumpet-like because of the way the pump (specially those with an analogue motor) adjusts its output. On the spindle that pushes the syringe is a displacement sensor. The output from this sensor is fed into a comparator that compares the displacement with the expected calculated displacement based on the installed rate. The difference than is used to adjust the motor current. The time constant of this control may vary between pumps. In the beginning there may be some oscillations around the ideal rate. These oscillations decrease and what rests is the offset or nominal error. Modern infusion pumps most likely will have an error of less than 5% from the ideal flow rate. Given the variability in drug concentration, the pharmacokinetic and pharmacodynamic variability between patients, it is not likely that the user will notice this on average less than 5% error of the infusion device. Very short deviations, for example, caused by the discrete steps of a stepper motor in the driving mechanism, or fast oscillations of the control loop as described above, will not influence the drug concentration in the target organ or the effect. Infusion pumps have mechanical parts that can wear out. Together with the above mentioned control loop this may cause oscillations with a larger time constant. Observations have been made in older infusion pumps where fluctuations in haemodynamic response where contributed to these type of oscillations.[2] For the determination of the accuracy it is therefore not enough to simply measure the output of the pump over a longer period of time at a given flow rate. Besides the infusion pump itself there are other sources of inaccuracies caused by the combination of syringe and infusion pump that may be of greater importance than the inaccuracy of the pump itself. To explain this it is important to first clarify another phenomenon related to the use of syringes.

Siphoning

When a 50-ml syringe with a loose hanging infusion line connected, is placed ±125 cm above the ground the syringe will empty itself within a few minutes. The physical principle behind this is simple: the pressure inside the syringe is -125 cm H_2O. This is independent of the diameter of the infusion line. A Becton Dickinson 60-ml syringe, for example, would empty itself in 5 min at a height of 130 cm. This is at a flow rate of 300 ml/h. If this happens with a patient connected, then obviously this would cause problems with most anaesthetic drugs that we use. It is difficult to predict what would be the critical height difference at which these phenomena will occur. It depends on the resistance between plunger and syringe wall. For the Becton Dickinson in the above example this critical level was around 110 cm. However, for a Diprifusor pre-filled syringe that is made of glass this value was 10 cm lower. The presence of silicon oil, present inside most syringes to lubricate the plunger and prevent 'sticking' of the syringe may also play a role. There are clinical scenarios thinkable in which siphoning can occur. For example when a patient is lifted from the bed onto the operating table often syringes are removed from the syringe pump. The mistake is than easily made by putting the syringe on a high piece of equipment. But even if the syringe is left in the pump siphoning may be a danger. Fitting of the syringe is not always tight and vertical displacements of the syringe pump can cause back-flow[3] dependant on the type of syringe and the pump.

Backlash and back flow

Backlash and back flow are completely different things. Backlash is called the phenomenon that, especially at a low flow rate, it may take a while after starting the infusion before actually fluid is leaving the syringe.[4, 5] By back flow is meant the fact that fluid may flow back into the syringe under circumstances. Both phenomena are caused by the same thing: loose fitting of the syringe in the syringe pump. A part of the backlash is also caused by the play in mechanical parts of the pump but with modern pumps this should be minimal.

The reason why the fitting in some pumps is so loose is that syringes differ in material thickness. So, to accommodate syringes from different manufactures there is deliberately some play in the clamp that holds the plunger and the space where the fingers of the syringe fit. For some syringe-pump combinations this can be more than 2 ml when a 50 ml syringe is used. Together with the siphoning phenomena this can cause back-flow when a syringe pump for example is placed from above the patient to below the patient.[3] Given the fact that the dead space in the infusion line is 0.5 ml it is clear that blood from the patient may contaminate the syringe. Using the same syringe for different patients is therefore not very prudent. One-way valves could theoretically prevent this contamination. Purging the system before connecting it to the patient should prevent backlash. However it should be kept in mind that backlash can occur after every syringe change.

Air in the syringe

It is almost impossible to fill the syringe without a small amount of air present in the syringe. In contrary to the volumetric pump the infusion pump has usually no air detection. Whether patients receive air from the syringe inside the infusion pump depends mostly on the point at which the end of infusion alarm is activated. This again depends on the pump/syringe combination and it is useful to test this locally because neither syringe manufacturer nor pump manufacturer will give detailed specifications for this. Air inside a syringe can cause more problems than accidentally being injected. Because air is compressible it will delay the occlusion alarm. Suppose there is 4 ml of air in a 50-ml syringe that runs on 10 ml/h. Suppose the occlusion alarm is activated at 1 Atm (760 mmHg). Then, the pressure is doubled and therefore, according to Boyle's law, the volume is halved. The volume of the air bubble will now be 2 ml and at 10

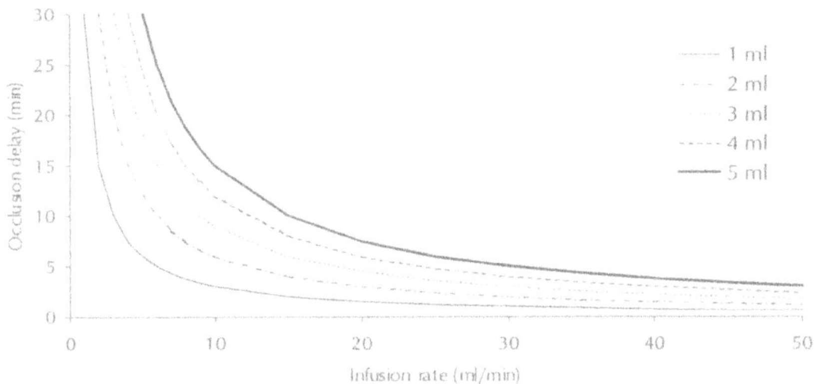

Figure 2
Relation between occlusion alarm delay and infusion rate. The curves are drawn for 1, 2, 3, 4 and 5 ml of air in the syringe. Occlusion pressure is assumed to be 1 atm.

ml/h this would take 12 min. Twelve min of no drug input would certainly be noticeable even when not so fast acting drugs are used. If the reason of the occlusion pressure is released a bolus of 2 ml will be delivered. Even automatic pressure release mechanisms that are available in some infusion devices will not be able to cover such a large volume. Expressed as a formula this time delay (T) is

$$T = \frac{V_{air}}{(1+P_{occlusion})*R_{ate}}$$

Graphically this relation between rate and occlusion time delay is represented in figure 2. It should also be noticed that in some infusion pumps the occlusion alarm is not adjusted to the size of a syringe. Because the pressure build up is inversely related to the surface of the plunger, 500 mmHg in a 50-ml syringe can become easily 1500 mmHg in a 20-ml syringe.

Dead space

One of maybe the most frequent causes of interrupted drug flow is when more pumps are connected to one infusion point. Especially when this is combined with a fluid infusion run by gravity. In the TCI part of this chapter an example is given of a running propofol TCI system where the theoretical stable infusion is disturbed by the dead space in the infusion line. The same is true for manual infusion.

Target controlled infusion

At the time of writing there is only one drug commercially available for target controlled infusion. This drug is propofol and it is delivered by Diprifusor TCI technology. It has been the joint effort of anaesthesiologists, an engineer and people from industry that made a technique that had itself proven to be of value for researchers, available to the clinical anaesthesiologists[6] who where asking for this technology after experiences with prototype systems. Although the technique itself is simple to use and the added functionality well protected against major mistakes by drug and dilution recognition of the ready to be used pre-filled syringe, the user has to know the principles with which the TCI principle works to avoid pitfalls[7].

Accuracy of TCI systems

The accuracy of the models that are used in the TCI systems is well described. Little research has been done on the TCI systems to check their accuracy when looking at drug outflow. Opposite to what has been published with volumetric pumps[9] the author found an extreme error of some infusion pumps when they were controlled by a computer. The error appeared to be caused by the fact that the control loop (see above) of the syringe pump was reset every time it received a command from the computer even when the actual infusion rate was not changed. The error was mainly found with infusion pumps that had an analogue motor like the Ohmeda 9000, the Welmed and the Graseby. The hypothesis that both the intervals at which the commands were send to the pump and the infusion rate influenced this error appeared to be true. As an example figure 3 relates the error to infusion rate and control interval for the Welmed pump. As a consequence one may expect that an experimental TCI system that does not correct for this error produces a large error at low drug targets when the infusion runs slowly.

Figure 4 shows such an experimental system. Drug outflow from the pump has been used to calculate the drug concentration with the same pharmacokinetic parameters as were used by the TCI system.

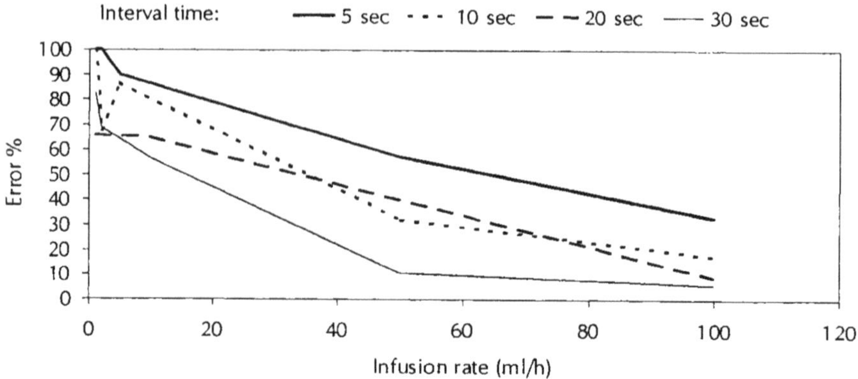

Figure 3
Error of a Welmed p4000 infusion pump when remotely controlled by a computer. Iteratively with an interval of 5, 10, 20 and 30 sec the same infusion rate is sent to the pump. This procedure has been repeated at several infusion rates. Note that at low infusion rates the pump stands still (100% error) without alarming!

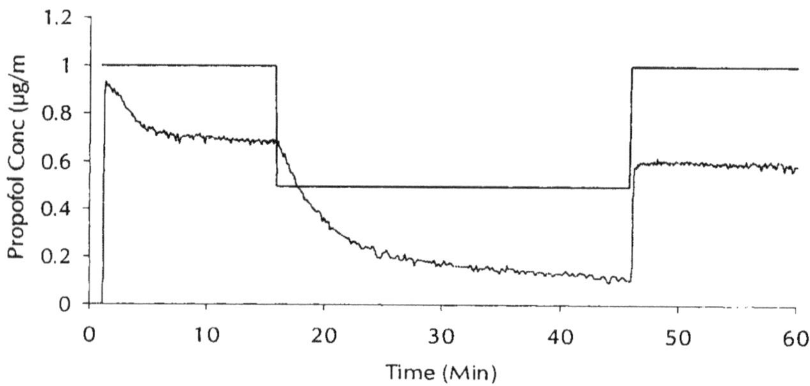

Figure 4
Consequence of the error caused by remote control when an experimental Target Controlled Infusion is developed that does not correct for the pump error.

It is obvious that there is a considerable error at these low targets although the system may perform reasonably well at normal targets. When the available commercial TCI systems are subjected to the same test one can see that they are not hampered by this problem but that the Diprifusor module corrects for this error by increasing the infusion rate from time to time (figure 5).

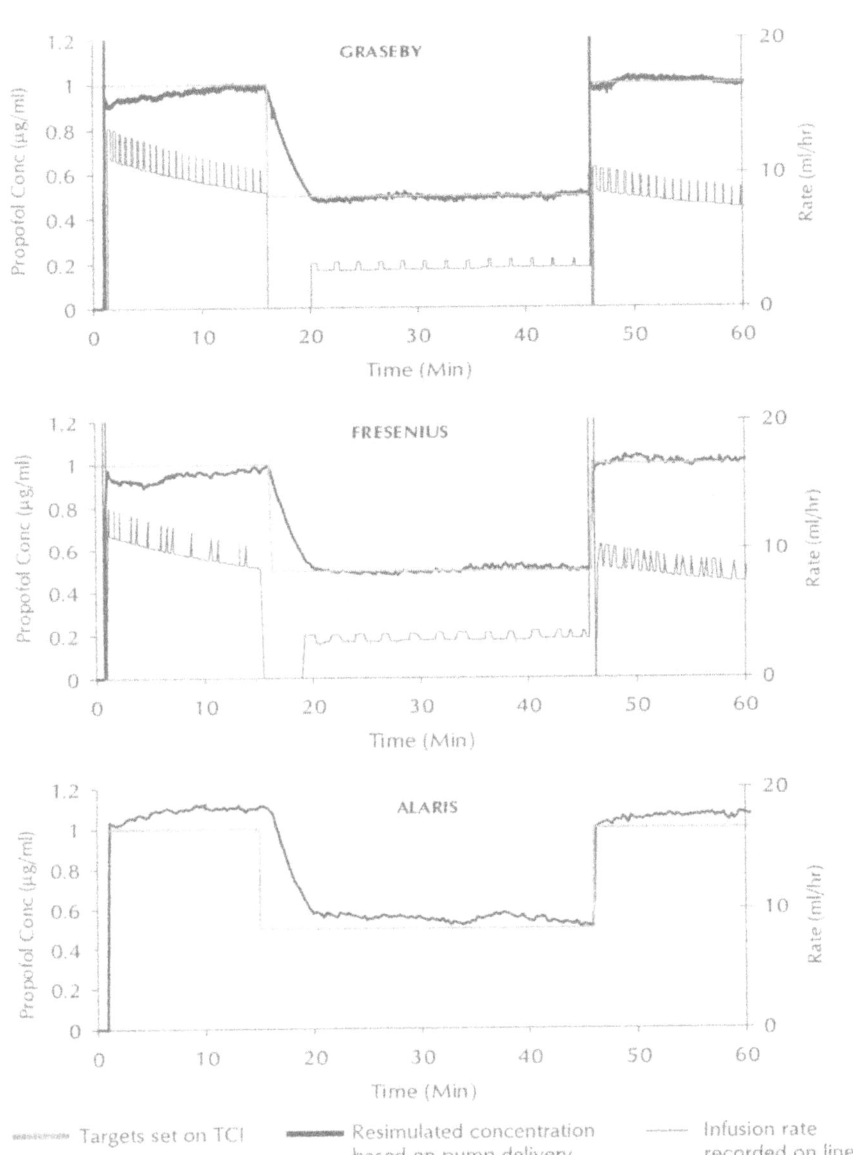

Figure 5
The accuracy of three TCI pumps with Diprifusor technology. Note the infusion rate changes with the Graseby and Fresenius pump to correct for pump errors. With the Alaris no infusion rate was recorded.
Test sequence: Target: 1 µg/ml for 30 minutes
Target: 0.5 µg/ml for 30 minutes
Target: 1 µg/ml for 30 minutes

Requirements of the infusion system

With target controlled infusion, an increase in the target will cause the pump to run at maximum speed of 1200 ml per hour. If the venous access is restricted by for example a narrow IV catheter this is the moment when an occlusion alarm will occur. If the intravenous drugs are connected via a T piece to an infusion running by gravity this may cause the drugs to run partially into the infusion line if no one-way valve prevents this. The white colour of propofol may help to prevent this, because the eye therefore can detect the back flow. With other, clear drugs this is more difficult. If for any reason no one-way valve is used it is advisable to connect propofol as the first drug on the infusion line between a gravity-forced infusion and the patient.

The dead space

Another problem with intravenous infusions connected to an infusion used for fluid replacement is the possible existence of dead space. If the iv drug is connected remote from the patient, for example to keep an eye on the connection, then the dead space between the T piece and the entrance in the body can be several ml. An infusion line with a length of 120 cm has a volume of 5 ml. During induction and thereafter the intravenous drugs will be transported through this dead space by the gravity running infusion. If the bottle of the infusion runs empty, the intravenous drug has to bridge this dead space. During several minutes the amount delivered to the patient will be almost zero. The speed at which this dead space is filled depends on the speed with which TCI pump runs at that moment. Although shortly after induction this is quite fast, the cessation of the drug delivery is at this moment the most dangerous for the patient as the compartments do not hold very much drug and the decrease in the blood concentration is quite fast because of the distribution of the drug. Furthermore, the more concentrated the drug the lower the infusion rate will be and the more extensive the drop in concentration will be, caused by the empty infusion bottle. When the intubation has been facilitated with a muscle relaxant then even when muscle relaxation is used modestly, full relaxation will still be present, obstructing the ultimate alarm against awareness: a moving patient. Added to this the possible start of surgical stimulation and the arousal caused by this stimulation, the scenario for a moment off unacceptable low level of anaesthesia is there, caused simply by the dead space in the infusion line and an empty

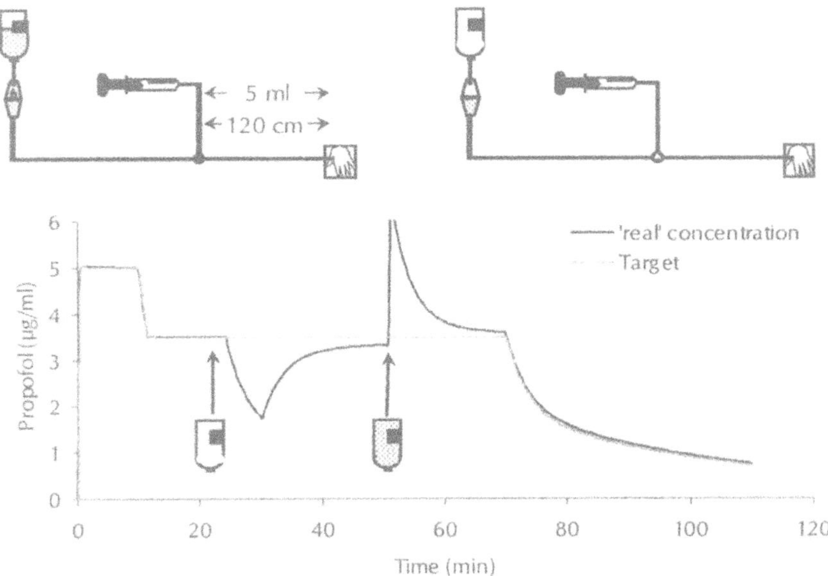

Figure 6
Effect the empty infusion bottle when a TCI system is connected to a infusion run by gravity and there is a deadspace between connection and patient.

infusion bottle. At the moment the empty infusion bottle is replaced by a full bottle, a bolus of 5 ml of propofol will increase the blood concentration significantly (see figure 6).

Practical consequences of using pharmacokinetic models

The pharmacokinetic model inside the Diprifusor is continuously calculating the concentration in the different compartments by taking into account the distribution and elimination of the drug. The concentrations are the result of all previously delivered infusions. The TCI system can recognise the fact that syringes are changed, but it can not recognise the change of the patient.

Suppose the Diprifusor has not been reset between two patients and the system is used for induction in the next patient then the concentrations in the compartments from the first patient will influence the infusion scheme for the second patient. The higher the concentration in the first patient and the longer this is maintained the more the influence will be. In figure 7 a simulation shows an example of what the effect can be on the expected concentration. From this

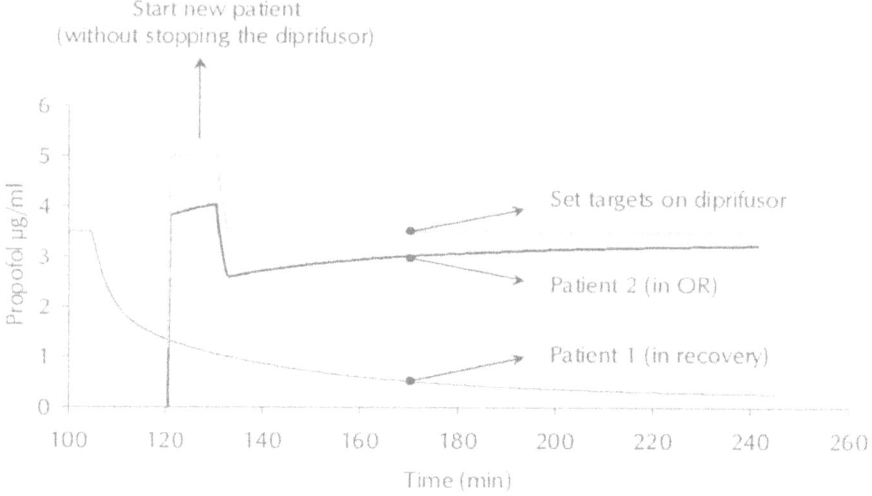

Figure 7
New patient started without resetting the Diprifusor. Concentrations in the new patient will be lower than predicted and slowly converge to the predicted concentration over time.

simulation it is clear that the effect of this error will decrease in time together with the drug decay in the previous patient. But this error will initially be significant.

The same but opposite is true if erroneously the system is restarted. This is even more likely to happen then the previous example. It may occur for example when the pump is damaged and fails and a new pump is brought into the operating theatre or when the patient is returning in the operating theatre after a short period. Because information on the concentration in the patient is lost the system will start with a bolus and infusion as if it was a new patient without residual drug concentrations in the body. If for whatever reason, TCI is restarted in a patient the anaesthesiologist has to be careful when selecting a target by gently increasing the target over time. There can be no real advise on the targets to be chosen in these circumstances because this is related to the time and targets that have been used before. In figure 8 simulations show what happens if a patient is re-induced with a TCI system 30, 60 and 90 min after an anaesthetic that lasted 105 min. In this example the influence of the previous

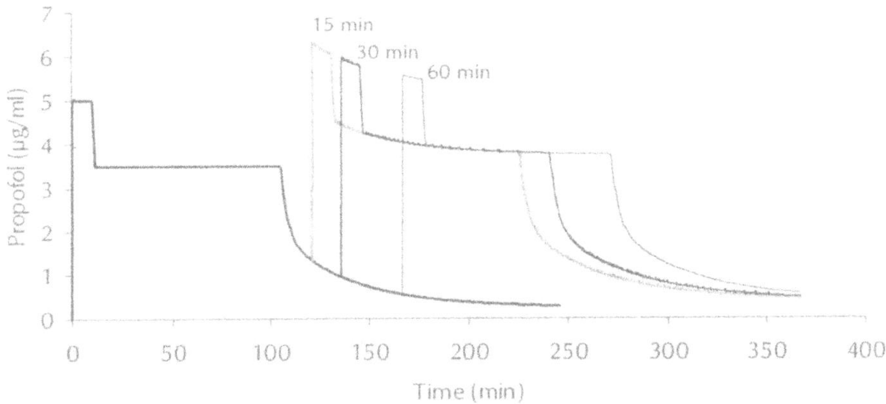

Figure 8
Effect of restarting a patient 15, 30 and 60 minutes after stopping the TCI system. 105 minutes of anaesthesia.

anaesthesia can be almost neglected after 1 h, if the previous anaesthesia lasted for about 2 h with comparable targets as in this simulation.

Recommendations and conclusion

- Avoid using high concentrated drugs that run at low speeds. This recommendation is especially important when using drugs with short context sensitive half-lives and short blood brain equilibration half-lives. One should realise that even fentanyl is a short acting drug when the duration of administration is short, e.g.15 min.
- Connect the drug infusion close to the patient. Avoid dead space. Do not combine vaso-active drugs with TCI on the same infusion line. If more drugs are connected use a carrier. There are special sets that can divide 1 line into 3 without increasing the dead space. The author found these very useful when applying TIVA/TCI techniques in children or neonates.
- Avoid air in the syringe.
- If you do not trust the accuracy of an infusion device, let it be thoroughly tested by qualified personnel. Simply checking the output over time is not enough.

- Avoid pumps that are too complex to use if their added functionality is not of a real advantage to you.
- Use one way valves, or use dedicated infusions for your TIVA if possible. Consider leaving out fluid replacement infusions if the patient does not need them.
- Avoid vertical displacements, if possible have your pumps at the same height of the infusion pump.
- Try a new (TCI) pump first without a patient connected.
- Purge your infusion system before commencing anaesthesia.
- Be careful with using one of the many available experimental TCI systems.

There is a lot of new functionality added to the current generation of infusion pumps. Unfortunately, not all of these enhancements lead to better and safer systems. In contrary, increased complexity in control may even expose the patient to a greater risk. It is a pity that medical devices are not as thoroughly tested as drugs before they are released on the market and that there is no report mechanism that records mishaps and accidents. There are however possibilities for the next generation of infusion pumps. When drug and dilution recognition become a more general implemented technique the pump could supply the user with intuitive help. Also more intelligent alarms, dependent on the type of drug and the expected calculated blood concentration, will in future be available.

References

1. Stokes DN, Peackock JE, Lewis R,Hutton P. The Ohmeda 9000 syringe pump. The first of a new generation of syringe drivers. Anaesthesia 45(12):1062-6;1990 Dec.
2. Schulze KF, Graff M, Schimmel MS, Schenkman A, Rohan P. Physiologic oscillations produced by an infusion pump. J Pediatr. 103(5):796-8;1983 Nov
3. Lonnqvist-PA;Lovqvist-B. Design flaw can convert commercially available continuous syringe pumps to intermittent bolus injectors. Intensive-care-Med 1998 Mar;24 (3):278.
4. O'Kelly SW;Edwards JC.A. Comparison of the performance of two types of infusion devices. Anaesthesia. 47(12): 1070-2;1992 Dec
5. Auty B, Infusion equipment for total intravenous anaesthesia. Monographs in Anaesthesiology 21 chapter 11: 205-223,1991 ISBN 0-444-81198-2
6. Gray JM, Kenny GN. Development of the technology for 'Diprifusor' TCI systems. Anaesthesia 53 Suppl 1:22-7,1998

7. Engbers F. Practical use of 'Diprifusor' systems. Anaesthesia 53 Suppl 1:28-34; 1998 Apr
8. Swinhoe CF, Peacock JE, Glen JB, Reilly CS.Evaluation of the predictive performance of a Diprifusor TCI system. Anaesthesia 53 Suppl 1:61-7; 1998 Apr
9. Connor SB, Quill TJ JacobsJR. Accuracy of drug infusion pumps under computer control. IEEE Trans Biomed Eng 39(9):980-2; 1992 Sep

Closed loop control of general anaesthesia

Anthony Absalom and Gavin N.C. Kenny

Glasgow, United Kingdom

Introduction

Why should we have a closed loop system?

Closed loop control of anaesthesia (CLAN) offers several benefits to the patient and the anaesthetist. Measurement of the anaesthetic depth variable is automated, so that more frequent measurements are possible, allowing more frequent and more accurate adjustments to the depth of anaesthesia. Thus better control of depth of anaesthesia is possible. The dose of drug administered is individualised for the specific patient, making allowances for variations in surgical stimuli, and for the large differences in pharmacokinetics and pharmacodynamics between patients. In this way feedback control systems may help to reduce the incidence of awareness under anaesthesia, while limiting the amount of drug administered to the exact requirements of the patient. Overdosing can thus be avoided, and recovery times optimised. Finally, feedback control systems, being automated, are likely to be more reliable than manual techniques performed by humans where fatigue and the distractions of the clinical environment can decrease performance.

In addition CLAN systems are useful research tools. The decisions on the amount of anaesthetic agent to be delivered are automated and therefore objective, making such systems ideal tools for studying the interactions between different drugs, and the effects of different anaesthetic techniques such as sup-

Table 1
Summary of closed loop anaesthesia systems

Author	Input signal	Control algorithm	Output	Year
Bickford[27]	EEG zero crossing	PID	Thiopentone bolus	1950
Schwilden[8]	Median frequency	PK-PD model, adaptive	Methohexitone infusion	1987
Schwilden[9]	Median frequency	PK-PD model, adaptive	Propofol infusion	1989
Schwilden[10]	Median frequency	PK-PD model, adaptive	Alfentanil infusion	1993
Robb[6]	Systolic blood pressure	PI controller	Isoflurane concentration	1993
Mortier[13]	BIS	PK-PD model, adaptive	TCI propofol	1998
Absalom	BIS	PI controller	TCI propofol	1999
Kenny[12]	AEP index	PI controller	TCI propofol	1999

plementary regional anaesthesia and surgical techniques on anaesthetic requirements.

Existing systems

The development of digital computers and of control theory has lead to a rapid increase in the use of feedback systems for the control of manufacturing and other non-medical processes. Since many of the homeostatic functions of the body are also controlled by feedback systems, these systems are well suited to the control of physiological variables in clinical practice. Feedback systems can be either open loop or closed loop, but in this paper we will focus on the application of closed loop feedback control systems to deliver general anaesthesia. Development of closed loop feedback systems for control of general anaesthesia has been hampered by the absence of an adequate input signal. However in recent years the auditory evoked potential index[1] and the bispectral index[2] have been developed and appear to be suitable for use as the control variable for feedback control of anaesthesia. Systems using these control variables will be discussed in greater detail. Other anaesthetic applications of feedback control such as regulation of blood pressure, muscle relaxation and ventilation have been reviewed by O' Hara and colleagues.[3]

Several systems for closed loop feedback control of anaesthesia have been described and these are summarised in table 1.

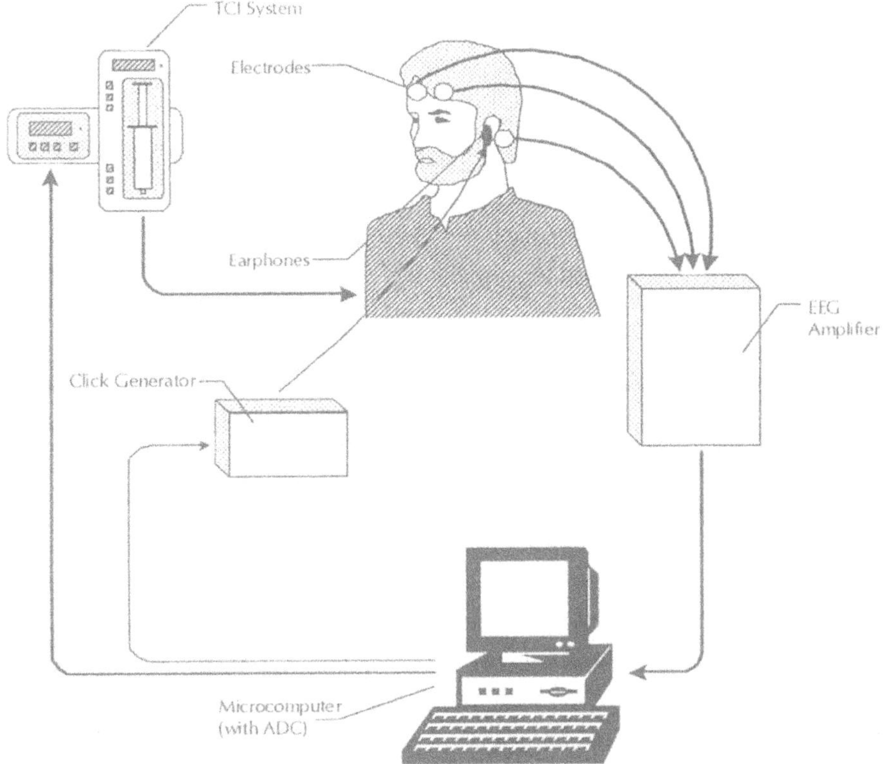

Figure 1
Diagram of a closed loop system using the auditory evoked potential (H Mantzaridis – PhD thesis - reproduced with permission).

Components of a closed loop system

All clinical closed loop control systems comprise the following basic components:

- The control variable - in the context of a closed loop anaesthesia system this will be a measure of depth of anaesthesia
- The set point or desired value of the control variable - chosen by the user/ anaesthetist
- An output variable such as the blood propofol concentration

- A control algorithm which applies the error (difference between set point and actual value of control variable) to a set of rules or equations to determine value of the output variable
- A control actuator (the drug delivery system)
- A computer to generate a user interface, retrieve the control variable, get the set point from the user, compare the control variable with the set point, run the control algorithm to calculate the value of the output variable, and pass this value to the control actuator (figure 1)

The control variable

In a closed loop system for administering general anaesthesia the control variable will be a measure of depth of anaesthesia. To date there is still no universally accepted gold standard measure of depth of anaesthesia. This is probably why most anaesthetists still rely on the traditional clinical signs to guide their administration of general anaesthetic agents, even though these signs are not completely reliable. Progress in this field has been hampered by a lack of understanding of what anaesthesia is, and when a patient is adequately anaesthetised. There is even debate of whether anaesthesia is a continuum or a binary phenomenon.[4, 5] Many of the clinical observations we make when assessing depth of anaesthesia are binary phenomena (such as patient movement, or the eyelash reflex). These are thus either present or absent under a specific set of circumstances. Most anaesthetists would agree that anaesthesia is a dynamic balance between hypnosis, analgesia and the noxious stimuli to which a patient is exposed.

At the moment, monitoring of clinical signs is the only routine method of determining depth of anaesthesia. When no neuromuscular blocking drugs are used, patient movement in response to surgical stimulation and the frequency and depth of respiration, accurately reflect the depth of anaesthesia. If adequate anaesthesia is schematically illustrated as a range of acceptable responses (figure 2), then the upper limit (insufficient anaesthesia) is determined by movement to surgical stimuli and the lower limit (excessive anaesthesia) by respiratory depression. If the patient's lungs are mechanically ventilated in a non-paralysed patient, then the lower limit is now determined by circulatory depression. A good measure of depth of anaesthesia should provide sufficient information to permit satisfactory anaesthetic and surgical conditions in a patient who is breathing

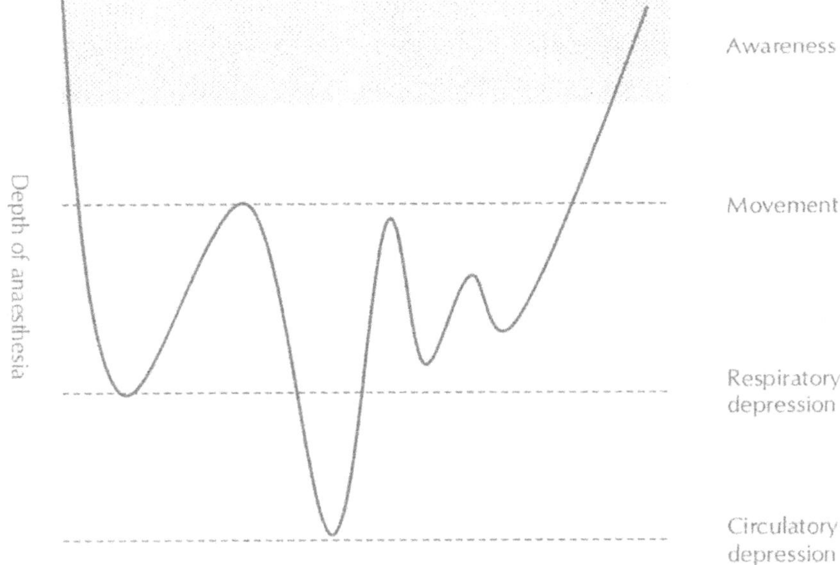

Figure 2
Signs relating to depth of anaesthesia in a spontaneously breathing patient.

spontaneously while undergoing a surgical procedure. Ideal surgical conditions include a lack of patient movement, and ideally for the patient there should be no incidence of awareness or recall (implicit or explicit) of intraoperative events.

The control variable for any closed loop system needs to be a reliable measure of the state of the system being controlled, and should vary monotonically with the state of the system. For example, a measure that first would increase and then decrease as anaesthesia is deepened would be an unreliable measure, because some values of the control variable could represent one of two states or depths of anaesthesia. Other criteria for a measure of depth of anaesthesia are:

- similar values for different anaesthetic agents at equipotent doses
- alter its signal appropriately during surgical stimulation
- similar value at induction of anaesthesia to that recorded at recovery
- unaffected by cardioactive drugs, hypotension or tachycardia
- obvious transition from conscious to unconscious and vice versa

Several variables have been used to control anaesthesia. Robb and colleagues used the systolic blood pressure to control an isoflurane and morphine anaesthetic, but when the system was tested, satisfactory control was achieved in only 31 out of 34 subjects [6]. There were no cases of awareness among the subjects in whom satisfactory control was achieved. In addition, all patients in this study were paralysed and the problem of assessing adequate depth of anaesthesia in such patients is well recognised.[7]

Much of the recent work to develop a measure of depth of anaesthesia has centred on the electroencephalogram (EEG). The raw (unprocessed) EEG is difficult to interpret, but techniques involving frequency analysis of the EEG have proved more useful. These techniques calculate the power within the different frequencies in the EEG and the results can be graphically represented as the compressed spectral array and the density spectral array. Further analysis of the distribution of the power within the frequencies allows calculation of the median and spectral edge frequencies (the frequencies below which 50% and 95% of the EEG power lie).

Schwilden and colleagues have used the median EEG frequency to control infusions of methohexitone[8], propofol[9] and alfentanil.[10] These systems were able to control anaesthesia effectively, but were only tested in small numbers of subjects (between 11 and 13 patients in each study), all of whom were paralysed, and some of whom still had corneal reflexes.

A study by Gajraj and colleagues[11] showed almost no separation between the MF and SEF values obtained in the awake and unconscious subjects casting serious doubt about the ability of these measurements to control anaesthesia and prevent awareness. The same study showed that the distinction between awake and unconscious values was better for the BIS and the best for the auditory evoked potential index. Kenny and Mantzaridis were able to effectively control anaesthesia in 100 non-paralysed subjects undergoing body surface surgery, using a closed loop system that used the AEPi to control a TCI propofol infusion.[12] This system produced good haemodynamic stability, few patients moved and there were no instances of recall of intraoperative events. The same system has also been used to control anaesthesia in several hundred paralysed patients (unpublished data).

More recently Mortier and colleagues have used the BIS to control propofol sedation[13], and Absalom and Kenny have developed a system that uses the BIS to control a TCI propofol infusion for anaesthesia in patients undergoing orthopaedic surgery under combined general and regional anaesthesia (unpublished data presented to May 1999 meeting of EuroSIVA, Amsterdam). The latter system is currently undergoing a trial in patients having body surface surgery under general anaesthesia supplemented by local anaesthesia.

Control algorithm

The control algorithm is an integral part of a closed loop system. It is a set of equations and/or rules that use the difference between the desired and actual value of the control variable to make an adjustment to the control actuator. Control algorithms used for controlling anaesthesia include the classical PID (proportional, integral, differential) controller that can be refined to be adaptive or self-tuning, and adaptive PK-PD (pharmacokinetic - pharmacodynamic) model-based controllers. Fuzzy logic and artificial neural networks (ANN) are particularly suited to non-linear systems, and as such would seem suitable for controlling physiological variables. Fuzzy logic is used in the controllers of a wide variety of consumer goods, industrial processes and even a subway system.[14, 15] Medical applications of fuzzy logic are rare, and so far fuzzy logic has not been used for control of general anaesthesia. However, Edwards and colleagues use a fuzzy logic controller in their system for automatic control of neuromuscular blockade[16] and Hanson and colleagues have developed a fuzzy control system for postoperative fluid resuscitation[17] and a neurofuzzy system for analysis of haemodynamic data[18].

Much work has been done on ANN analysis of the EEG, for example recognition of the patterns associated with dementia and epilepsy.[19, 20] So far, little has been published on the use of ANNs for predicting depth of anaesthesia from the EEG, although the work that has been done shows some promise. Kochs and colleagues subjected bispectral EEG analysis and MLAEP data to wavelet transform and were able to train an ANN to classify these data and correctly predict movement in 80% of cases [21]. Watt trained an ANN to recognise the EEG spectral signatures associated with three different MAC levels of volatile anaesthetic agent in dogs[22] and in humans.[23] The ANN was able to correctly predict the anaesthetic level of unknown data with an overall accuracy of 80% in dogs and 83% in humans. They also trained a network to recognise the patterns in a bispectral EEG analysis, and this correctly predicted anaesthetic level of unknown data in humans with an overall accuracy of 89%. In New York, Veselis trained a neural network to recognise EEG patterns associated with different levels of sedation[24], and the EEG patterns associated with different sedative drugs.[25] Attempts have also been made to teach neural networks how to control depth of anaesthesia by observing the actions of anaesthetists.[26]

One of the basic problems with ANNs is that although they can be trained to learn complex tasks, they do not use conventional logic to do so (which is why they work well with non-linear systems). It is therefore difficult to document the logic used, and to verify the safety of neural network-based systems. Hybrid system may thus be more acceptable - e.g. an ANN with a rule-based safety "shell".

Output

Closed loop systems aim to keep the control variable at a desired level by making frequent changes to the output or control actuator. If there is a long delay between an alteration in the control actuator and the effect of that change on the system, then the efficiency of the system will suffer, as it will be longer before the loop can truly be closed. Currently reported closed loop anaesthesia systems have had as control actuator either the inspired isoflurane concentration or a blood concentration of anaesthetic (either by means of a target-controlled infusion system or by means of a "BET" infusion system). A system that administered simple infusions, and altered the rate of the infusion according to the error in the control variable would not be very efficient because after making an adjustment there would be a long delay before steady state blood concentrations were reached. Target controlled infusions eliminate these delays, but nonetheless there is still a delay in transfer of the drug from the blood to the active site of the drug (the "effect site"). The rate of transfer of the drug from blood to brain will depend on the pharmacokinetic properties of the drug. With systems that administer a volatile anaesthetic agent there are further delays because there first has to be equilibration between the breathing system and the lungs before blood and brain equilibration. The ideal control actuator is thus probably a system designed to deliver a specific effect site concentration of drug.

Conclusion

The lack of a "gold standard" means of monitoring depth of anaesthesia has hampered progress in this field, and continues to leave our patients exposed to the risk of awareness under anaesthesia. An ideal monitor should not be agent specific, and should not be affected by vasoactive drugs or by the haemodynamic status of the patient. More importantly there should be clear separation between the values given by the monitor for the awake and the unconscious state. The ability of a measure of depth of anaesthesia to be able to control anaesthesia in a closed loop system is an "acid test" of the significance of the measure. At present the AEPi is the only measure to have been able to provide satisfactory anaesthesia in a large number of subjects in this manner.

References

1. Mantzaridis H, Kenny GN: Auditory evoked potential index: a quantitative measure of changes in auditory evoked potentials during general anaesthesia. Anaesthesia 52:1030-1036, 1997
2. Rampil I: A Primer for EEG Signal Processing in Anesthesia. Anesthesiol. 89:980-1002, 1998
3. O'Hara DA, Bogen DK, Noordegraaf A: The Use of Computers for Controlling the Delivery of Anesthesia. Anesthesiol. 77:563-581, 1992
4. Prys-Roberts C: Anaesthesia: a practical or impractical construct? Br.J.Anaesth. 59: 1341-1345, 1987
5. Kissin I: General Anesthetic Action: An Obsolete Notion? Anesth.Analg. 76:215-218, 1993
6. Robb HM, Asbury AJ, Gray WM, Linkens DA: Towards a standardized anaesthetic state using isoflurane and morphine. Br.J.Anaesth. 71:366-369, 1993
7. Russell IF: Midazolam-alfentanil: an anaesthetic? An investigation using the isolated forearm technique. Br.J.Anaesth. 70:42-46, 1993
8. Schwilden H, Schüttler J, Stoeckel H: Closed-loop feedback control of methohexital anesthesia by quantitative EEG analysis in humans. Anesthesiol. 67:341-347, 1987
9. Schwilden H, Stoeckel H, Schüttler J: Closed-loop feedback control of propofol anaesthesia by quantitative EEG analysis in humans. Br.J.Anaesth. 62:290-296, 1989
10. Schwilden H, Stoeckel H: Closed-loop feedback controlled administration of alfentanil during alfentanil-nitrous oxide anaesthesia. Br.J.Anaesth. 70:389-393, 1993
11. Gajraj RJ, Doi M, Mantzaridis H, Kenny GN: Analysis of the EEG bispectrum, auditory evoked potentials and the EEG power spectrum during repeated transitions from consciousness to unconsciousness. Br.J.Anaesth. 80:46-52, 1998
12. Kenny GNC, Mantzaridis H: Closed-loop control of propofol anaesthesia. Br.J. Anaesth. In Press:1999
13. Mortier E, Struys M, De ST, Versichelen L, Rolly G: Closed-loop controlled administration of propofol using bispectral analysis. Anaesthesia 53:749-754, 1998

14. Sangalli A: Fuzzy logic goes to market. New Scientist 36-39, 1992
15. Kosko B, Isaka S: Fuzzy logic. Scientific American 62-67, 1993
16. Edwards ND, Mason DG, Ross JJ: A portable self-learning fuzzy logic control system for muscle relaxation. Anaesthesia 53:136-139, 1998
17. Hanson CW, Weiss Y, Frasch F, Marshall C, Marshall BE: A Fuzzy Control Strategy for Postoperative Volume Resuscitation. Anesthesiology 85:B131996
18. Hanson CW, Weiss Y, Frasch F, Marshall C, Marshall BE: Neurofuzzy Analysis of Haemodynamic Data. Anesthesiology 85:B61996
19. Baxt WG: Application of artificial neural networks to clinical medicine. Lancet 346: 1135-1138, 1995
20. Miller AS, Blott BH, Hames TK: Review of neural network applications in medical imaging and signal processing. Medical & Biological Engineering & Computing 30: 449-464, 1992
21. Kochs E, Kalkman C, Thornton C, Bischoff P, Kuppe E, Abke J, Stockmanns G: Classification of inadequacy of anesthesia by spontaneous and evoked electroencephalogram using neural net and wavelet transform. Anesthesiology 85: A4711996
22. Watt RC, Samuelson H, Navabi MJ: A comparison of artificial neural networks and classical statistical analysis. Anesthesiology 75:A4511991
23. Watt RC, Sisemore CS, Kanemoto A, Malan TP, Frink EJ: Neural networks applied to bispectral analysis of EEG during anesthesia. Anesthesiology 83:A5031995
24. Veselis RA, Reinsel R, Sommer S, Carlon G: Use of neural network analysis to classify electroencephalographic patterns against depth of midazolam sedation in intensive care unit patients. J.Clin.Monit. 7:259-267, 1991
25. Veselis RA, Reinsel R, Wronski M: Analytical methods to differentiate similar electroencephalographic spectra: neural network and discriminant analysis. J.Clin. Monit. 9:257-267, 1993
26. Rehman HU, Linkens DA, Asbury JA: Neural networks and nonlinear regression modelling and control of depth of anaesthesia for spontaneously breathing and ventilated subjects. Comput Methods Programs Biomed 40:227-247, 1993
27. Bickford RG: Automatic electroencephalographic control of general anesthesia. Electroencephalogr.Clin.Neurophysiol. 2:93-96, 1951

THE EFFECT OF OPIOIDS ON THE PHARMACOKINETICS AND PHARMACO-DYNAMICS OF PROPOFOL

Jaap Vuyk

Leiden, The Netherlands

Introduction

In contrast to approximately a decade ago when the pharmacokinetics and dynamics of intravenous anaesthetic agents were almost exclusively determined when given as sole agent, increasingly data are gathered on interactions between the agents we administer on a daily basis. We combine anaesthetic agents because the provision of anaesthesia on the basis of a single agent is associated with significant side effects compromising haemodynamic and/or respiratory function, reducing operating conditions, or postponing postoperative recovery. Because of the small therapeutic window a detailed characterisation of the concentration-effect relationships of anaesthetic agents is required to allow a proper selection of the various intravenous agents and the combinations thereof to an optimal therapeutic pharmacological effect in the absence of significant side effects. During the past decade, for propofol and the various opioids fentanyl, alfentanil, sufentanil, and remifentanil considerable progress has been made in the characterisation of the pharmacokinetics and pharmacodynamics of these agents and of the combinations thereof.

Terminology and characterisation of drug interactions

Recently, Bovill reviewed the methodology of the study of drug interaction and described 4 ways of interaction analysis; fractional analysis, isobolographic analysis, method of Plummer and Short and the parallel line assay[1]. The response surface modelling technique as presented at the SIVA 1996 meeting is the latest branch on the modelling tree. In general all these modelling techniques use more or less the same terminology. When given as single agent the relationship between the concentration of a drug in the blood and the effect can be described on the basis of 4 modalities. These are potency, efficacy, slope and variability. Potency reflects the sensitivity of the organ or tissue to the drug, and is defined by the location of the curve on the x-axis of the concentration-effect relationship. Potency is often described in terms of the EC_{50} or the MAC, the median effective concentrations of intravenous and inhalational anaesthetic agents. With this parameter the effectiveness of different agents with respect to a specific effect, and the effectiveness with which a single agent exerts various effects can be determined. Efficacy, or maximum efficacy, is the (maximum) effect that a drug can produce. With this parameter agonists and partial agonists can be differentiated. The slope of the curve is related to the mechanism of action of the drug, e.g. receptor binding. The steepness of a curve describes the concentration range between almost no effect and maximum effect. Finally, the interindividual variability in concentration-effect relationships is reflected by the standard deviation or standard error of the EC_{50} or the MAC.

The MAC is defined as the minimum alveolar concentration of a volatile anaesthetic agent at which 50% of patients do not respond to a standard stimulus. In man, MAC is determined by examining the absence or presence of a purposeful motor response to skin incision at different alveolar (end-tidal) anaesthetic concentrations. In animal studies tail-clamping is the standard stimulus. The potency of intravenous agents is, by analogy to that of volatile agents, described in terms of the EC_{50}. In general 4 classes of drug interactions are defined. Zero-interaction is said to occur when the effect of the combination of two drugs is exactly the sum of the effects of the individual agents. This is more often referred to as an additive interaction. This occurs when two agents do not really interact but simply provide their action next to one another without influence. When the effect of the combination is greater than that expected as based on the concentration-effect relationships of the individual agents, the interaction is said to be synergistic. Supra-additivity or potentiation are often used as synonyms for synergism. In this case one needs relatively less of the combination to obtain a certain effect compared to when one of the agents is given as single agent. Finally, an infra-additive interaction is said to occur when the effect of the combination is less than the sum of the effects of the individual agents. One then needs relatively more of the combination to obtain a certain effect compared to when one of the agents is given as single agent. Lastly, antagonism is the situation where the effect of the combination is less than that of one of its constituents; e.g. the combined effect of alfentanil and naloxone is less than that of alfentanil alone.

Do opioids and propofol affect each other's distribution and/or clearance?

The pharmacokinetics of propofol when given as sole agent have been described thoroughly. After intravenous administration propofol distributes and redistributes rapidly to a large volume of distribution at steady state, and finally is mainly cleared from the body by hepatic metabolism. During target controlled infusion (TCI) intravenous anaesthetic agents are administered not on the basis of mg per kg body weight, but on the basis of the concentration in the blood. The concentration in the blood is continuously calculated by the computer on the basis of a population pharmacokinetic parameter set. On the basis of the concentration desired by the anaesthesiologist the computer communicates with the infusion pump and controls the infusion rate required to maintain the desired concentration. The performance of a target controlled infusion device is a measure of the difference between the measured blood concentrations and those predicted by the computer. For most PK-parameter sets that were tested[2, 3], with increasing target propofol concentration the measured concentrations increasingly exceeded those predicted. This suggests that propofol affects its own distribution and/or elimination. Propofol has been shown to reduce cardiac output and liver blood flow. This haemodynamic effect may result in a reduced clearance of propofol as well as in a slower distribution to peripheral compartments. If this is true, when increasing propofol concentrations are required, the change in the infusion rate of propofol should be made proportional to its depressant effect on haemodynamic function. With higher blood propofol concentrations a smaller step in the infusion rate would be required to increase the concentration in the blood with a certain amount than at lower blood propofol concentrations. It should be noted, however, that other studies suggest that the pharmacokinetics of propofol are linear over a wide concentration range[4].

Besides the fact that propofol may affect its own pharmacokinetics, increasingly data suggest that opioids influence the distribution and elimination of propofol as well. Schüttler et al.[5] already in 1993 using a NONMEM population pharmacokinetic analysis revealed that fentanyl and alfentanil both increased the volume of the central compartment and the clearance of propofol. More recently, Pavlin et al.[6] showed that alfentanil at plasma concentrations of 40 ng/ml, at which patients still breathed spontaneously, blood propofol concentrations were increased by 20% during a study on the combined sedative effects of these agents. Vuyk and Mertens et al.[7] then showed that alfentanil reduced both the distribution and clearance of propofol. Plasma alfentanil concentrations of about 80 ng/ml increased the blood propofol concentrations by 15%. Furthermore, Matot et al.[8] showed that the first-pass pulmonary uptake of propofol in cats was reduced from 60% to 40% after pre-treatment with fentanyl. A reduced first-pass pulmonary uptake of propofol may indeed increase the initial blood propofol concentration after a bolus dose administration. Vice versa both Gepts et al.[9] and Pavlin et al.[6] report on the increased plasma alfentanil concentrations in the presence of propofol. This may be the result of the, thus far only in vitro described, inhibition of the oxidative metabolism of alfentanil by the cytochrome P450 enzyme after administration of propofol.[10, 12] Also sufentanil metabolism appears to be inhibited in the presence of propofol. Other sedative agents that interfere with the metabolism of opioids are midazolam and dexmedetomidine that have been shown to inhibit the metabolism of alfentanil and pregnenolone that has been shown to induce alfentanil metabolism in vitro. In conclusion, evidence is increasing that many sedative/hypnotic agents and the opioids affect each other's distribution and/or elimination. Further studies are necessary to evaluate the precise mechanisms that cause these pharmacokinetic interactions.

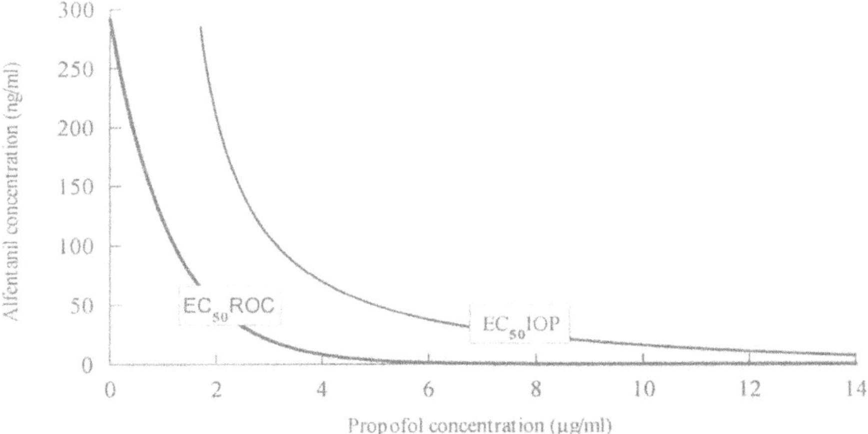

Figure 1
The interaction between propofol and alfentanil for suppression of responses to lower abdominal surgery (IOP) and return of consciousness (ROC) postoperatively. The lines show blood propofol and alfentanil concentrations that assure these effects in 50% of the patients. The higher the plasma alfentanil concentration, the lower the requirered intraoperative blood propofol concentration. In the presence of still high plasma alfentanil concentrations at the end of the procedure, the blood propofol concentration has to decrease much further to allow return of consciousness than when no alfentanil is present. The shape of the curves show that the interaction is strongly synergistic (supraadditive) for both end points (with permission)[15,16].

Do opioids affect the concentration-effect relationship of propofol?

Pharmacodynamic interactions between propofol and the various opioids can be characterised in many different ways[12-19]. According to Berenbaum[12] the most valid way to do so is by means of an isobolographic analysis. With an isobolographic analysis concentration combinations are connected that exert a similar effect. If these iso-effective concentration combinations lie on a straight line the interaction is judged to be additive. A concave-up shaped isobole corresponds with a synergistic (supraadditive) interaction (figure 1), whereas a concave-down shaped isobole is characteristic of an infraadditive interaction.

Combinations of propofol in concentrations of 0.1 to 1 µg/ml and alfentanil (40 ng/ml) increase one another's sedative and analgesic properties. Furthermore, propofol offsets the emetic effects of alfentanil, whereas the alfentanil-induced pruritus persists.[6] With these concentrations ventilation is affected only moderately. Resting minute ventilation decreases by approximately 25% in the presence of a somewhat smaller reduction in the CO_2 production of approximately 15%, resulting in a moderate increase in the end-tidal partial pressure of CO_2 of 41 mmHg to 46 mmHg.

Both fentanyl and alfentanil have been shown to decrease the propofol requirements for induction of anaesthesia in a synergistic manner.[13, 14] A plasma fentanyl concentration of 3 ng/ml, and a plasma alfentanil concentration of 122 ng/ml both reduce the blood propofol concentration associated with loss of consciousness in 50% of patients (EC_{50}) by 40% (figure 1). Although alfentanil reduces propofol requirements, the reduced dose requirements of propofol do not assure a more haemodynamically stable induction of anaesthesia because alfentanil potentiates the haemodynamically depressant effects of propofol to a similar degree as is potentiates its sedative effects.
Intraoperatively, propofol is potentiated by opioids as well.[13-15] Propofol concentrations required to blunt motor responses to skin incision in 50% of patients (EC_{50INC}) diminished greatly with plasma fentanyl concentrations increasing from 0 to 3 ng/ml. Higher plasma fentanyl concentrations did not reduce the EC_{50INC} of propofol any further demonstrating the ceiling effect in the propofol dose reduction of fentanyl requirements. Intraoperatively, with a five-fold increase in the propofol concentration from 2 to 10 μg/ml the alfentanil requirements were reduced by over tenfold in female patients undergoing gynaecological surgery (figure 1). For both fentanyl and alfentanil the magnitude of the interaction with propofol increases with the strength of the stimulus (the concavity of the isobole for loss of eyelash reflex or consciousness < skin incision < intraabdominal surgery). Lastly, alfentanil has been shown to affect the propofol concentration at which patients awake postoperatively. In the presence of still significant plasma alfentanil concentrations of 150 ng/ml the blood propofol concentration has to decrease to as far as 0.5 to 1 μg/ml before patients regain consciousness (figure 1). Whereas, in the presence of plasma alfentanil concentrations below 50 ng/ml, patients already awake at blood propofol concentrations of 2–3 μg/ml. By PK/PD modelling the optimal propofol-alfentanil concentration combination that is defined as the propofol and alfentanil concentrations that assure adequate anaesthesia and result in the most rapid possible recovery in 50% of patients, has been determined.[16] This

optimal propofol-alfentanil concentration combination occurs with a blood propofol concentration of 3.5 μg/ml combined with 85 ng/ml of alfentanil. After termination of a 5-h target controlled infusion with these concentrations 50% of patients will regain consciousness after 16 min. With the use of PK/PD computer simulations it was recently found that this optimal propofol concentration is affected both by the choice of the opioid as well as by the infusion duration. The steeper the decay in the opioid concentration relative to the decay in the propofol concentration the more the optimal propofol-opioid concentration shifts to a lower propofol and a higher opioid concentration. As a consequence, the optimal propofol concentration is much lower when combined with remifentanil compared to fentanyl, sufentanil, or alfentanil. Whereas the optimal propofol concentration when combined with alfentanil is in the order of 3.5 μg/ml, when combined with remifentanil the optimal propofol concentration is in the order of 2.5 μg/ml[16] (figures 2 and 3). The optimal propofol-opioid concentrations are the result of the pharmacokinetics of propofol relative to those of the opioid as well as of the position of the interaction curves associated with a 50% or 95% probability of no response to surgical stimuli relative to the position of the interaction curve associated with a 50% probability of return of consciousness postoperatively. The decay in the effect site propofol-opioid concentration relative to the decay in the opioid concentration to achieve return of consciousness is affected to a great extent by the selection of the opioid and only marginally by the duration of infusion. For infusion durations of 15-600 min the context-sensitive halftimes of the opioids decrease in the order of fentanyl > alfentanil > sufentanil >> remifentanil. The longer the context-sensitive halftime of the opioid relative to propofol, the more the opioid delays the return of consciousness and the more the propofol-opioid combination shifts to higher propofol concentrations and correspondingly lower opioid concentrations. As a result, the optimal propofol concentration decreases in the order of fentanyl > alfentanil > sufentanil >> remifentanil. The duration of infusion is the second factor of influence on the decay of the two agents and thereby on the optimal propofol-opioid concentrations. With increasing duration of infusion the optimal effect site propofol-opioid concentrations change only marginally. This is explained by the fact that for return of consciousness the concentrations of fentanyl, alfentanil, and sufentanil only have to decrease by 15-25%, while that of remifentanil decreases approximately by 60%. Because the effect site propofol concentration decreases more rapidly than that of alfentanil, fentanyl and sufentanil, return of consciousness is mainly caused by a reduction in the effect site propofol concentration (by 50%), and less by alfentanil, fentanyl or sufentanil (15-25%). In contrast, after propofol-remifentanil anaesthesia the effect site propofol concentration drops much slower than that of remifentanil. As a result, return of consciousness after propofol-remifentanil anaesthesia is much more caused by a decrease in the effect site concentration of the opioid (by 60%) than that of propofol (by 25%). The 15 % decrement curve of fentanyl and the 25% decrement curve of alfentanil and sufentanil, run almost parallel to the 50% context-sensitive halftime curve of propofol. Furthermore, the 60% decrement curve of remifentanil runs more or less parallel to the 25% decay curve of propofol. Consequently, infusion duration has little effect on the value of optimal concentrations. Although the concept of the context-sensitive halftime has improved our understanding of the clinical implications of the pharmacokinetics of anaesthetic agents, much more than the elimination half-life, one should keep in mind that concentrations not always need to decrease by as much as 50% to achieve return of consciousness or spontaneous breathing. It is clear that at suboptimal concentrations, as often will occur in clinical practice due to the interindividual variability in pharmacokinetics, recovery is much more postponed after propofol-fentanyl anaesthesia than when propofol is combined with alfentanil and sufentanil. It is also clear that the optimal propofol-remifentanil concentrations are less important than for the other propofol-opioid combinations because even at suboptimal propofol-remifentanil concentrations recovery after prolonged infusion still is rapid. To avoid a delayed return of consciousness these data suggest that intraoperative responses can be best counteracted by additional propofol in the combination with fentanyl, alfentanil or sufentanil and by additional remifentanil during propofol-remifentanil anaesthesia. Furthermore, when spontaneous breathing is desired, lower than optimal effect site opioid concentrations (e.g. effect site alfentanil concentrations < 50 ng/ml) in the presence of correspondingly higher than optimal effect site propofol concentrations should be given. Whereas, in contrast, in the cardiovascular compromised patient, the haemodynamic function may become less depressed in the presence of higher than optimal effect site alfentanil and correspondingly lower than optimal effect site propofol concentrations. In

Table 1
Infusion schemes of propofol and the opioids required to maintain effect site concentrations of these agents, when given in combination, within +/- 15% of the effect site concentrations that are associated with a 50% and 95% probability of no response to surgical stimuli and the most rapid possible return of consciousness after termination of the infusions (with permission)[16].

Opioid	Alfentanil EC_{50}-EC_{95} (90-130 ng/ml)	Fentanyl EC_{50}-EC_{95} (1.1-1.6 ng/ml)	Sufentanil EC_{50}-EC_{95} (0.14-0.20 ng/ml)	Remifentanil EC_{50}-EC_{95} (4.7-8.0 ng/ml)
Bolus	25-35 μg/kg in 30 sec	3 μg/kg in 30 sec	0.15-0.25 μg/kg in 30 sec	1.5-2 μg/kg in 30 sec
Infusion 1	50-75 μg/kg/h for 30 min	1.5-2.5 μg/kg/h for 30 min	0.15-0.22 μg/kg thereafter	13-22 μg/kg/h for 20 min
Infusion 2	30-42.5 μg/kg/h thereafter	1.3-2 μg/kg/h up to 150 min		11.5-19 μg/kg/h thereafter
Infusion 3		0.7-1.4 μg/kg/h thereafter		
Propofol	Propofol EC_{50}-EC_{95} (3.2-4.4 μg/ml)	Propofol EC_{50}-EC_{95} (3.4-5.4 μg/ml)	Propofol EC_{50}-EC_{95} (3.3-4.5 μg/ml)	Propofol EC_{50}-EC_{95} (2.5-2.8 μg/ml)
Bolus	2.0-2.8 mg/kg in 30 sec	2.0-3.0 mg/kg in 30 sec	2.0-2.8 mg/kg in 30 sec	1.5 mg/kg in 30 sec
Infusion 1	9-12 mg/kg/h for 40 min	9-15 mg/kg/h for 40 min	9-12 mg/kg/h for 40 min	7-8 mg/kg/h for 40 min
Infusion 2	7-10 mg/kg/h for 150 min	7-12 mg/kg/h for 150 min	7-10 mg/kg/h for 150 min	6-6.5 mg/kg/h for 150 min
Infusion 3	6.5-8 mg/kg/h thereafter	6.5-11 mg/kg/h thereafter	6.5-8 mg/kg/h thereafter	5-6 mg/kg/h thereafter

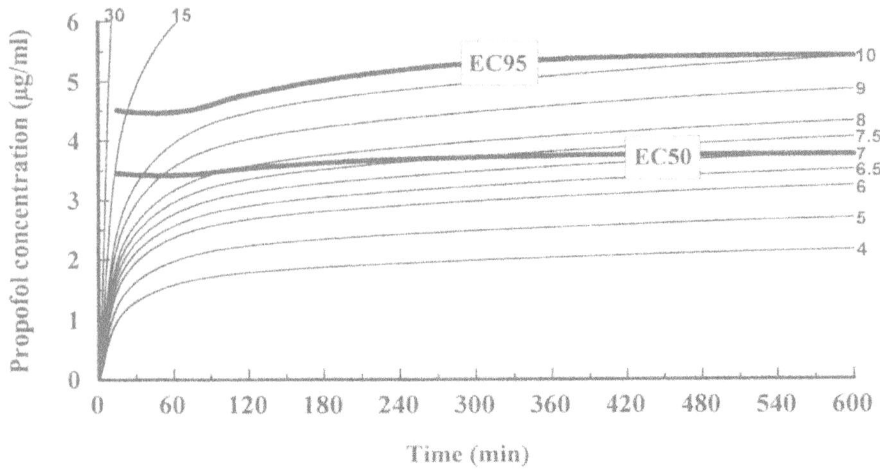

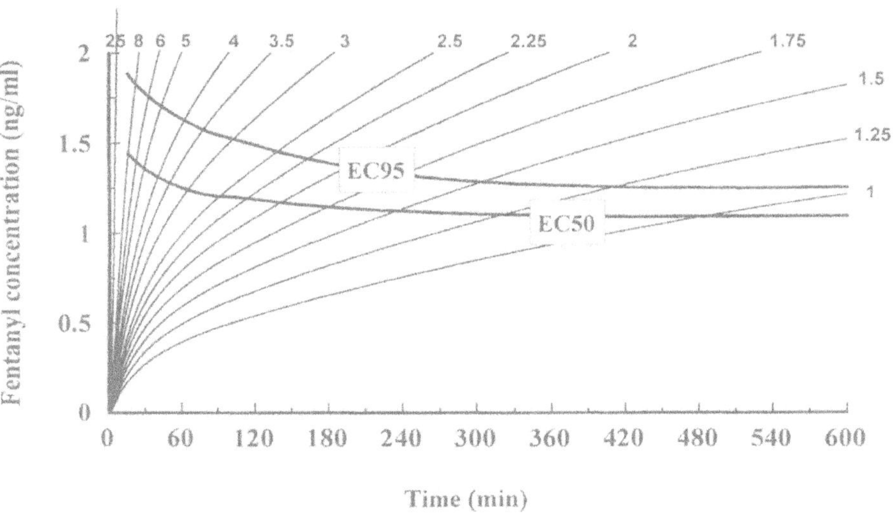

Figure 2
Nomograms defining the optimal EC_{50}-EC_{95} infusion regimens (infusion regimens that assure adequate anaesthesia and, after termination of the infusion, the most rapid possible return to consciousness) when propofol and fentanyl are combined. In the presence of an optimal propofol EC_{95} of about 5 µg/ml (to be reached with propofol infusion rates of 10-16 $mg.kg^{-1}.h^{-1}$) plasma fentanyl concentrations of 1-1.6 ng/ml are needed. These plasma fentanyl concentrations are reached with fentanyl infusion rates of 1-2 $µg.kg^{-1}.h^{-1}$ (see also table 1). On the right hand side of the figure infusion rates of propofol are diplayed in $mg.kg^{-1}.h^{-1}$ and of fentanyl in $µg.kg^{-1}.h^{-1}$.

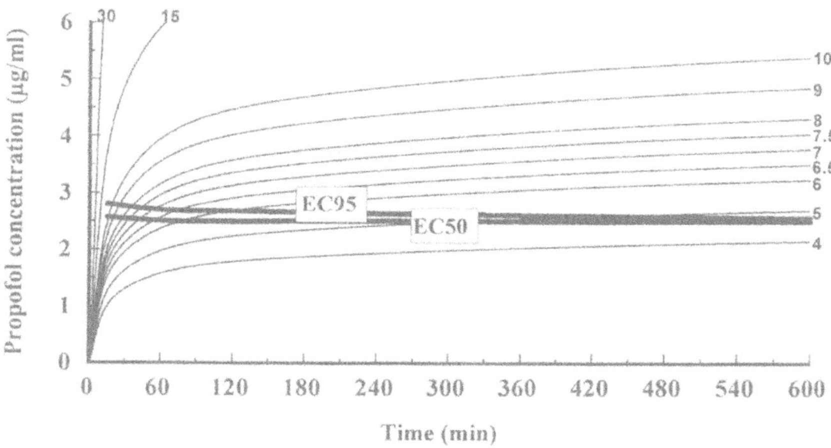

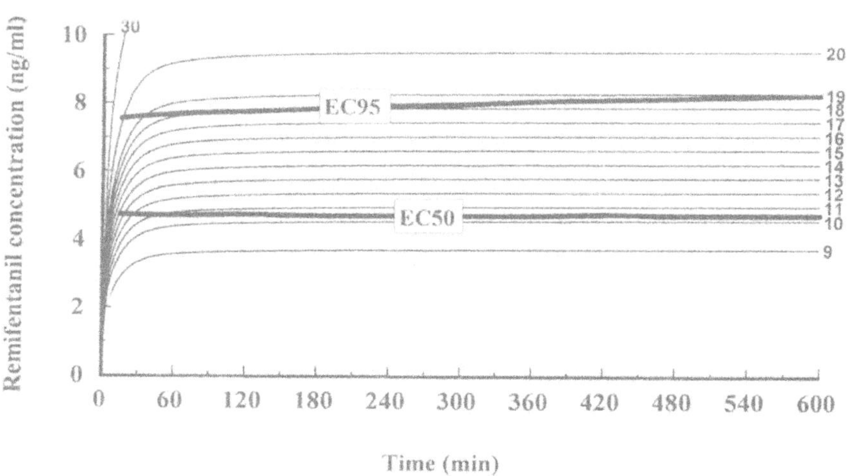

Figure 3
Nomograms defining the optimal EC_{50}-EC_{95} infusion regimens regimens (infusion regimens that assure adequate anaesthesia and, after termination of the infusion, the most rapid possible return to consciousness)when propofol and remifentanil are combined. In the presence of an optimal propofol EC_{95} of about 2.5 µg/ml (to be reached with propofol infusion rates of 5-7 $mg.kg^{-1}.h^{-1}$) plasma remifentanil concentrations of 5-8 ng/ml are needed. These plasma remifentanil concentrations are reached with remifentanil infusion rates of 10-20 $\mu g.kg^{-1}.h^{-1}$ (see also table 1). On the right hand side of the figure infusion rates of propofol are diplayed in $mg.kg^{-1}.h^{-1}$ and of remifentanil in $\mu g.kg^{-1}.h^{-1}$.

spontaneously breathing and cardiovascularly compromised patients suboptimal propofol-opioid concentrations thus are indicated intraoperatively at the expense of a prolonged recovery.

From the optimal propofol-opioid concentrations optimal propofol and opioid infusion schemes can be derived that assure adequate anaesthesia and the most rapid return of consciousness after termination of the infusion when propofol is combined with one of the opioids fentanyl, alfentanil, sufentanil or remifentanil (table 1, figures 2 and 3). These infusion schemes should be used as guidelines and adjustments should be made to the individual needs of the patient and in anticipation of factors such as age, sex and stimulus intensity related to the type of surgery.

Conclusion

Propofol and the opioids affect each other's distribution and elimination resulting in increased concentrations of both agents, when combined. Furthermore, the pharmacodynamic synergistic interaction strengthens the action of both agents even more. Optimal propofol-opioid concentration combinations have been defined that allow an adequate anaesthesia to be given followed by the most rapid possible recovery. Optimal propofol concentrations are affected by the choice of the opioid; the longer acting the opioid, the lower the concentrations of the opioid one should provide in the presence of equivalently higher propofol concentrations. Fentanyl, therefore, should be combined with a relatively high propofol dosage scheme, alfentanil and sufentanil with an intermediate propofol dosage scheme, whereas remifentanil, in relatively high concentrations, should be combined with a low propofol infusion regimen (see table 1).

References

1. Bovill J.G. Analysis of drug interactions. In Baillière's clinical anaesthesiology 1998, Vol. 12, No. 2, 153-168.
2. Coetzee JF, Glen JB, Wium CA, Boshoff L: Pharmacokinetic model selection for target controlled infusion of propofol. Anesthesiology 199 5; 82: 1328-1345.

3. Vuyk J, Engbers FHM, Burm AGL, Vletter AA, Bovill JG. Performance of computer-controlled infusion of propofol: an evaluation of five pharmacokinetic parameter sets. Anesth Analg 1995; 81: 1275-1282.
4. Schnider TW, Minto CF, Gambus PL, Andresen C, Goodale DB, Shafer SL and Youngs EJ. The influence of method of administration and covariates on the pharmacokinetics of propofol in adult volunteers. Anesthesiology 1998; 88 (5): 1170-82.
5. Schüttler J, Ihmsen H. Population pharmacokinetics of propofol. Anesthesiology 1993; 79: A331.
6. Pavlin DJ, Coda B, Shen DD, Tschanz J, Nguyen Q, Schaffer R, Donaldson G, Jacobson RC, Chapman CR. Effects of combining propofol and alfentanil on ventilation, analgesia, sedation, and emesis in human volunteers. Anesthesiology 1996; 84: 23-37.
7. Vuyk J., Mertens M.J., Vletter A.A., Burm A.G.L., Bovill J.G. Alfentanil modifies the pharmacokinetics of propofol in volunteers. Anesthesiology 1997; 87, A 300
8. Matot I, Neely CF, Katz RY, Neufeld GR. Pulmonary uptake of propofol in cats. Anesthesiology 1993; 78: 1157-1165.
9. Gepts E, Jonckheer K, Maes V, Sock W, Camu F. Disposition kinetics of propofol during alfentanil anaesthesia. Anaesthesia 1988; 43 (suppl): 8-13.
10. Janicki PK, James FHM, Erskine WAR. Propofol inhibits enzymatic degradation of alfentanil and sufentanil by isolated liver microsomes in vitro. Br J Anaesth 1992; 68: 311-312.
11. Baker MT, Chadam MV, Ronnenberg WC. Inhibitory effcets of propofol on cytochrome P450 activities in rat hepatic microsomes. Anesth Analg 1993; 76: 817-821.
12. Berenbaum MC. What is synergy? Pharmacological Reviews 1989; 41: 93-141.
13. Smith C, McEwan AI, Jhaveri R, Wilkinson M, Goodman D, Smith R, Canada A, Glass PSA. The interaction of fentanyl on the CP50 of propofol for loss of consciousness and skin incision. Anesthesiology 1995; 81: 820-828.
14. Vuyk J, Engbers FHM, Burm AGL, Vletter AA, Griever GER, Olofsen E, Bovill JG. Pharmacodynamic interaction betqween propofol and alfentanil when given for induction of anesthesia. Anesthesiology 1996; 84: 22-33.
15. Vuyk J, Lim T, Engbers FHM, Burm AGL, Vletter AA, Bovill JG: The pharmacodynamic interaction of propofol and alfentanil during lower abdominal surgery in female patients. Anesthesiology 1995; 83: 8-22.
16. Vuyk J, Mertens MJ, Olofsen E, Burm AGL, Bovill JG. Propofol anesthesia and rational opioid selection. Anesthesiology 1997; 87:1549-1562.
17. Kazama T, Ikeda K , Morita K, Katoh T, Kikura M. Propofol concentration required for endotracheal intubation with a laryngoscope or fiberscope and its interaction with fentanyl. Anesth-Analg. 1998; 86(4): 872-9
18. Kazama T, Ikeda K, Morita K, Sanjo Y. Awakening propofol concentration with and without blood-effect site equilibration after short-term and long-term administration of propofol and fentanyl anesthesia. Anesthesiology. 1998; 88(4): 928-34
19. Kazama T, Ikeda K, Morita K. Reduction by fentanyl of the Cp50 values of propofol and hemodynamic responses to various noxious stimuli. Anesthesiology. 1997 ; 87(2): 213-27

Strategies to prevent awareness

Michel Struys, Eric Mortier and Linda Versichelen

Gent, Belgium

Introduction

The objective of any intravenous anaesthetic drug administration is to obtain the desired clinical level of anaesthesia or sedation. Nowadays, in clinical practice, most anaesthetic drugs are given using standard dosing guidelines without applying the knowledge of their pharmacokinetics and dynamics to control their administration. Drugs are sometimes administered with the rationale: "Give some drug and observe your patient to see what happens". The ultimate goal when administering a particular dose of a drug is to obtain the desired clinical effect, for which a specific therapeutic concentration of the drug at the site of action (= the receptor) is necessary. For most anaesthetic agents, this effect-site (or bio-phase) is not the plasma but the central nervous system and the effect-site concentration is not measurable. Therefore, the relation between the therapeutic plasma concentration and the clinical effect can be considered instead. Based on this concentration-effect relationship, it is possible to select a target plasma concentration. This target concentration can be defined as the plasma concentration which, on the basis of available information, is most likely to yield the desired effect[1].

The problem of defining "depth of anaesthesia"

By using the classical theories of anaesthesia based on unitary non-specific mechanisms of anaesthetic actions, one anaesthetic may be replaced freely by another, and in the case of anaesthetic combinations, the anaesthetic effect of mixtures is expected to be additive [2-6]. In this classic concept of anaesthesia, the state of general anaesthesia is a multifeatured phenomenon with one underlying mechanism, and, to be common for all general anaesthetics with diverse chemical structures, this mechanism is supposed to be non-specific. The problem with the classic concept of the state of anaesthesia became obvious when neuromuscular blocking agents, opioids and barbiturates began to be widely used in combination with inhaled anaesthetics. In 1987, Prys-Roberts[7] suggested that if pain is considered a "conscious perception of a noxious stimulus", then "a state of anaesthesia" can be defined as drug-induced unconsciousness in which the patient neither perceives nor recalls pain. According to his theory surgery causes noxious stimuli resulting in a series of somatic (i.e., pain and movement), autonomic and haemodynamic responses that may be modified by different drugs. Kissin further refined the definition of anaesthesia[6,8]. He stated that a wide spectrum of pharmacological actions via different drugs can be used to create a general anaesthetic state. These pharmacological actions could include analgesia, anxiolysis, amnesia, unconsciousness and suppression of somatic, motor, cardiovascular and hormonal responses to the stimulus of surgery. He mentioned that the spectrum of effects that constitutes the state of general anaesthesia should not be regarded as the sum of several components but should be regarded as the sum of separate pharmacological actions, even if the anaesthesia is produced by one drug. Following his hypothesis, recent data suggest that our understanding of depth of anaesthesia will advance only when there is more information available on the interaction of different anaesthetic drugs. In a recent editorial Glass[9] stated that the interaction between hypnotics and opioids for achieving two major endpoints in general anaesthesia (loss of consciousness and inhibition of movement at skin incision) is based on the evidence that loss of consciousness and response to skin incision are not part of a single continuum of increasing "anaesthetic depth" but rather two separate phenomena. Combining these observations he proposed the following hypothesis of general anaesthesia. General anaesthesia is a process requiring a state of unconsciousness of the brain (produced primarily by the intravenous or volatile anaesthetic-hypnotic drug). If only unconsciousness is achieved, a noxious stimulus needs to be inhibited from reaching higher central nervous system centres. This is achieved by the action of the opioid at opioid receptors within the spinal cord (or local anaesthetics at peripheral nerves, or volatile anaesthetics at the spinal cord when administered at concentrations equal to their minimum alveolar concentration (MAC)).

Available measures for controlling depth of anaesthesia

Various parameters to measure and predict the depth of the anaesthetic component of anaesthesia are proposed in the literature. Depth of anaesthesia is nowadays judged clinically by the observation of somatic (patient movement) and autonomic reflexes (increased heart rate and blood pressure, tears and pupil dilation). Recently, several studies have suggested that movement and autonomic changes during anaesthesia do not necessarily represent the effect of anaesthetics on the central nervous system[10,11], since it has been demonstrated that the structures of the forebrain are not essential in mediating movement to surgical stimulation[12]. The usefulness of measured and/or calculated (= predicted) drug concentration to predict the time course of anaesthetic effect has been demonstrated by several authors[13-17]. In contradiction with the inhalation anaesthetics, where the inspired and end-tidal concentration can be measured on-line and displayed, the actual plasma concentration of an intravenously administered drug is not measurable in clinical practice. Therefore, it is impossible to steer an intravenous infusion regimen to maintain a stable (and on-line measured) blood concentration. Thanks to the development of new short-acting drugs, the availability of advanced computers, electronic devices and syringe pumps, in combination with a better understanding of the pharmacokinetics and dynamics, it is possible to administer intravenous hypnotic drugs to achieve and maintain a desired concentration by applying target controlled infusion (TCI). The basic idea behind the TCI technique is the use of pharmacokinetic modelling and to predict a drug concentration in one of the pharmacokinetic compartments, e.g. the central compartment or the theoretical effect-site compartment. These TCI devices will rapidly achieve and maintain this desired predicted concentration in the specific compartment. The availability of these TCI techniques may increase the quality of anaesthesia. Therefore, a proper understanding of therapeutical drug concentrations has to become a basic knowledge of the anaesthetist. Multiple articles have been published on therapeutic drug concentrations in a variety of surgical situations. We will only give a few examples. For the intravenous anaesthetics, Ausems et al.[18] described the relationship between plasma alfentanil concentrations and the likelihood of response to a noxious stimulus. Here, the autonomic and somatic changes on noxious stimuli were correctly used as analgetic endpoints. For propofol, various authors described the relationship of plasma concentrations and drug effect. Chortkoff et al.[19] found a good correlation between plasma concentrations of propofol and the suppression of response to command (Cp50-awake = 2.69 ± 0.56 μg/ml). In the same study, they defined a MAC-awake for desflurane of 2.60% ± 0.46 %. Similar reports for all kinds of drugs can be found in the literature. Nevertheless, for anaesthetics, the blood compartment is not the site of drug effect. The site at which the drug exerts its effect is termed the biophase or effect-site. In an attempt to further improve these TCI techniques, Shafer and Greg [20] described an algorithm to control the target concentration in the theoretical effect-site. It now becomes clear that for the intravenous anaesthetics effect compartment controlled target controlled infusion increases the quality of anaesthesia[14,21,22].

While the MAC, as developed by Eger et al. in 1965[23], has been a powerful scientific and clinical tool for understanding depth of inhalational anaesthesia, Zbinden et al.[10,11] have shown that when isoflurane is given as the sole anaesthetic agent and both movement and haemodynamic responses are examined in relation to defined noxious stimuli, increasing concentrations can prevent purposeful movement but can not prevent significant haemodynamic (hypertension, tachycardia) responses, even at high end-tidal concentrations of isoflurane. Haemodynamic control with high isoflurane concentrations occurs from a decrease of the prestimulation baseline. Thus, while haemodynamic responses are the clinical measures most commonly used to judge the depth of inhalational anaesthesia and adjust dosage, the scientific basis for this is less than clear. These variables might be modified by disease, drugs and surgical techniques[24]. In clinical practice, opioids and other drugs are added routinely to inhalational anaesthetics, making the clinical evaluation of depth of anaesthesia even more difficult. Therefore, there is a need to introduce newer and more precise measures of the depth of anaesthesia. The following techniques are well described in the literature: the isolated forearm technique (IFT), frequency of lower oesophageal contraction (LOC) spontaneous surface electromyography (SEMG), electroencephalography (EEG) and evoked potentials (EP). The use of

LOC and IFT to measure depth of anaesthesia is hampered by many drawbacks, we will therefore only focus on the SEMG, EEG and EP[25,26].

Measuring the hypnotic drug effect

Spontaneous surface EMG (SEMG)

In patients who are not paralysed by neuromuscular blocking agents, a SEMG can be recorded from various muscle groups. Especially facial, abdominal, and neck muscles are used. It has been shown that increasing SEMG activity of facial and neck muscles reflects both recovery from the effect of neuromuscular blocking agents and a reduced depth of anaesthesia, induced either by increased intensity of surgical stimulation or reduced anaesthetic concentrations. Unfortunately, the SEMG offers no accurate information on the depth of anaesthesia when the patient lost has consciousness and the signal is saturated[26-30].

Electro-encephalogram (EEG)

The interpretation of subtle changes in the raw EEG requires a neurophysiologist. Therefore, computerisation of EEG monitoring is essential when this technique is used continuously in the operating room (OR) or intensive care unit (ICU). Two analysis techniques for analysing the three-dimensional (amplitude or voltage, frequency and time) EEG data exist: one in the time domain and one in the frequency domain. Time domain refers to a display of time versus a specific physiological variable. The conventional EEG, electrocardiogram (ECG), and arterial pressure waveforms are examples of time domain recordings. Frequency domain refers to a method of EEG spectral analysis that displays the separate frequencies of a complex waveform against another variable, such as amplitude or power. Some of the early methods of EEG analysis are time domain analyses. The "burst suppression ratio" is the only time domain processing technique still used in clinical practice. It evaluates the proportion of a given epoch representing electrical suppression. These changes typically occur at deep levels of anaesthesia. Therefore, this method is not appropriate for monitoring levels of light sedation[31].

Signal processing in the frequency domain represents the original complex EEG waveforms transformed into voltage (or power = voltage ^{2}) as a function of frequency. "Power spectrum analysis" is the best known example of EEG analysis in the frequency domain. The transformation from time to frequency domain is performed in several steps. First, the data are digitised at several intervals. A number of these intervals (usually representing 2 to 30 seconds of EEG) comprise an epoch, which is then subjected to a complex mathematical manipulation known as Fast Fourier Transformation (FFT). The details of this analysis and the underlying assumptions can be found in the engineering literature[39]. For the purpose of this discussion, the FFT of an EEG may be considered to be a mathematically equivalent description of the EEG, composed of regularly spaced frequency components whose amplitude and relationship to each other are defined by the transformation. The size of the frequency steps is defined by the duration of the epoch, and the bandwidth is related to the number of samples in the epoch. The advantage of this transformation is that mathematical manipulations can be performed with substantially greater ease on the transformed EEG than on the original signal.

The power spectrum is the most common used computation of the FFT. This computation provides an estimate of the amplitude of the EEG for each component in the original transformation. It is repeated for each epoch transformed, and plotted using one of the three-dimensional techniques. Because the power spectrum is inherently a complex representation of the EEG, there have been numerous attempts to further simplify this "three-dimensional" information by computing a one-dimensional (univariate) descriptor of the power spectra. Examples are the spectral edge frequency (= frequency below which 95% of the power exists), the median frequency (= frequency below which 50% of the power spectrum exists) and peak power frequency[33]. By using power spectrum analysis to study the EEG, not all information provided by the EEG is used. Power spectrum analysis assumes a Gaussian, stationary, and first-order (linear) model of frequencies within the EEG. This means that the amplitudes of the EEG are supposed to be normally distributed, the stationary properties assume that this does not change over time and the frequency constituents are uncorrelated[34]. Under this assumption, the EEG is considered to be made up by a linear superimposition of statistically independent sinusoidal wave components. Only frequency and power estimates are considered, whereas phase information is generally ignored. In reality, however, biologic systems exhibit significant non-linear complexities that do not conform to the assumption of conventional power spectrum analysis[34].

Bispectral analysis (BIS) is an advanced signal processing technique that is capable of tracking non-linear as well as linear changes in signals. The mathematical approach of bispectral analysis relies on the expansion of the widely used Fourier Transformation method of signal decomposition into simpler component waves, however, it is computationally much more intensive than power spectrum analysis. The BIS incorporates information of quadrate interactions between the different components of the EEG. It does so by quantifying the phase coupling between two frequencies and a third frequency (= harmonic) and their sum (or difference). The extent of coupling between two frequencies (bicoherence) can vary from 0 % (if no harmonic is generated) to 100 % (if a harmonic is generated for the duration of the period analysed).

Because the standard power spectral analysis of the EEG does not take into account the phase information of the constituent sinusoids, two very different complex waveforms with different phase structures can have identical power spectra. Thus, even though two such signals represent two different phenomena (i.e. different EEG patterns), the difference will not be evident. Phase coupling of the constituent frequencies is a characteristic feature of nonlinear systems. The identification of the phase relation in the EEG signal may provide additional information about the properties of the EEG, especially about certain EEG patterns in which there is phase locking between harmonic frequency components. Although bispectral analysis is a classic method of analysing waveforms, it has only recently been incorporated in a commercial device (Aspect, Natick, MA, USA) for monitoring the EEG during anaesthesia.

Evoked potentials

A sensory evoked potential is the electrical response of the nervous system to a sensory stimulus and can be recorded along the sensory pathway to the cerebrum[27,28]. Three types of stimulation are commonly used: somatosensory (electrical) stimulation of peripheral nerves; auditory stimulation by clicks or tones; visual stimulation by alternating visual patterns[29]. The potentials that are evoked are generally very low in amplitude (0.1 to 20 μV) and hence it is not possible to distinguish them from the background electroencephalogram (100 μV)[27]. To extract the evoked potential from the background brain wave activity, signal-averaging techniques are used. These techniques are based on repetitive stimulation with the corresponding signal time-locked to the stimulus[28]. Since the background noise varies at random and each evoked response has essentially the same morphology, time-locking and averaging will improve the signal (evoked potential) to noise (electroencephalogram) ratio[27]. This will allow extraction of the evoked potential from the underlying electroencephalogram. Evoked potentials can be divided into near-field and far-field[30]. Near-field potentials arise in structures adjacent (2 to 2.5 cm) to the detecting electrode whereas far-field potentials arise in structures further away[30]. With recordings from scalp electrodes, cortical responses are near-field potentials and brain stem responses are far-field potentials[27,30].

Far-field potentials are propagated by volume conduction (brain, cerebrospinal fluid), which occurs immediately. On the other hand, near-field potentials are propagated by nerve transmission. Generally, near-field responses are affected more by anaesthetic agents, than far-field responses[27]. The morphology of the evoked potential can be described by measuring the latency and amplitude of the generated waveforms[27]. Deflections below the baseline are termed positive (P) and those above the baseline negative (N)[30]. To identify a waveform, the letter designating the direction of the deflection is followed by a number indicating the nominal poststimulus latency (expressed in ms)[30]. Somatosensory evoked potentials are mainly used for monitoring the spinal cord during procedures that carry a risk of ischaemia, or disruption of the conducting pathways[28]. Visual evoked potentials seldom are used, because the flash evoked response is so variable that some consider it not reproducible enough[28,29].

Auditory evoked potentials are monitored during surgical procedures in the posterior cranial fossa[30]. Furthermore, some groups use them to assess depth of anaesthesia[28]. This is not surprising, since it has been shown that in some cases auditory information can be recalled in the postoperative period. The auditory evoked response can be divided in three series of positive and negative waves. The brain-stem response is obtained in the first 10 ms after stimulation (brainstem auditory evoked potentials, BAEP). The early cortical response occurs 10 to 100 ms post-stimulus (mid-latency auditory evoked potentials, MLAEP). The late cortical response is obtained later (late latency auditory evoked potentials, LLAEP). These series of waves represent propagation and processing of auditory information from the cochlea to the brainstem, the primary auditory cortex and the association areas in the frontal cortex[35]. Brainstem evoked potentials remain for the greater part unchanged during general anaesthesia. Late latency evoked potentials are almost impossible to obtain during general anaesthesia[28]. However, the early cortical responses can be provoked in a reproducible way and are susceptible to the effects of anaesthetic agents[36]. Therefore, they can be used to assess the processing of information in the primary auditory cortex during general anaesthesia[35]. The mid-latency auditory evoked potentials consist of five waves that are labelled as No, Po, Na, Pa and Nb[29]. The corresponding power spectra (obtained by Fast Fourier Transformation (FFT) and rank-correlation procedure (RCF)) reveal that the periodic waveform of the mid-latency evoked potentials has its maximal energy in the 30 to 40 Hz frequency range[37]. Another approach to detect unintentional conscious awareness is the use of the auditory steady state response (ASSR)[38]. This steady state response is evoked following repeatedly presented auditory stimuli, delivered so rapidly that they cause overlapping of the responses[38]. The frequency of stimulus delivery that produces the largest auditory steady state response in the conscious individual is about 40/sec. However, frequencies between 35 and 45 Hz are suitable[39]. The amplitude of the steady state response is reduced during sleep and during anaesthesia. Furthermore, it correlates well with recovery from anaesthesia[38-42].

Which measure should we choose for monitoring depth of anaesthesia?

Various approaches to neurophysiological monitoring for measuring adequacy of anaesthesia have been used in clinical practice with varying degrees of success[43]. Controversy exists on the use of these measures to monitor loss and return of consciousness, depth of anaesthesia and hypnotic drug effect. An adequate measure of depth of anaesthesia or sedation should be one that provides information on loss and return of consciousness as well as on the anaesthetic drug effect and allow us to prevent a too deep level of anaesthesia. Initial reports on the classical univariate EEG measures (MF and SEF 95% and RDELTA) have concluded that these correlate well with anaesthetic adequacy[44,45]. All these investigators used haemodynamic or somatic (movement) response to surgical stimuli as the clinical end-point to assess the accuracy of the different indicators of anaesthetic depth[46], but it has been shown that this clinical end-point is inaccurate for this purpose[47]. In a more recent study, Dwyer et al. found that these univariate measures do not predict depth of isoflurane anaesthesia as defined by the response to surgical incision, the response to verbal command or the development of memory[48]. This was also demonstrated by others[49]. A large number of prospective studies have demonstrated the clinical utility of BIS monitoring in surgical patients[50-57]. BIS provides information on drug-effect during propofol sedation and hypnosis[56] and predicts the probability of recovery of consciousness after a single injection of propofol[43]. BIS shows a good correlation with intra-operative recall and depth of propofol-induced sedation[52]. Leslie et al.[58] found a mathematical correlation between the BIS and the plasma concentration of propofol within a range of 1 - 4 µg/ml, but did not find a correlation between SEF 95 % and propofol plasma concentration; higher concentrations were not tested. In a comparative trial[26], we have evaluated the usefulness of SEMG, MF, SEF 95%, RDELTA and BIS as measures of depth of anaesthesia and hypnotic drug effect during propofol sedation in combination with spinal anaesthesia for orthopaedic surgery on the lower extremities. The BIS is the only one among those tested that provided information on those two criteria. The univariate measures (MF, SEF 95% and RDELTA) provided no reproducible information and the SEMG is only useful for detecting loss and return of consciousness, without any predictive value. The SEMG is not good for measuring depth of anaesthesia after loss of consciousness. BIS has also been validated for midazolam, thiopental, isoflurane, sevoflurane, nitrous oxide , and opioids[50,54,58-63]. Using the large ASPECT® database, Shafer et al.[64] calculated the relation between BIS, blood pressure, drug concentrations (measured plasma and predicted plasma and effect-site concentrations of propofol) and probability of recall. He concluded that there was no correlation between the haemodynamics and the probability of recall. When the effect-site concentration of propofol was lower than 1.5 µg/ml, he found a significant correlation between BIS, predicted effect-site concentration and the probability of recall. At higher concentrations, he concluded that the BIS revealed no additional information when using the predicted effect-site concentration to predict recall. Nevertheless, when looking to implicit awareness, our group[65] found that the addition of the BIS to standard clinical practice can be useful in titrating the propofol effect-site concentration, resulting in an improved stability of depth of

sedation and prevention of awareness even at effect-site concentration higher than 1.5 µg/ml.
Regarding the evoked potentials, halothane, enflurane, isoflurane, sevoflurane and desflurane all increase the latency and decrease the amplitude of the mid-latency evoked potentials in a reversible, dose- and concentration - related way[37,66-69]. In contrast to the volatile anaesthetics, nitrous oxide has little effect on mid-latency evoked potentials when given to supplement these agents[35]. The change in latency and amplitude of mid-latency evoked potentials after administration of intravenous anaesthetics such as thiopentone, etomidate and propofol is similar to that observed with inhaled agents[25, 35,70]. Opioids, even at high doses, have no effect on the morphology of the mid-latency evoked potentials[71,72]. The amplitudes and latencies of mid-latency evoked potentials are not changed by ketamine in induction doses[73]. The same holds true for benzodiazepines such as diazepam, flunitazepam and midazolam[35].

To evaluate and quantify depth of anaesthesia on-line with the aid of auditory evoked potentials, an auditory evoked potential index has been devised[74]. The latter is a mathematical derivative which reflects the morphology of the auditory evoked potential[74]. Recently, it has been compared with 95 % spectral edge frequency, median frequency and the bispectral index during repeated transitions from consciousness to unconsciousness by target controlled infusion of propofol[75]. In comparison with the other three electrophysiological variables, the auditory evoked potential index scored better at distinguishing the transition from unconsciousness to consciousness but the BIS correlated better correlated with increasing drug concentration[75]. Recently, it has been shown that while BIS is able to predict recovery from unconsciousness to consciousness, the auditory evoked potential index is better at detecting this transition[76].

Conclusion

Because the prevention of awareness is an important objectives during our clinical anaesthetic drug delivery, the optimalisation of hypnotic anaesthetic drug administration should be guided by a better understanding of the principles of pharmacokinetics and dynamics (e.g. such as in TCI techniques) combined with an accurate measure of "depth of anaesthesia". Among the many available measures the auditory evoked potentials and bispectral index seem to be the most promising techniques.

References

1. Danhof M: Does variability explain (all) variability in drug effects? Topics in pharmaceutical science. Edited by: Breimer DD, Crommelin DJA, Midha KK. Noordwijk: Amsterdam Med. Press BV, 1989, pp 573-86
2. Vermon M, Sebel PS: Memory and awareness in anaesthesia. Seminars in Anesthesia 1993;12:123-31
3. Plombey F: Operations upon the eye. Lancet 1847;1:1847
4. Guedel AE: Inhalational anaesthesia: a fundamental guide. New York: Macmillan, 1937
5. Artusio JF, Jr., Corssen G, Dornette WH, Reves JG: Monitoring depth of anesthesia. Clin Anesth 1973;9:211-22
6. Kissin I: A concept for assessing interactions of general anesthetics. Anesth Analg 1997;85:204-10
7. Prys-Roberts C: Anaesthesia: a practical or impractical construct? Br J Anaesth 1987; 59(11):1341-5
8. Kissin I: General anesthetic action: an obsolete notion? [editorial] [see comments]. Anesth Analg 1993;76:215-8
9. Glass PS. Anesthetic drug interactions: an insight into general anesthesia--its mechanism and dosing strategies [editorial; comment]. Anesthesiology 1998;88:5-6
10. Zbinden AM, Petersen-Felix S, Thomson DA: Anesthetic depth defined using multiple noxious stimuli during isoflurane/oxygen anesthesia. II. Hemodynamic responses [see comments]. Anesthesiology 1994;80:261-7
11. Zbinden AM, Maggiorini M, Petersen-Felix S, Lauber R, Thomson DA, Minder CE: Anesthetic depth defined using multiple noxious stimuli during isoflurane/oxygen anesthesia. I. Motor reactions [see comments]. Anesthesiology 1994;80:253-60
12. Rampil IJ, Mason P, Singh H: Anesthetic potency (MAC) is independent of forebrain structures in the rat. Anesthesiology 1993;78:707-12
13. Kenny GN: The development and future of TCI. Acta Anaesthesiol Belg 1997;48: 229-32
14. Struys M, Versichelen L, Thas O, Herregods L, Rolly G: Comparison of computer-controlled administration of propofol with two manually controlled infusion techniques. Anaesthesia 1997;52:41-50
15. Struys M, Versichelen L, Rolly G: Propofol target-controlled infusion in clinical practice. Acta Anaesthesiol Belg 1997;48:207-11
16. White P: Target-controlled infusion (TCI): a critical analysis. Eur J Anaesthesiol Suppl 1995;10:87
17. Coetzee JF, Glen JB, Wium CA, Boshoff L: Pharmacokinetic model selection for target controlled infusions of propofol. Assessment of three parameter sets. Anesthesiology 1995;82:1328-45
18. Ausems ME, Hug CC, Jr., Stanski DR, Burm AG: Plasma concentrations of alfentanil required to supplement nitrous oxide anesthesia for general surgery. Anesthesiology 1986;65:362-73.
19. Chortkoff BS, Eger EI, 2nd, Crankshaw DP, Gonsowski CT, Dutton RC, Ionescu P: Concentrations of desflurane and propofol that suppress response to command in humans. Anesth Analg 1995;81:737-43

20. Shafer SL, Gregg KM: Algorithms to rapidly achieve and maintain stable drug concentrations at the site of drug effect with a computer-controlled infusion pump. J Pharmacokinet Biopharm 1992;20:147-69
21. Jacobs JR, Reves JG: Effect site equilibration time is a determinant of induction dose requirement [editorial; comment]. Anesth Analg 1993;76:1-6
22. Jacobs JR, Williams EA: Algorithm to control "effect compartment" drug concentrations in pharmacokinetic model-driven drug delivery. IEEE Trans Biomed Eng 1993;40:993-9
23. Eger Eld, Saidman LJ, Brandstater B: Minimum alveolar anesthetic concentration: a standard of anesthetic potency. Anesthesiology 1965;26:756-63
24. Moerman N, Bonke B, Oosting J: Awareness and recall during general anesthesia. Facts and feelings. Anesthesiology 1993;79:454-64
25. Thornton C, Konieczko KM, Knight AB, Kaul B, Jones JG, Dore CJ, et al.: Effect of propofol on the auditory evoked response and oesophageal contractility. Br J Anaesth 1989;63:411-7
26. Struys M, Versichelen L, Mortier E, Ryckaert D, De Mey JC, De Deyne C, et al.: Comparison of spontaneous frontal EMG, EEG power spectrum and bispectral index to monitor propofol drug effect and emergence. Acta Anaesthesiol Scand 1998;42:628-36
27. Sebel PS: Evoked Potentials, Monitoring the central nervous system. Edited by Sebel PS, Fitch W. Oxford, London, Edingburgh, Cambridge MA, Carlton Victoria Australia: Blackwell Science, 1994, pp 267-93
28. Kalkman CJ: Monitoring the central nervous system. Anesth Clin North Am 1994;12:173-76
29. Thornton C, Jones JG: Evaluating depth of anesthesia: review of methods. Int Anaesth Clin 1993;31:67-88
30. Grundy BL: Evoked potential monitoring, Monitoring in Anesthesia and Critical Care Medicine. Edited by Blitt CD. New York: Churchill Livingstone, 1990: pp 461-524.
31. Avramov MN, While PF: Methods for monitoring the level of sedation. Critical Care Clinics 1995;11:803-826
32. Blackman RB, Tukey JW: The measurement of Power Spectra. New York, Dover, 1958
33. Levy WJ, Shapiro MM, Maruchak G, Meathe E: Automated EEG processing for intraoperative monitoring: a comparison of techniques. Anesthesiology 1980;53: 223-36
34. Sigl JC, Chamonn NC: An introduction to bispectral analysis for the EEG. J Clin Monit 1994;10:392-404
35. Schwender D, Klasing S, Madler C, Pöppel E, Peter K: Midlatency auditory evoked potentials and cognitive function during general anesthesia. Int Anesth Clin 1993; 31:89-106
36. Stanski DR: Monitoring depth of anesthesia. Anesthesia. Edited by Miller RD. New York: Churchill Livingstone, 1990, pp1001-29
37. Madler C, Keller I, Schwender D, Poppel E: Sensory information processing during general anaesthesia: effect of isoflurane on auditory evoked neuronal oscillations. Br J Anaesth 1991;66:81-7
38. Plourde G, Picton TW: Human auditory steady state response during general anaesthesia. Anesthesia and Analgesia 1990;71:460-468
39. Plourde G: Clincal use of the 40 Hz auditory steady state response. International Anesthesiology Clinics 1993; 31:107-120
40. Plourde G, Boylan JF: The auditory steady state response during sulfentanil anaesthesia. British Journal of Anaesthesia 1999;66:683-691

41. Plourde G, Villemeer C: Comparison of the effects of enflurane/N2O on the 40 Hz auditory steady state response versus the auditory middle-latering response. Anesthesia and Analgesia 1996;82:75-83
42. Plourde G: The effect of propofol on the 41 Hz auditory steady state response and on the electroencephalogram in humans. Anesthesia and Analgesia 1996;82:1015-22
43. Flaishon R, Lang E, Sebel PS: Monitoring the adequacy of intravenous anesthesia. Textbook of intavenous anesthesia. Edited by White PF. Baltimore: Williams & Wilkins, 1996, pp 545-63
44. Schwilden H, Stoeckel H, Schuttler J: Closed-loop feedback control of propofol anaesthesia by quantitative EEG analysis in humans [see comments]. Br J Anaesth 1989;62:290-6
45. Rampil IJ, Matteo RS: Changes in EEG spectral edge frequency correlate with the hemodynamic response to laryngoscopy and intubation. Anesthesiology 1987;67: 139-42
46. Smith WD, Dutton RC, Smith NT: Measuring the performance of anesthetic depth indicators. Anesthesiology 1996;84:38-51
47. Antognini JF, Schwartz K: Exaggerated anesthetic requirements in the preferentially anesthetized brain [see comments]. Anesthesiology 1993;79:1244-9
48. Dwyer RC, Rampil IJ, Eger EI, 2nd, Bennett HL. The electroencephalogram does not predict depth of isoflurane anesthesia. Anesthesiology 1994;81:403-9
49. Traast HS, Kalkman CJ: Electroencephalographic characteristics of emergence from propofol/sufentanil total intravenous anesthesia. Anesth Analg 1995;81:366-71
50. Glass PS, Bloom M, Kearse L, Rosow C, Sebel P, Manberg P: Bispectral analysis measures sedation and memory effects of propofol, midazolam, isoflurane, and alfentanil in healthy volunteers. Anesthesiology 1997;86:836-47
51. Gan TJ, Glass PS, Windsor A, Payne F, Rosow C, Sebel P, et al.: Bispectral index monitoring allows faster emergence and improved recovery from propofol, alfentanil, and nitrous oxide anesthesia. BIS Utility Study Group. Anesthesiology 1997; 87:808-15
52. Liu J, Singh H, White PF: Electroencephalographic bispectral index correlates with intraoperative recall and depth of propofol-induced sedation. Anesth Analg 1997; 84:185-9
53. Song D, Joshi GP, White PF: Titration of volatile anesthetics using bispectral index facilitates recovery after ambulatory anesthesia. Anesthesiology 1997;87:842-8
54. Rampil IJ, Kim JS, Lenhardt R, Negishi C, Sessler DI: Bispectral EEG index during nitrous oxide administration. Anesthesiology 1998;89:671-7
55. Katoh T, Suzuki A, Ikeda K: Electroencephalographic derivatives as a tool for predicting the depth of sedation and anesthesia induced by sevoflurane. Anesthesiology 1998;88:642-50
56. Kearse LA, Jr., Rosow C, Zaslavsky A, Connors P, Dershwitz M, Denman W: Bispectral analysis of the electroencephalogram predicts conscious processing of information during propofol sedation and hypnosis. Anesthesiology 1998;88:25-34
57. Flaishon R, Windsor A, Sigl J, Sebel PS: Recovery of consciousness after thiopental or propofol. Bispectral index and isolated forearm technique. Anesthesiology 1997; 86:613-9
58. Leslie K, Sessler DI, Schroeder M, Walters K: Propofol blood concentration and the Bispectral Index predict suppression of learning during propofol/epidural anesthesia in volunteers. Anesth Analg 1995;81:1269-74.
59. Sebel PS, Bowles SM, Saini V, Chamoun N: EEG bispectrum predicts movement during thiopental/isoflurane anesthesia. J Clin Monit 1995;11:83-91

60. Iselin-Chaves IA, Flaishon R, Sebel PS, Howell S, Gan TJ, Sigl J, et al.: The effect of the interaction of propofol and alfentanil on recall, loss of consciousness, and the Bispectral Index [In Process Citation]. Anesth Analg 1998;87:949-55
61. Liu J, Singh H, White PF: Electroencephalogram bispectral analysis predicts the depth of midazolam-induced sedation. Anesthesiology 1996;84:64-9
62. Billard V, Gambus PL, Chamoun N, Stanski DR, Shafer SL: A comparison of spectral edge, delta power, and bispectral index as EEG measures of alfentanil, propofol, and midazolam drug effect. Clin Pharmacol Ther 1997;61:45-58
63. Hoffman WE, Zsigmond E, Albrecht RF: The bispectral index during induction of anesthesia with midazolam and propofol. J Neurosurg Anesthesiol 1996;8:15-20
64. Shafer SL: Proceedings of the SIVA, New Orleans, October 1996
65. Struys M, Versichelen L, Byttebier G, Mortier E, Moerman A, Rolly G: Clinical usefulness of the bispectral index for titrating propofol target effect-site concentration. Anaesthesia 1998;53:4-12
66. Thornton C, Catley DM, Jordan C, Lehane JR, Royston D, Jones JG: Enflurane anaesthesia causes graded changes in the brainstem and early cortical auditory evoked response in man. Br J Anaesth 1983;55:479-86
67. Thornton C, Heneghan CP, James MF, Jones JG: Effects of halothane or enflurane with controlled ventilation on auditory evoked potentials. Br J Anaesth 1984;56: 315-23
68. Schwender D, Conzen P, Klasing S, Finsterer U, Poppel E, Peter K: The effects of anesthesia with increasing end-expiratory concentrations of sevoflurane on midlatency auditory evoked potentials. Anesth Analg 1995;81:817-22
69. Schwender D, Klasing S, Conzen P, Finsterer U, Poppel E, Peter K: Midlatency auditory evoked potentials during anaesthesia with increasing endexpiratory concentrations of desflurane. Acta Anaesthesiol Scand 1996;40:171-6
70. Thornton C, Heneghan CP, Navaratnarajah M, Bateman PE, Jones JG: Effect of etomidate on the auditory evoked response in man. Br J Anaesth 1985;57:554-61
71. Schwender D, Rimkus T, Haessler R, Klasing S, Poppel E, Peter K: Effects of increasing doses of alfentanil, fentanyl and morphine on mid- latency auditory evoked potentials. Br J Anaesth 1993;71:622-8
72. Schwender D, Weninger E, Daunderer M, Klasing S, Poppel E, Peter K: Anesthesia with increasing doses of sufentanil and midlatency auditory evoked potentials in humans. Anesth Analg 1995;80:499-505
73. Schwender D, Klasing S, Madler C, Poppel E, Peter K: Mid-latency auditory evoked potentials during ketamine anaesthesia in humans. Br J Anaesth 1993;71:629-32
74. Mantzaridis H, Kenny GN: Auditory evoked potential index: a quantitative measure of changes in auditory evoked potentials during general anaesthesia. Anaesthesia 1997;52:1030-6
75. Gajraj RJ, Doi M, Mantzaridis H, Kenny GN: Analysis of the EEG bispectrum, auditory evoked potentials and the EEG power spectrum during repeated transitions from consciousness to unconsciousness. Br J Anaesth 1998;80:46-52
76. Gajraj RJ, Doi M, Mantzaridis H, Kenny GN: Comparison of bispectral EEG analysis and auditory evoked potentils for monitoring depth of anaesthesia during propofol anaesthesia. Br J Anaesth 1999;82:672-8

Patient Controlled Sedation during Locoregional Anaesthesia

Nick Sutcliffe and Daniel Amutike

Glasgow, United Kingdom

Introduction

The use of locoregional anaesthesia for a variety of surgical procedures is increasing as it provides not only satisfactory operating conditions and good intra- and post- operative analgesia, but also has advantages in terms of health economics. The important advantages offered by locoregional anaesthesia include low cost, ease of administration, avoidance of the risks associated with general anaesthesia, including decreased risk of deep vein thrombosis, and good postoperative recovery. The major disadvantage of locoregional anaesthesia alone is that many patients are anxious and find being awake during the operation to be an uncomfortable and stressful experience. In order to improve patient acceptability, comfort and reduce stress it is common practice to provide some form of sedation during the operation. Ideally, the patient should be relaxed, comfortable and co-operative throughout the procedure. Increasingly, procedures which were once undertaken as open surgical operations can now be achieved by less invasive techniques. Many procedures that required general anaesthesia in the past can now be performed under locoregional anaesthesia and sedation. This has led to an increase in the requirement for conscious sedation for such procedures.

Conscious sedation is a technique in which drugs are used to depress the central nervous system, to allow treatment or examination to be performed while verbal contact is maintained throughout the sedation. The aim of con-

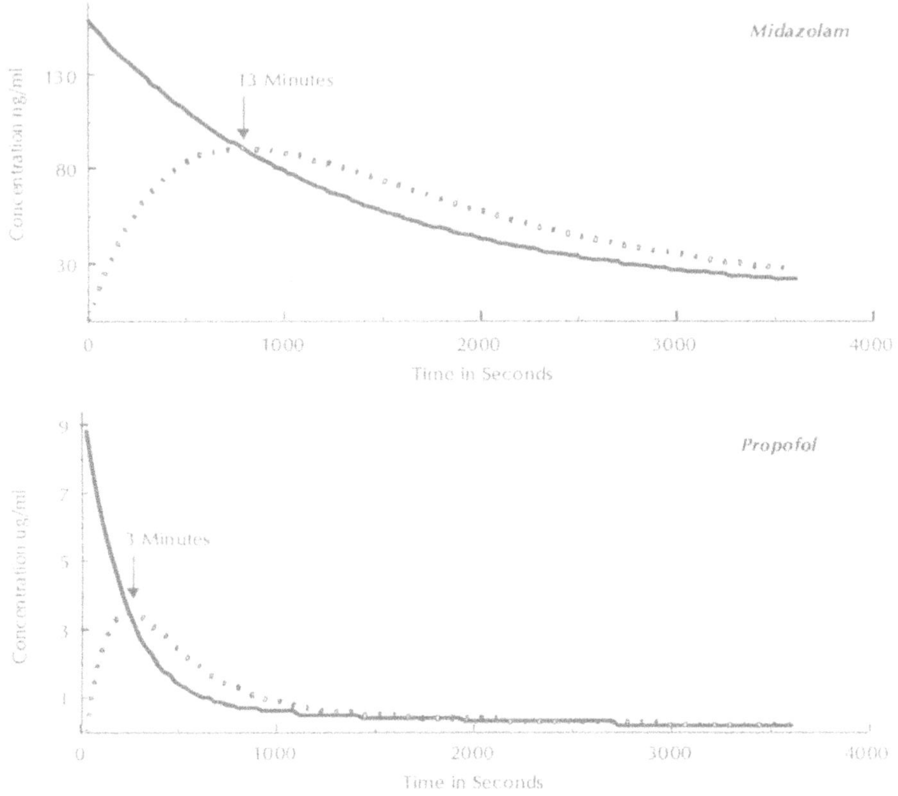

Figure 1
Blood (———) and effect site (□□□) concentration of propofol and midazolam following a bolus dose.

scious sedation is to minimise anxiety and discomfort of the patient while providing a maximum degree of safety. In practice, achieving this ideal is often more challenging than providing general anaesthesia

Traditionally physicians will provide sedation with intravenous boluses of hypnotic agent titrated to the point at which the physician thinks that the patient is "adequately sedated". Often combinations of opiate and hypnotic agents are employed for procedures associated with noxious stimuli not easily ameliorated by local anaesthesia. The aim of this technique is to produce a state of calm in a patient who is comfortable and maintains his or her own airway, and may sleep but will still be easily roused by command. Unfortunately, such a state is not easily achieved and maintained in a circumstance of variable surgical stimulus. Firstly, the therapeutic window for acceptable sedation is narrow when compared to anaesthesia. Secondly, there is a delay between administration of a drug an its peak effect on the patient. This delay differs between drugs and is described by the k_{e0} of the drug. Drugs with a rapid k_{e0} such as propofol have a relatively short time to peak effect. However, drugs such as midazolam have a slower k_{e0} and a longer time to peak effect. Figure 1 shows the simulated blood and effect site concentrations for both midazolam and propofol after a bolus dose (for a full explanation of the concept of effect site concentration; see the manuscript by Bovill). It can be readily appreciated that the longer the time to peak effect of a drug then the more the potential to give further doses before the peak effect of each dose is reached. Thus, there is more the potential for eventual over-sedation once the cumulative effect of all these doses reaches a peak. It is therefore all too easy to over-sedate a patient in an effort to achieve sedation within a reasonable time frame. This may lead to loss of airway and in an inadequately monitored and supervised situation can result in serious complications and even fatality. Further, the wide pharmacodynamic variation between patients makes it impossible to predict an appropriate dose for each individual patient.

The concept of patient controlled sedation

Such difficulties have led a number of researchers to assess techniques which allow the patient to self-administer sedative agents. The term Patient Controlled Sedation (PCS) is used when self-administered sedation is utilised to allow procedures to be undertaken. It appears that this form of sedation is strongly preferred by the patients.[1] The technique allows the patient to self-administer sedative agent by pressing a button in a similar manner to patient controlled analgesia (PCA). In this way the patient can titrate his or her own sedation to the point at which they are satisfied. Such an approach has the potential to overcome the pharmacodynamic variation between individual patients. PCS appears to be safe and acceptable to patients, surgeons and anaesthetists. In addition, patients may derive psychological benefit by being able to modify the level of sedation and thus maintain some degree of control over their circumstances. Using a well-designed PCS system, with a suitable dose and lock out schedule, patients can generally titrate themselves to an appropriate level of sedation without the risk of over-sedation.

Sedative Agents

An ideal sedative agent should produce a rapid and smooth onset of action with easy control of the level and duration of sedation. The drug should have a wide therapeutic ratio with minimum cardiorespiratory depression. The metabolites must be inactive, non-cumulative and metabolism should not be affected by reduced hepatic or renal function. It should have a rapid offset and recovery without rebound or emergence effects to enable rapid discharge from recovery area and hospital. Unfortunately we currently do not have an agent which exactly fits this ideal profile but a number of drugs have been used successfully to provide PCS. Most commonly Propofol and Midazolam have been used for PCS. Short acting opioids like alfentanil and fentanyl have been used as adjuncts to propofol and midazolam or occasionally alone.

The pharmacokinetics properties and recovery characteristics of propofol make it the most suitable agent currently available for PCS. The short half-life and rapid clearance and rapid k_{e0} of propofol ensure a rapid and predictable onset of effect and easy dose adjustment. Recovery from propofol sedation is rapid and clear-headed with little post sedation nausea or vomiting. Propofol has a significant intra-operative amnesic effect that may be beneficial for some procedures. Midazolam is a water-soluble benzodiazepine which is often used for sedation both by anaesthetists and non-anaesthetists in preference to diazepam. It is a sedative hypnotic with good anxiolytic, profound amnesic and muscle relaxation properties. Midazolam offers advantages over older benzodiazepines, in terms of its more rapid onset and offset and is thus more suitable for short team sedation. However, compared to propofol, midazolam has a slow onset and offset time and the recovery time and quality are inferior.

Studies on Patient Controlled Sedation

Over the past decade around 30 studies on patient controlled sedation have been published. One third have been for procedures not requiring regional anaesthesia; the remainder have involved PCS combined with regional anaesthesia. The two commonly used sedative agents in the studies were propofol and midazolam, either alone or in combination with opioids. Two methods of administration of sedative agents for PCS were used. The majority describes the use of a modified Patient Controlled Analgesia (PCA) pump that delivers a set amount of a bolus of the sedative agent with or without a lockout time. Two studies describe the use of a relatively new method that uses a modified Target Controlled Infusion (TCI) device with the patient being able to increase the target concentration for sedation by pressing a demand button.

Studies Using Modified PCA Equipment

Drugs Used

A variety of drugs have been used for PCS in various studies; propofol and midazolam have been the most common agents although successful techniques using methohexitone[2], diazepam[3], droperidol[4] and alfentanil[5] have been described. Four studies have directly compared PCS with propofol and PCS with midazolam.[6-9] These studies demonstrated a faster onset, less over-sedation and better recovery in the patients receiving propofol. There were more respiratory complications in the midazolam groups as evidenced by lower SaO_2 and higher $PaCO_2$ values.[6, 7] Rudkin and colleagues compared midazolam-PCS, 0.5 mg bolus, with propofol, 20 mg bolus, with both a lockout period of 1 min in patients having dental procedures. They observed that midazolam may be associated with deeper sedation scores as compared to propofol. The proportion of unsuccessful to successful patient request for drug delivery in a single lockout period was greater in the midazolam group (17.8 : 14 in the midazolam group; 2.8 : 8 in the propofol group). Memory recall was less impaired in the propofol group as compared to midazolam and the accuracy of recall was also more impaired in the midazolam group. There was no significant difference between groups for patient satisfaction elicited on the day after surgery and the patients liked the idea of self-administration of sedation. The study indicated that propofol is more suitable than midazolam for PCS because of its more rapid response to fluctuating patient requirements, as shown by a more favourable ratio of successful to unsuccessful demands without over-sedation. Propofol also appears to have a more beneficial effect on patient mood. The investigators found PCS to be a safe technique, which provided good intra-operative conditions and a high level of patient satisfaction.

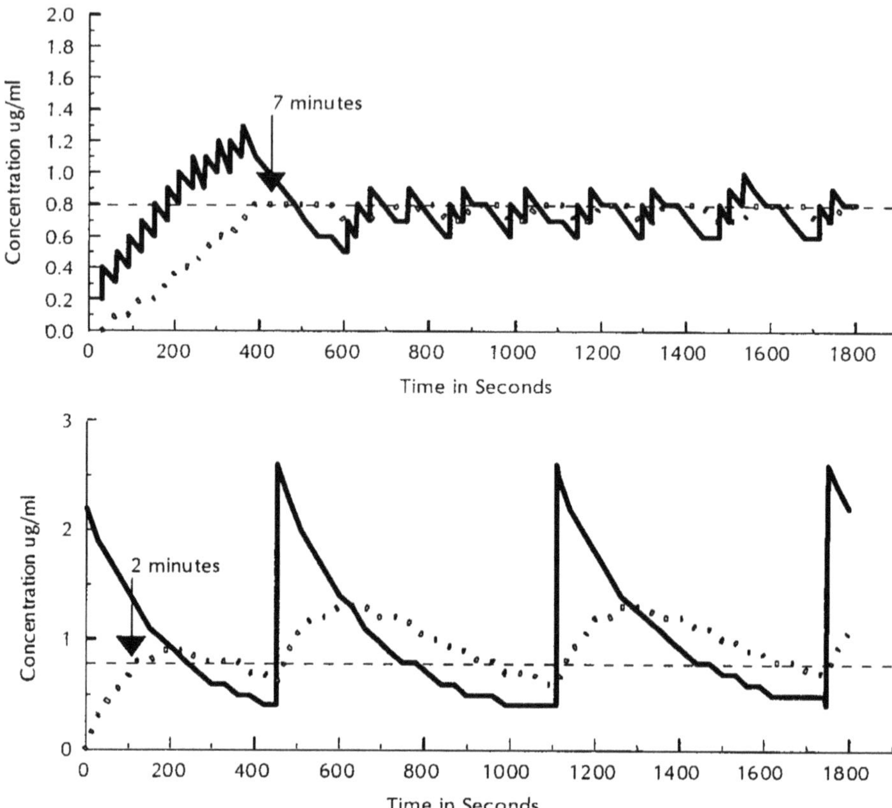

Figure 2
Blood (———) and effect site (□□□) concentration of propofol for two different PCS regimens. Top graph shows a simulation of a bolus dose of 3 mg with no lockout period assuming the patient makes a demand every 30 sec until an effect site concentration of 0.8 μg/ml is reached. Bottom graph shows a simulation of a bolus dose of 0.7 mg/kg with a lockout time of 3 min. Dashed line at 0.8 μg/ml.

Drug Regimens for PCS

Patient controlled sedation followed naturally from the acceptance of patient controlled analgesia. The landmark paper, which first described PCS using propofol and a PCA device, was by Rudkin and co-workers in Adelaide.[10] They initially used a standard Graseby PCA pump modified to deliver propofol 0.7 mg/kg at a rate of 16.7 mg/min. with a lockout interval of 1 min. At the standard infusion rate of 100 ml/h, it took over 2 min to deliver a demand dose to a 70 kg patient and this was followed by a lockout interval of 1 min giving an effective lockout time of 3 min. They observed that when demand rates were high at the beginning of the procedure, the long delivery times and the short lockout interval meant that the patients were effectively receiving an interrupted infusion rather than an intermittent dose of sedation as intended. In a subsequent study, they modified an Ohmeda 9000 PCA pump to infuse the demand dose of 0.7 mg/kg at 1200 ml/h.[11] The higher infusion rates increased the ratio of successful to unsuccessful demands, presumable due to a faster onset of action with the higher rate of delivery. Compared with the previous study the total amount of propofol consumption per patient was reduced significantly. Cook and colleagues introduced the concept of zero lockout interval for patient controlled sedation.[9] They used a modified Graseby PCA pump to delivery propofol in 3 mg aliquots with an infusion rate of 200 ml/h and a zero lockout interval. The aim of their study was to provide an infusion system that could deliver enough of the drug at the beginning of the procedure for the patients to be able to establish their own level of sedation without requiring an initial loading dose administered by the anaesthetist. This according to Cook et al. was true patient controlled sedation. Figure 2 illustrates these two approaches; the upper figure shows a simulation of a low bolus dose (3 mg) with no lockout period, the lower figure shows a higher bolus (0.7 mg/kg) with a 3 min lockout. For the purposes of the simulation two assumptions have been made; one that in the zero lockout time illustration the patient presses the button every 30 sec until satisfied with the sedation. Secondly, that the window of patient satisfaction lies within effect site concentrations of 0.7-0.8 μg/ml propofol. The simulations demonstrate that the low bolus method has the potential to achieve a very stable effect site concentration with little potential for overdose. The down side is that it takes longer to achieve an effective concentration and the patient has to press his button repeatedly during the onset phase and regularly thereafter to maintain a sedative effect site concentration. The higher bolus technique has a more rapid onset, in this theoretical example an effective concentration is reached within 2 min with just one button press. However, there is more potential for oversedation because of the relatively large variation in effect site concentration with the larger bolus. The effect site concentration will vary over a wider range and thus the level of sedation will be more variable with this technique. Our own experience suggests that small changes in the

Table 1
Comparison of patient controlled sedation (PCS) and anaesthetist controlled sedation (ACS) from (12).

	ACS	PCS	p
Dose rate ($mg.kg^{-1}.h^{-1}$	6.5 (4.9-8.2)	5.4 (1.6-8.7)	ns
Duration of induction (min)	2 (1-6)	7 (4-16)	0.0018*
Duration of recovery (min)	2 (1-20)	2 (0-5)	ns
Median propofol C_b (μg/ml)	1.8 (0.8-2.5)	1.1 (0.2-2.3)	ns

calculated effect site concentration can result in clinically relevant changes in sedation level, and particularly in elderly patients may be the difference between adequate sedation and airway compromise.

PCS versus Anaesthetist controlled sedation (ACS)

Seven studies have compared PCS with ACS. Osborne and co-workers compared propofol PCS with ACS using an infusion of propofol in a randomised crossover study.[1] There were no detectable differences between the groups in terms of recovery, operating conditions and total dose of propofol. However, patients in the PCS group had lower sedation scores and expressed a stronger preference for the PCS technique. Oei-Lim and colleagues compared ACS using TCI propofol (arguable the most controllable form of physician controlled sedation) with PCS propofol.[12] They studied 11 patients for dental surgery under local anaesthesia, in a randomised crossover design. The PCS regimen consisted of a 4 mg propofol bolus with no lockout period, ACS was provided with TCI propofol with an initial target of 2.5 μg/ml, which was adjusted in 0.2 μg/ml steps until the desired level of sedation was achieved. Table 1 shows a comparison of the two techniques. Although ACS produced a faster onset, PCS resulted in a lower total dose of propofol and a tendency towards faster recovery. Both techniques were well tolerated, although one patient became oversedated during ACS. In general, drug usage and level of sedation were lower and respiratory depression was less in the PCS groups. Patient satisfaction tended to be higher in the PCS groups, although, since a variety of drugs were used in the ACS groups and mainly propofol in the PCS groups, this may have been due to a beneficial effect on mood with propofol.

A further seven studies have combined opioids with the PCS, either as a pre-medication or as part of each PCS bolus. The combination of propofol and alfentanil has been advocated and the very short acting opioid remifentanil may be useful for this purpose as well. Alfentanil has been successfully used alone for PCS.[5] In general, the addition of opioids into any PCS regimen is associated with a higher incidence of nausea and respiratory complications. However, differences in PCS regimen and study design make direct comparison between the studies difficult.

Studies Using Modified TCI Equipment

The limitation of a standard bolus type PCS is that blood and effect site concentrations will never be stable. Each new bolus produces a peak concentration with the potential for over sedation, the blood concentration then decays with time until a new bolus is initiated at which point the patient must be uncomfortable in order to initiate a new bolus. Recently, Kenny and colleagues have described a modified propofol Target Controlled Infusion (TCI) system for patient controlled sedation that allows the patient to modify the set target concentration of propofol by using a push button. The term Patient Maintained Sedation (PMS) has been used to describe this technique.[13] This approach was used to provide PCS for 36 patients undergoing general surgical procedures under regional anaesthesia. A TCI infusion of propofol was started at a target of 1 µg/ml. The patient was then able to increase the target propofol concentration in 0.2 µg/ml increments by pressing a demand button. There was a lockout interval of 2 min to allow some equilibration between blood and effect site concentration. Over the first 20 min, if there were no button presses in any 6 min period, the system automatically cut back the target by 0.2 µg/ml. From 20 min onwards the system decreased the target after 12 min without demand. The maximum permissible target concentration was 3 µg/ml. In the study there was considerable inter-individual variability in propofol consumption. Optimum sedation was provided at median target concentration of 0.8 - 0.9 µg/ml. The investigators observed that there was no cardiovascular instability and little over-sedation. Respiratory rate decreased with the onset of sedation but the lowest recorded rate was 10 breaths/ min. There were no instances of airway obstruction requiring intervention. However, 8 patients (ASA I and II) required supplementary nasal oxygen therapy because of oxygen saturation readings below 92% and oxygen supplementation was effective in all cases. Recovery was rapid following the cessation of the infusion and there were no delays in discharge from the recovery room.

This technique combines the benefits of TCI with patient controlled feedback and produces safe intra-operative sedation during loco-regional anaesthesia with rapid recovery and high patient satisfaction. Further study may provide data that, given the fact that the patients were cardiovascularly stable and that respiratory rate was not reduced below 10/min, may question the requirement of the direct presence an anaesthetist in all cases.

With this in mind Kenny's group undertook a number of volunteer studies in which the volunteer was asked to try to anaesthetise themselves using the same TCI patient controlled system.[14] In the first study the same regimen was used as in the paper described above. Two volunteers required the intervention of the supervising anaesthetist to maintain the airway. In a second study the system was modified to give 0.1 µg/ml step increases with a 4 min lockout, and the initial target was set at 0.5 µg/ml. The longer lockout time would allow 75% equilibration between blood and effect site concentrations rather than the 40% which occurs with a lockout time of 2 min. Using this more gentle regimen none of the volunteers required the intervention of the supervising anaesthetist. However, the time to onset of sedation was increased because of the combination of the lower starting target the smaller step changes and the longer lockout time. Figure 3 shows the two regimens simulated. If again we assume adequate sedation at an effect site concentration of 0.8 µg/ml we can see that this is achieved in 4 min with the original regimen but it may take 18 min with the modified regimen.

Although apparently safer, would the modified regimen provide adequate sedation in the clinical setting? With this question in mind we used this system to provide sedation for patients undergoing joint replacement under locoregional anaesthesia. Twenty four patients have been studied to date, informed consent was obtained at the pre-operative assessment and the patient was instructed in the use of the equipment and a pre-medication of 10 mg of temazepam was prescribed. All patients had spinal anaesthesia induced with 20-22.5 mg of bupivacaine; epidural anaesthesia was instituted postoperatively.

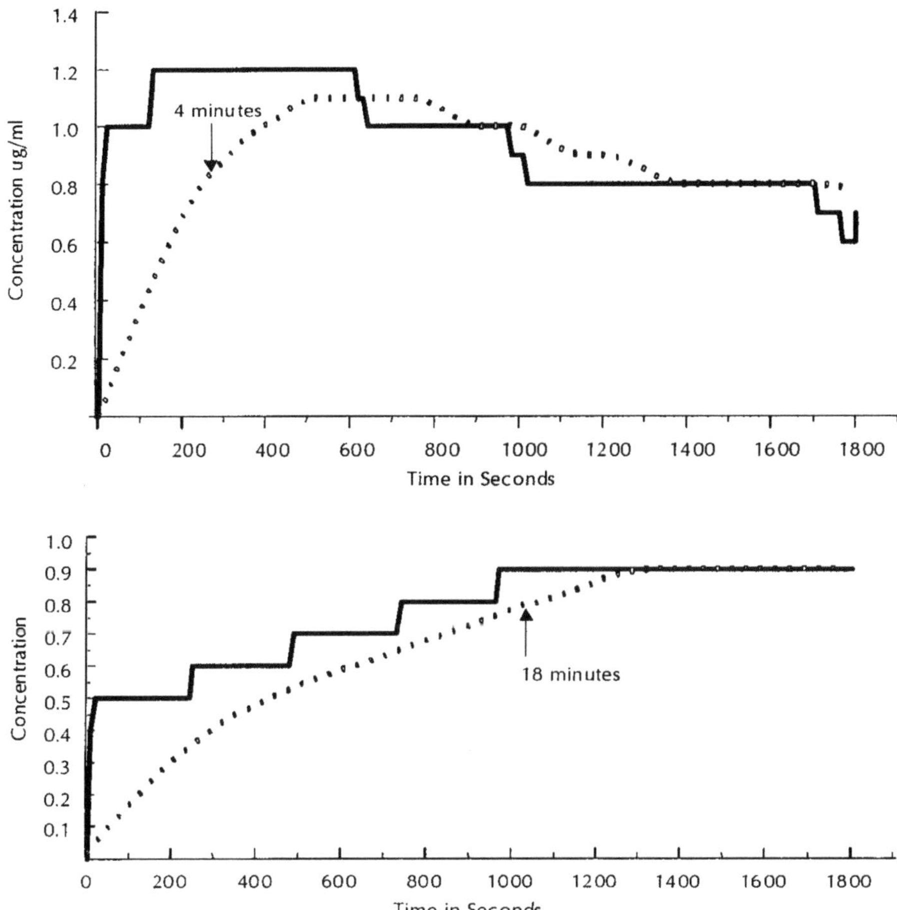

Figure 3
Blood (▬▬) and effect site (▫▫▫) concentration of propofol for two different TCI PCS regimens. See text for an explanation of the two regimens.

Once the block was established the patient was taken into theatre and the TCI propofol was commenced at a target of 0.5 µg/ml. The patient was positioned for surgery and then given the "patient button" and allowed to control their sedation as they wished, all patients received 2 L/min 0_2 via a nasal cannula after positioning. Blood pressure, $Sa0_2$, and a sedation assessment was noted every 5 min along with the calculated effect site and blood concentration of propofol. Five patients had to be converted to general anaesthesia

Table 2
Sedation score.

• a	awake eyes open
• v	eyes closed responds to speech
• s	eyes closed responds to mild stimulus
• p	eyes closed responds to pain
• u	unresponsive

because of an inadequate regional block. The bispectral index (BIS) was monitored in 7 patients. The need for vasopressors was noted and the surgeon was asked to grade the surgical field and general operating conditions on a visual analogue scale from 0-10. The patients were interviewed the evening of surgery and asked about their experience and whether they would have the same type of anaesthetic if they required a second joint replacement in the future. In general, the technique provided good conditions for the procedure. Adequate sedation was achieved within the time taken to position the patient for surgery; no patient became over-sedated requiring intervention from the supervising anaesthetist.

Table 2 shows the sedation scoring system, no patient was graded as deeper than "S" (eyes closed responding to mild stimulus). Most patients titrated themselves to a relatively deep level initially, but appeared to be happy with a lower level of sedation later in the operative period, presumable when they had developed more confidence with the technique. Three patients did not press the button at all, two of these had had regional anaesthesia before and were happy with a minimal level of sedation. The third patient achieved adequate sedation with the initial target of 0.5 μg/ml. The lowest SaO_2 recorded was 93 % in one patient prior to commencement of oxygen therapy. Patient satisfaction was high with all patients scoring the technique excellent or good.

Table 3
Mean target blood and effect site concentrations, total dose, surgical scores and mean ephedrine dose for the group compared with those for the 5 patients converted to GA ().

- Mean calculated propofol concentration: 0.45 ug/ml (2.53 GA)
- Mean effect site propofol concentration: 0.44 ug/ml (2.50 GA)
- Mean propofol dose: 135 mg (70 GA)
- Mean ephedrine dose: 1.8 mg (10.5 GA)
- Mean surgical scores: 7.85 (7.8 GA)

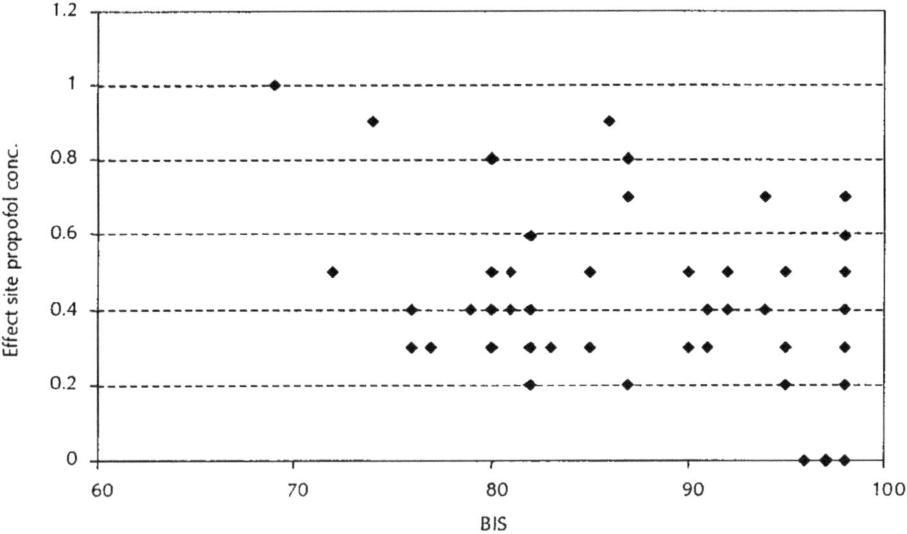

Figure 4
Calculated effect site concentration of propofol versus BIS value in 7 patients.

Nineteen out of 20 patients would have the technique again for a future procedure, one patient had nausea postoperatively which he attributed to the epidural and would therefore not have the technique in the future.

Table 3 shows the mean target blood and effect site concentrations, total dose, surgical scores and mean ephedrine dose for the group compared with those for the 5 patients converted to GA. Figure 4 shows the BIS values for the whole group plotted against the effect site concentration of propofol. There is a tendency for the BIS value to be lower at higher blood propofol concentrations but there was no clear relation demonstrated in this small group of patients at this relatively light level of sedation.

Future Developments

All the PCS regimens presented to date have been a compromise between safety and efficacy. The lower the doses or step changes and the longer the lockout times, then the more safe are the regimens. A small dose or step reduces the chance that each single dose will result in overdosing. The longer the lockout time, then the more the effect site concentration will equilibrate with

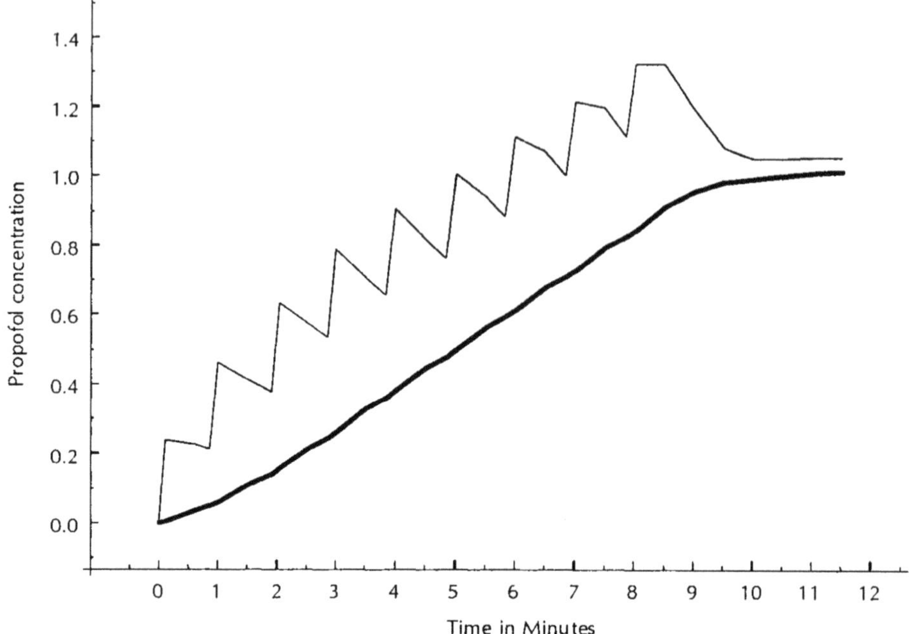

Figure 5
The calculated blood (thin line) and effect site (bold line) concentrations as provided by an effect site target controlled patient controlled sedation TCI system.

the blood concentration, thus the less chance of dose stacking. The problem with such an approach is that an effective level of sedation takes a long time to achieve, and with small doses the patient needs to repeatedly press the button to maintain an adequate level of sedation, which may make the technique unsuitable for clinical practice. The modified TCI technique helps in this respect by using an initial target set by the anaesthetist and will maintain a level of sedation with relatively few button presses. However, the variation between patients makes it impossible to predict exactly what the initial target should be for an individual patient. Moreover, this will not help if the patient needs to significantly increase their level of sedation to cope with an increase in stimulus during the procedure. Purists would also argue that this is not true PCS, as it requires the anaesthetist's input in order to initiate sedation.

Another approach is to use effect site target controlled infusions. With this algorithm mathematical modelling is used to target and control the effect site rather than the blood propofol concentration. This allows the target effect site concentration to be reached as rapidly as possible without overshoot (for a description see the manuscript by Bovill). With such a technique, modified for patient control, it should be possible for patients to titrate relatively rapidly to an effective and stable effect site concentration, and thus level of sedation starting from zero with small step changes. Figure 5 shows the calculated blood and effect site concentration of such a system. If again we assume a patient will be adequately sedated at an effect site propofol concentration of 0.8 μg/ml, this will be achieved in less than 8 min, even with a step increase set at 0.1 μg/ml and a 1 min lockout. We have used such a system with 6 healthy volunteers who have been asked to try to anaesthetise themselves. To date no subject has needed intervention by the supervising anaesthetist, and none had de-saturated below 96%. All six subjects have been able to be easily roused by voice throughout the study period. The subjects appear to forget the purpose of the study before they are able to render themselves unconscious. This technique requires further evaluation before being introduced into clinical practice.

Conclusions

Patient Controlled Sedation during locoregional anaesthesia has been shown by several studies to be effective and highly acceptable to patients. The technique offers the advantage of being able to accommodate the wide variations in sedation requirements of individual patients. PCS may also confer psychological benefit to the patients from the sense of retaining control that PCS allows. Patient maintained sedation using a modified TCI device has potential benefits but requires further assessment. Despite the use of various regimens and different drugs all the studies to date report success with patient controlled sedation. It appears propofol is theoretically the most suitable agent available for PCS and the literature supports this. All the regimens used to date have been a compromise between efficacy and safety. Lower bolus regimens with long lockout times are safer but can lead to an unacceptably long time to adequate sedation. The use of effect site targeted infusions for PSC may offer a better alternative allowing small step changes in the effect site to be achieved as rapidly as possible without the potential for over-shoot. Unfortunately, such equipment is not currently available commercially. Whether any of these techniques will allow unsupervised PCS is a matter of debate. However, this may be preferable to current practice in some centres where non-anaesthetists administer multiple bolus doses of agents such as midazolam, and then commence the procedure themselves without adequate supervision of the patient and before the peak effect of the administered drugs has been reached.

References

1. Osborne GA, Rudkin GE, Jarvis DA. Patient controlled sedation. A crossover comparison of patient preference for patient controlled propofol and propofol by continuous infusion. Anaesthesia 1994;49(4) :287-292.
2. Hamid SK, Mc Cann N, Mc Ardle L, Asbury AJ. Comparison of patient controlled sedation with either Methohexitone or Propofol. British Medical Journal 1996;77(6): 727-730.
3. Roseveare C, Patel P, Seavell C, Criswell J, Kimble J, Jones C, Shepherd H. Patient Controlled Sedation using propofol, Alfentanil during colonoscopy. A prospective randomised controlled trial. Gastroenterology 1998;114(4) suppl.part 2 :a36 Ab G0148.
4. Herrick IA, Craen RA, Gelb AW, Miller LA, Kubu CS, Girvin JP et al. Propofol sedation during awake craniotomy for seizures: Patient controlled administration versus neurolept analgesia. Anaesthesia & Analgesia 1997;84(6):1285-1291
5. Kortis HI, Amory DW, Wagner BK, Levin R, Wilson E, Pitchford DE, Pollak P. Use of patient controlled analgesia for extracorporeal shock wave lithotripsy. Journal of clinical Anaesthesia 1995;7(3):205-210.
6. Pac-Soo CK, Deacock S, Lockwood G, Carr C, Whitwam JG. Patient Controlled Sedation for cataract surgery using Peribulbar block. British Journal of Anaesthesia 1996; 77(3):370-374
7. Uyar M, Ugur G, Bilge S, Ozyar B, Ozyurt C. Patient controlled sedation and analgesia during shockwave lithotripsy (SWL). Journal of Endourology 1996;10(%):407-410.
8. Rudkin GE, Osborne GA, Finn BP, Jarvis DA, Vickers D. Intraoperative patient controlled sedation. Comparison of patient Controlled propofol with patient controlled midazolam. Anaesthesia 1992;47(5) 376-381.
9. Cook LB, Lockwood GG, Moore CM, Whitwam JG. True patient controlled sedation. Anaesthesia 1993;48:1039-1044.
10. Rudkin GE, Osborne GA, Curtis NJ. Intraoperative patient controlled sedation. Anaesthesia 1991;46:90-92.
11. Osborne GA, Rudkin GE, Curtis NJ, Vickers D, Craker AJ. Intraoperative patient controlled sedation. Anaesthesia 1991;46:553-556.
12. Oei-Lim VBL, Kalkman CJ, Makkes PC, Ooms WG. Patient controlled versus Anaesthesiologist controlled sedation with propofol for dental treatment in anxious patients. Anaesthesia and Analgesia 1998;86(5):967-972.
13. Irwin MG, Thompson N, Kenny GNC. Patient maintained propofol sedation. Anaesthesia 1997;52(6):525-530.
14. Kenny GNC. Personal communication. University Department of Anaesthesia, Glasgow University.

TARGET CONTROLLED SEDATION IN THE INTENSIVE CARE UNIT

Sandra M. Groen-Mulder

The Hague, The Netherlands

Introduction

Intensive care treatment has evolved significantly in the past decades. With intensive treatment patients suffering from critical illnesses or severe trauma can now be cured. Intensive care would not be possible without adequate analgesic and sedative regimens. In fact, sedation is essential to modern intensive care medicine. The fundamental goal of critical care medicine is to support organ function and maintain homeostasis until healing can occur. Sedation and analgesia may blunt the physiologic and psychological sequelae of ICU stress and may support homeostasis. Although most drugs given in the intensive care unit are titrated to the individual needs of the patient, administration of sedative drugs is still usually done on the basis of fixed infusion regimens. A commonly used regimen is the administration of midazolam at a rate of 2-5 mg/h, which is switched off when sedation is no longer considered necessary. Whether or not the patient suffers from renal or liver failure is often not taken into account. The presence of these and other factors, however, may strongly influence the pharmacological behaviour of the drug, and thus the response of the patient to the drug. Adjustment of the sedative regimen to the presence of stimuli is also done rarely. The physicians providing ICU care often do not realise that the interindividual variability in sedating patients is considerable. Obviously appropriate analgesic regimens should be administered when necessary, in particular for postoperative patients. This chapter will focus on sedation.

Target Controlled Infusion

Target controlled infusion (TCI) techniques are increasingly used and accepted in anaesthetic practice in the OR setting. The Diprifusor for target controlled delivery of propofol is now available in most European countries, as well as in some South American and Asian countries. With this device TCI has become more readily available. With the increasing experience in using TCI, there is growing interest in the application of TCI in other fields of care. One of its newer applications is sedation of patients undergoing surgery under regional anaesthesia and sedation for patients undergoing diagnostic procedures outside the operating rooms (e.g. MRI scan). There is also increasing interest in the application of TCI for drug administration in the intensive care unit.

Sedation

Sedation can be defined as a technique in which the use of a drug produces a state of depression of the central nervous system to evoke a level of reduced consciousness. This state represents a continuum. At one end is the patient who is very lightly sedated, well responsive to verbal commands and in possession of his protective reflexes. At the other end is the unconscious, unresponsive patient in a state of general anaesthesia. ICU sedation generally applies to a state of responsiveness somewhere in the middle of this spectrum.

As with any therapeutic intervention, when sedating patients the physician acts on the basis of a therapeutic decision tree. This includes the assessment of a condition, the therapeutic intervention and the reassessment after the intervention. Interventions should be titrated to a given end-point on the basis of a well-defined parameter. Preferably, this end point should be sensitive, reproducible and objective. For sedation the most commonly used assessment is the sedation scale according to Ramsay[1] or a modified version of this scale. It is very easy to determine in patients and with experience a consistent scoring of the sedative level can be achieved. As yet, it is still the most commonly used scale. However, this scale has some limitations. Some argue that it is very subjective. With a nursing shift change, one may find a change in the Ramsay score. Furthermore, the score does not provide for a patient who is sedated yet agitated, although such patients are not uncommon. In heavily sedated patients

Table 1
Ramsay sedation scale.

1.	Awake, agitated, restless
2.	Co-operative, oriented, tranquil
3.	Drowsy or asleep, responds to commands
4.	Asleep, brisk response to loud stimulus
5.	Asleep, slow response to loud stimulus
6.	Asleep, no response to loud, or painful stimulus

a painful stimulus, e.g. nail-bed pressure, may be given, where a response may relate more to the level of analgesia, then to the actual sedation score.

Various neurophysiological monitors are currently being developed and assessed to provide a more objective parameter for the evaluation of the level of sedation. The electroencephalogram (EEG) in its raw or processed form offers possibilities. The bispectral index is currently being assessed for use in the ICU. The presence of muscle activity however seems to interfere with a reliable signal.[2] Other parameters as the median frequency and auditory evoked potentials are under investigation.[3] However, all these techniques are cumbersome, still under investigation and not very widely used in general ICUs. So far, that leaves the Ramsay sedation scale as still the best monitor for sedation.

Sedative agents for ICU sedation

The ideal sedative agent should have a rapid on- and offset, enabling the physician to achieve a rapid change in effect if desired. When administered for longer periods of time it should not accumulate and it should not have active metabolites. Cardiovascular or respiratory depression should be avoided. Interference with other drugs should be absent. It should be easy to administer, and preferably be cheap. Administration should be by continuous infusion to avoid the hills and valleys associated with intermitted bolus administration. Currently available drugs are the benzodiazepines, of which midazolam is the most commonly prescribed, and other intravenous anaesthetics of which propofol is most commonly used. How do these most commonly used agents, midazolam and propofol, compare to the ideal sedative agent? Midazolam when administered for short periods of time has a short duration of action; it works relatively fast because of its fast equilibration with the brain. In low dose ranges it has little haemodynamic or respiratory effect. It has a relatively wide therapeutic index. It is easy to use and cheap. For benzodiazepines a reversal agent is available, flumazenil. The negative effects include accumulation, especially in patients with compromised liver and/or kidney function. Midazolam's metabolism depends on hepatic capacity and blood flow. One of its metabolites, α-hydroxymidazolam, in its glucuronidated form, is excreted solely by the kidney. It has distinctive sedative properties and in patients with renal failure can account for a significantly prolonged sedation. The duration of the effect of midazolam can therefore be unpredictable in critical ill patients. Tolerance for midazolam has been reported. Furthermore, midazolam has a synergistic interaction with opioids.[4]

The other agent most commonly used for sedating intensive care patients is propofol. It has a rapid onset of action because it has a relatively short blood-brain equilibration half-life.[5] After termination of an infusion of propofol, even a longer lasting one, a rapid offset of effect occurs. This can be explained by its relatively short context-sensitive half-time.[6] This means, that even after a long infusion, a relatively fast decline in the plasma concentration can still be seen after stopping the infusion. In lower dose ranges propofol has little respiratory effects. However, with a rapid increase in the plasma concentration severe respiratory depression does occur, and precautionary measures should be taken. Propofol does not accumulate, and has no active metabolites. The availability of prefilled syringes makes it easy to use. Especially at higher blood concentrations it does have haemodynamic side effects. Propofol causes pain on injection. It comes in a lipid emulsion, which facilitates bacterial growth, and care should be taken to ensure asepsis. When given for longer periods of time the lipid load may become high and should be taken into account. An infusion rate of 3-4 mg/kg/h equals a lipid load of 500 kCal/24 h; hyperlipidaemia has been described.[7] With the now available 2% solution this problem is in fact halved. Propofol's synergistic interaction with opioids is well known and has been extensively studied.[8] Development of tolerance cannot be ruled out, although studies are not conclusive.[9] Lastly, propofol has some specific effects, which may add to its favourable profile for sedating ICU patients; it has significant anti-emetic properties[10], it has an anti-pruritus effect[11] and it may be beneficial due to its anti-oxidant effects.[12]

Pharmacokinetics for ICU sedation

When discussing the optimal pharmacological characteristics for sedatives in the ICU, two pharmacokinetic/dynamic parameters are of importance. A short $t_{1/2}k_{e0}$ is desired because the effect will then become evident rapidly after starting the administration of the drug. The $t_{1/2}k_{e0}$ is shorter for propofol compared to midazolam. With respect to the termination of the infusion, it is desirable for the effect to wear off quickly, independent of the duration of infusion. In other words, especially in the ICU, drugs with a short context-sensitive half-time are desirable. Most data addressing these issues for propofol and midazolam are derived from studies done in volunteers, in an operating room setting, at higher concentrations and shorter duration of infusion than generally applied in the ICU. These data therefore may not be applicable to ICU patients. One may expect the pharmacological characteristics of a given drug to be different in ICU patients for a number of reasons. The pharmacokinetics of sedative drugs may change when drugs are administered for longer periods of time. With long-term infusions the three compartments will fill up, an equilibrium will be reached within the compartments. Renal and liver function may be impaired in critically ill patients, which may affect drug metabolism and elimination. Body fluid distribution may be altered. ICU patients are often in a catabolic state resulting in a low plasma albumen content, which can contribute to a higher free fraction of the drug. This in turn may affect the distribution and the effect of the drug. Co-medication may also exercise an influence on drug characteristics. These considerations have led to a number of investigations regarding the pharmacological behaviour of propofol and midazolam in ICU patients. The results of these studies vary. For midazolam studies indicate highly variable pharmacokinetic parameters with elimination half-lives of 1.5 - 50 h.

This may in part reflect the large interindividual variability in ICU patients. In one specific subgroup (post CABG patients), Zomorodi et al. have described the pharmacokinetics extensively.[13] These findings indicate a rather long context-sensitive half-life of midazolam in the ICU setting. Figure 1 shows two decay curves of midazolam. This shows that after an infusion of midazolam for 24 h to a deep level of sedation, where it may take a reduction of 80% in the plasma concentration for a patient to wake up, it may take up to 20 h after termination of the infusion, before the patient will regain consciousness. Most

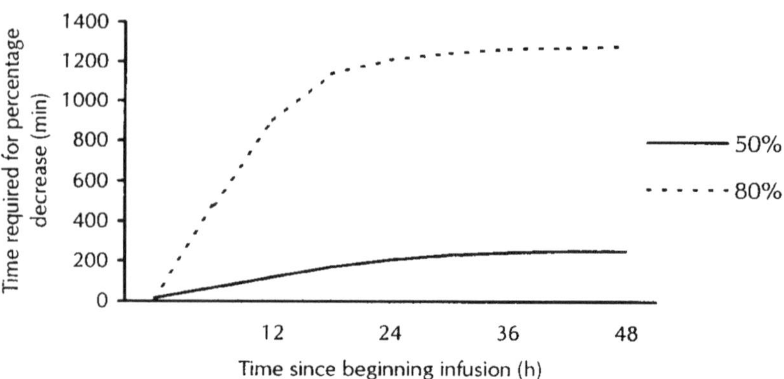

Figure 1
The influence of infusion duration on the time required after termination of the infusion to reach 50% or 80% of the initial plasma midazolam concentration (with permission).[13]

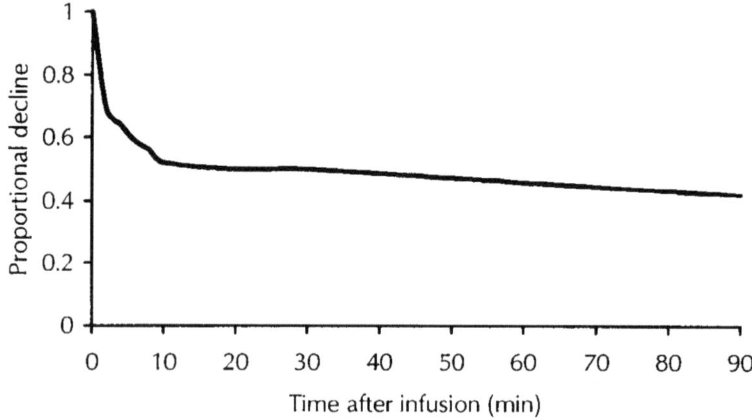

Figure 2
Proportional decline in the blood propofol concentration after termination of an infusion of 85 h (with permission).[14]

studies done with propofol show a fast decrease in the plasma concentration after stopping drug administration, even after prolonged infusion.

Figure 2 shows the proportional decline in the propofol concentration after an infusion of 85 h.[14] The time for the plasma concentration to decrease by 50% is approximately 10 min.

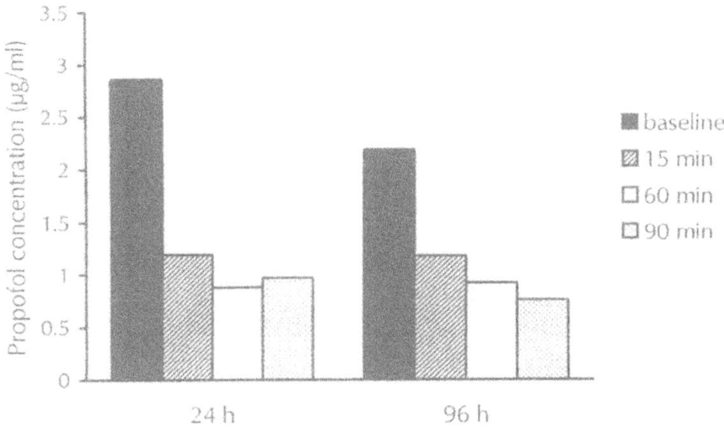

Figure 3
Decrease in the blood propofol concentration after 24 h and 96 h of propofol infusion (with permission).[15]

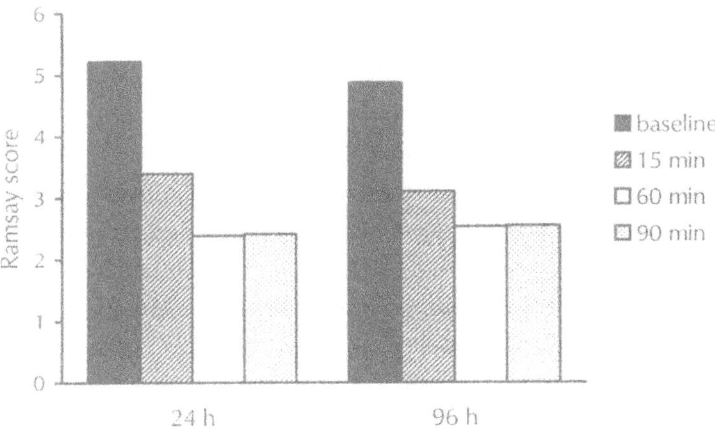

Figure 4
Ramsay scores after 24 h and 96 h of propofol administration (with permission).[15]

Beller et al. administered propofol as a continuous infusion for 4 days and discontinued the infusion every 24 h.[15] Figure 3 shows the decrease in the plasma concentration after 1 day of administration and after 4 days. This figure

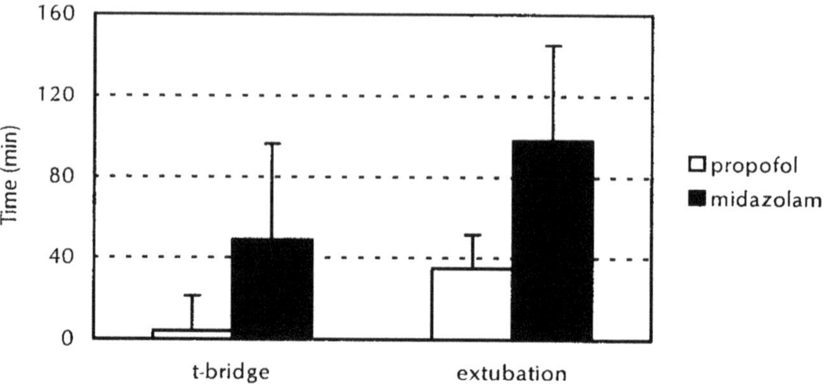

Figure 5
Weaning times after mean propofol and midazolam infusions of 6 days (with permission).[16]

shows the rapid decline in the blood propofol concentrations, associated with an increase in patient's arousal, as determined by the decrease in Ramsay sedation scores shown in figure 4. Even after an infusion of propofol for 4 days, this steep decay maintains. This quick decrease in the blood concentration is found in all studies done with ICU patients, although it is unclear how to explain this pharmacokinetically. From a practical point of view, the most important thing is that patients wake up fast after switching off a prolonged propofol infusion.

When looking at times to wean ICU patients from ventilatory support, the rapid offset of effect of propofol compared to midazolam can be expected to have favourable effects on weaning times and therefore on the cost of the ICU stay. In one study Barrientos-Vega and colleagues sedated patients for a mean period of 6 days using either midazolam or propofol.[16] They studied the time from stopping the drug infusion to extubation. Figure 5 shows the time until the first T-bridge trial (i.e. no more ventilatory support), and the time to extubation. They found those time intervals to be less then half for propofol as compared to midazolam. They also showed the variability in recovery times to be larger for midazolam than for propofol. Propofol was also found to be more cost-effective. When assessing the studies comparing midazolam to propofol for sedating ICU patients, the general view is that both provide adequate sedation, that awakening times are shorter for propofol, and, however debatable this may be, that the quality of sedation seems to be better with propofol.

When administering sedation in an ICU, it is very important to be aware that the huge inter-individual variability, which we are used to in the operating theatre, may be even more pronounced in ICU patients. Titrating the drug to the desired effect is therefore very important. Nevertheless, it is uncommon to see e.g. the midazolam 2-5 mg/h regimen being adjusted for interventions. Tailoring the sedative regimen to the changing individual needs of the patient requires very close attention and an effort from both nursing staff and ICU physicians. Being able to titrate drugs to the desired effect is one of the major advantages of target controlled drug administration. The increasing experience with these types of drug delivery systems has led to the use of these systems outside the operating room. Recently, there have been publications on the use of TCI systems for the administration of patient controlled analgesia, with alfentanil or remifentanil.[17] Also there is increasing interest in using TCI to sedate patients, both inside and outside the operating room. This has led to the use of TCI for delivery of sedative drugs in ICU patients. So far, although probably many academic anesthesiologists have used TCI systems in this way, not many data have are available on this topic. This is most likely due to the difficulties in analysing the pharmacokinetics of the drugs and the lack of a good measurable clinical end-point. Zomorodi and Somma and colleagues from Stanford published two studies last year on the pharmacokinetics and pharmacodynamics of midazolam using target controlled drug delivery in ICU patients.[11,18] They found that using a TCI system to administer midazolam was useful, as sedation scores could be predicted on the basis of the predicted plasma concentrations. However, they found the correlation between effect and concentration to be best, if they took into account the residual effects of anaesthesia. This was called the "virtual drug concentration". Figure 6 shows how midazolam concentrations combined with the effect of this virtual drug concentration correlated with sedation scores. Even after adding this virtual drug effect, there is still considerable interindividual variability. At a plasma concentration of around 200 ng/ml a patient can have a sedation score of 3 to 5. From a clinical point of view this is important: at a Ramsay score of 5 you would probably not extubate a patient, whereas at 3 you possibly could. The predictability of the sedation score in correlation with a given plasma concentration is therefore not very high.

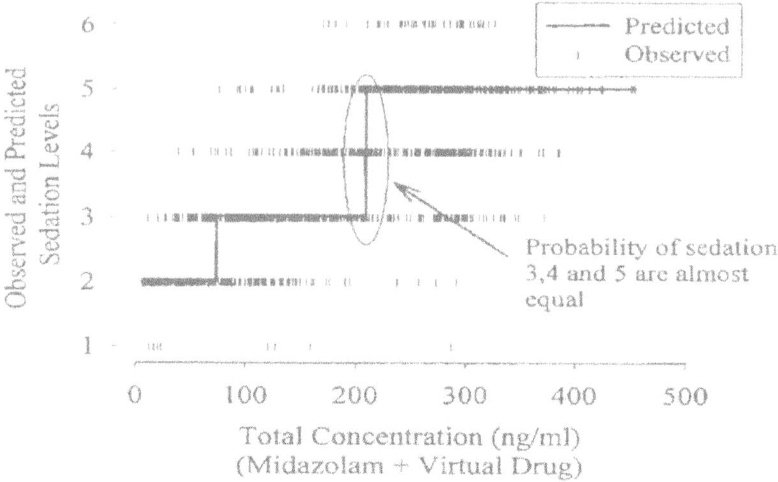

Figure 6
Plasma midazolam concentrations and sedation scores (with permission).[11,18]

The therapeutic window for propofol is not as large as for midazolam. Concentrations associated with sedation lie in the range of 0.2-2 μg/ml. Barr and colleagues from Stanford published some preliminary data, suggesting the concentration range should be between 0.3 and 1.5 μg/ml. They found an EC_{50} for sedation of 0.47 μg/ml.[19] This seems to correlate well with other studies. Maybe with the use of a TCI system for administration of propofol some of the problems described above could be overcome.

The currently commercially available TCI system, the Diprifusor, is programmed with the pharmacokinetic model according to Marsh.[20] This model may or may not be appropriate for ICU patients. Using TCI propofol one can adjust the level of sedation faster and better than when using a conventional infusion device. The pharmacological model incorporated in the TCI device can help sedative management in the ICU as is illustrated in figure 7.

After surgery the patient is transferred to the ICU with a TCI device for propofol still running. After arrival in the ICU the target concentration is lowered to allow the patient to wake up, which occurs at a target propofol concentration of 1 μg/ml. After a short period he needs to rest, and the target is set at 1.5 μg/ml. After this is reached, the Ramsay sedation score is 3. Eventually he needs endotracheal suction, and for that purpose the target concentration is

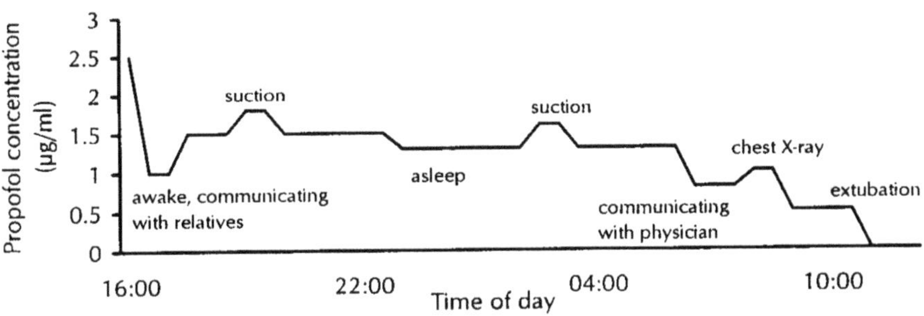

Figure 7
An example of the blood propofol concentrations over time in a surgical ICU patient.

shortly raised to 1.8 µg/ml. During the night he is kept comfortable at a target propofol concentration of 1.5 µg/ml. This is adjusted downward when his Ramsay score is 5. At one point he once again needs endotracheal suction and the target is again shortly increased. Toward the morning the target is lowered again to allow the patient to wake up. During morning rounds he can communicate with the physician. Chest X-ray is performed with a slightly higher target to minimise discomfort. Once this is done, the infusion is stopped (target is 0 ug/ml) and the patient is extubated soon thereafter. Research in this field is necessary to establish the place of TCI propofol in the ICU. In the future TCI techniques may enable ICU physicians to tailor their sedative regimen in this manner to the exact needs of their patients.

References

1. Ramsay MAE, Savege TM, Simpson BR, Goodwin R. BMJ 1974;2(920):656-59.
2. O'Connor M, Kress JP, Pohlman A, Tung A, Hall J. Pitfalls of monitoring sedation in the ICU with the bispectral index (abstract). Anesthesiology 1998, A461, V89, No 3A.
3. Frenkel C, Schüttler J, Ihmsen H, Heye H, Rommelsheim K. Pharmacokinetics and pharmacodynamics of propofol/alfentanil infusions for sedation in ICU patients. Int Care Med 1995;21:981-88.
4. Shafer A. Complications of sedation with midazolam in the intensive care unit and a comparison with other sedative regimens. Crit Care Med 1998;26:947-56.
5. Dyck JB, Shafer SL. Effects of age on propofol pharmacokinetics. Semin Anesth 1992;11:2-4.

6. Hughes MA, Glass PSA, Jacobs JR. Context-sensitive half-time in multicompartment pharmacokinetic models for intravenous anaesthetic drugs. Anesthesiology 1992; 76:334-41.
7. Carrasco G, Molina R, Costa J et al. Propofol versus midazolam in short-, medium-, and long-term sedation of critically ill patients. Chest 1993;103:557-64.
8. Vuyk J, Lim T, Engbers FHM et al. The pharmacodynamic interaction of propofol and alfentanil during lower abdominal surgery in women. Anesthesiology 1995;83:8-22.
9. Buckley PM. Propofol in patients needing long-term sedation in intensive care: an assessment of the development of tolerance. Int Care Med 1997;23:969-74.
10. Borgeat A, Wilder-Smith OHG, Saiah M, Rifat K. Subhypnotic doses of propofol possess direct antiemetic properties. Anesth Analg 1992;74:539-41.
11. Torn K, Tuominen M, Tarkkila P, Lindgren L. Effects of subhypnotic doses of propofol on the side effects of intrathecal morphine. Br J Anaesth 1994;73:411-12.
12. Murphy PG, Myers DS, Davies MJ, et al. The antioxidant potential of propofol. Br J Anaesth 1992;68:613-18.
13. Zomorodi K, Donner A, Somma J, Barr J, Sladen R, Ramsay J, Geller E, Shafer SL. Population pharmacokinetics of midazolam administered by target controlled infusion for sedation following coronary artery bypass grafting. Anesthesiology 89;1414-29, 1998.
14. Bailie GR, Cockshott ID, Douglas EJ, Bowles BJM. Pharmacokinetics of propofol during and after long term continuous infusion for maintenance of sedation of sedation in ICU patients. Br J Anaesth 1992;68:486-91.
15. Beller JP, Pottecher T, Lugnier A, et al. Prolonged sedation with propofol in ICU patients: recovery and blood concentrations during periodic interruptions in infusion. Br J Anaesth 1988;61:583-88.
16. Barrientos-Vega R, Mar Sanchez-Soria M, Morales-Garcia C, Robas-Gomez A, Cuena-Boy R, Ayensa-Rincon A. Prolonged sedation of critically ill patients with midazolam or propofol: impact on weaning and costs. Crit Care Med 1997;25:33-40.
17. Van den Nieuwenhuyzen MCO, Engbers FHM, Burm AGL et al. Target Controlled Infusion of alfentanil for postoperative analgesia. Br J Anaesth 1997;78:17-23.
18. Somma J, Donner A, Zomorodi K, Sladen R, Ramsay J, Geller E, Shafer SL. Population pharmacodynamics of midazolam administered by target controlled infusion in SICU patients after CABG surgery. Anesthesiology 1998;89:1430-43.
19. Barr J, Egan TD, Feeley T, Shafer SL. The pharmacokinetics and pharmacodynamics of computer-controlled propofol infusions in ICU patients (abstract P II-62)). Clin Pharmacol and Ther 1994;55(2):185.
20. Marsh B, White M, Morton N, Kenny GNC. Pharmacokinetic model driven infusion of propofol in children. Br J Anaesth 1991;67:41-8.

State of the art on neuromuscular blockade

COMPUTER-CONTROLLED INFUSION OF NEUROMUSCULAR BLOCKING AGENTS

Valérie Billard and Philippe Mavoungou

Villejuif and Nantes, France

Introduction

Neuromuscular blocking agents are useful in anaesthesia and in intensive care medicine to paralyse patients for anaesthetic (intubation and ventilation) or surgical procedures. The level of neuromuscular blockade required depends on the procedure. When it is insufficient, neuromuscular blocking agents become useless, movement or coughing may occur and may be harmful to the patient e.g. during eye- or neurosurgery, or during peritoneal closure. On the other hand, overdose of neuromuscular blocking agents has few side effects as long as amnesia is provided and artificial ventilation is controlled. Its main consequences are a delayed recovery and a useless increase of drug consumption and costs.

The level of neuromuscular blockade can be estimated by measuring the evoked muscular response to a well-defined electrical stimulus like the single twitch, the train of four (TOF), the post-tetanic count (PTC) and the double burst suppression (DBS).[1] Response is often assessed visually or manually as the number of responses to the TOF or the DBS. From the musculus adductor pollicis a quantitative measure can be obtained by measuring either the current corresponding to the action potential by electromyography (EMG), by the force developed by a force transducer, or by measuring the acceleration of the thumb by accelerometry.

Per se, paralysing peripheral muscles such as the adductor pollicis is not clinically relevant, except as a reflection of the intensity of blockade of all muscles in the body. Years of experience and research have defined quite accurately the relationship and the discrepancies between the monitored blockade at the musculus adductor pollicis, or orbicularis oculi and the desired blockade of the larynx, diaphragm and abdominal wall.[2, 3] Consequently, anaesthesiologists now are used to describe neuromuscular blockade directly in terms T_4/T_1, or $T_1/T_{initial}$ ratios and all know which level of measured blockade corresponds to an adequate level of paralysis for surgical procedures. Since patients are different from each other, the same dose doesn't induce the same blockade in all patients. To achieve a desired neuromuscular blockade, the doses should be adjusted according to the measured effect.

This could be done manually. After having given a first dose, often a bolus dose, the anaesthesiologist determines what the next dose should be according to the desired time course of the blockade. This method, that is widely used in clinical practice, is simple, has only low costs related to the medical devices, but is rather time consuming, for the anaesthesiologist should frequently verify the level of blockade to avoid both over- and underdosage. Because the measured blockade on the musculus adductor pollicis is reliable and the adequacy of the blockade for surgery well defined, it did make sense to try to administer neuromuscular blocking agents automatically through a computer-controlled infusion, connected to both the pump and the monitor, and designed to maintain a chosen level of blockade.

As for other controlled-processes in medicine, computer-controlled infusion of neuromuscular blocking agents requires several conditions; the effect of the neuromuscular blocking agent should be quantitative and measurable, the intensity of the effect should be dose-dependant and the measured effect should be related as few as possible to other factors than the concentration of the neuromuscular blocking agent.

Several techniques were proposed during the past 10 years in clinical studies whom methods and results will be discussed in this chapter. All these techniques require a common set of equipment including a pump with a 2-way serial port to receive remote commands and send back information on the infusion status, a neuromuscular function monitor to measure evoked responses and to automatically compute the parameter used as the target effect parameter (most often the T_4/T_1 ratio), and a microprocessor with an algorithm designed to convert the difference between the measured and the target effects into the new dose or infusion rate. Because those techniques are still at a research level, the devices used are separate pieces. As none of the available algorithms has until now a CE mark for clinical use, they should be used in clinical studies having IRB approval.

Two main classes of algorithms have been described: the direct close-loop systems and the pharmacokinetic/pharmacodynamic (PK/PD) approach. The direct closed-loop systems are based on iterative adjustment of the dose in order to minimise the difference between the target and the measured blockade without any assumption about a mathematical relationship between dose and effect. The PK/PD approach calculates the dose or infusion rate according to a mathematical model that describes the relationship between dose, concentration and effect. The dosage is adjusted in order to minimise the difference between the target blockade and the predicted blockade. When the intensity of the neuromuscular blockade is also measured, the model can be improved by adjusting some of its parameters in order to minimise the difference between the predicted and the measured blockade.

Direct closed-loop systems

These are based on regular measurements of effect and adjustment of the infusion rate in order to minimise the difference e between the target effect and the measured effect (figure 1).

$$e = \textit{measured blockade} - \textit{target blockade}$$

This error influences the rate of infusion through a mathematical equation (P, PI and PID controllers) or a logical equation (fuzzy logic).

The mathematical approach

The simplest algorithm would be just proportional:

$$v = k_p.e \quad \text{or} \quad v = k_p.weight.e$$

This algorithm may have a poor performance, either because of a steady state offset, or because the changes are too rough around the target. For those reasons, other algorithms have been proposed including:

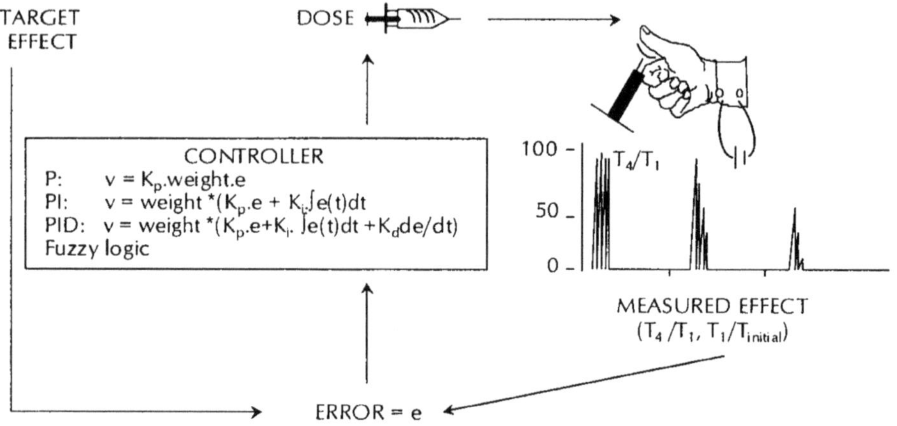

Figure 1
The organisation of a direct closed-loop system for the infusion of neuromuscular blocking agents with its various controllers.

an integrative component (proportional-integral algorithm, P.I.):

$$v(t) = weight.[\ k_p.e(t) + k_i.\int e(t)dt]$$

or a derivative component (proportional-integral-derivative algorithm, P.I.D.):

$$v(t) = weight.[\ kp.e(t) + ki.\int e(t)dt+kd.de/dt]$$

The fuzzy logic approach

In the fuzzy logic approach the inputs are qualitative data derived ("fuzzified") from the time course of the measured effect compared with a target. A controller processes the input according to some rules, and returns a qualitative output, which needs to be "defuzzified" to become a command for the infusion pump. In a simple controller, inputs are usually the error and the change in the error, qualified as "small", "big", going "up" or "going down" [4], but other data as the onset of blockade and the rate of recovery from initial blockade can also be used.[5] The output is processed by a set of "if then" statements like "if error is 0 and change in error is positively small, then output is negatively small".[4] When all the rules are predefined, the controller is called fixed-rule based, as has been described for atracurium.[6] Those controllers often require

Table 1
Performance of various closed-loop neuromuscular agent administration devices.

Reference	Drug	Measure	Controller	Error (mean)
7	Atracurium	EMG	P.I.D.	3%
7	"	Force/EMG	P.I.D.	11%
8	"	EMG	P.I.	1.3%
9	"	EMG	P.I.D.	8.5-13%
10	Atracurium/vecuronium	EMG/accelerometry	P.	10-50%
11	Atracurium	Accelerometry	P.	negl.
5	Atracurium	EMG	Fuzzy (SOFLC)	0.5%

numerous statements to reach good performance. More sophisticated controllers use the inputs at two levels. The first level returns an output. The second level calculates the performance of the first level processing and may modify the rules in order to improve it. Those controllers are called self-learning or self-organising fuzzy logic controller (SOFLC). They require less *a priori* statements, since they improve over time, and result in less erratic infusion rates, less oscillations or diverging of the system, compared to the simple controllers. The performances obtained with mathematical or fuzzy logic closed-loop systems during surgery are summarized in table 1.

With the fuzzy as well as with the mathematical approach, all direct closed-loop systems require numerous and regular measures of effect and may diverge when the error between target and measured effect can not be calculated. That is why the main problems described in studies using these devices were due to electrodes coming unstuck, or loss of signal during diathermic use. Instability after changing the syringe has also been described.

The pharmacokinetic/pharmacodynamic relationship approach

From PKPD model to TCI

The second technique to administer neuromuscular blocking agents by computer controlled infusion is based on pharmacokinetic/pharmacodynamic

(PK/PD) modelling. This approach assumes that the effect is related to the concentration at the effect site, which is related to the plasma concentration with a lag time due to blood/neuromuscular junction transfer. Furthermore, the plasma concentration depends on the dose and on a set of constant parameters.

For neuromuscular blocking agents as for most intravenous anaesthetic agents, the plasma concentration-time relationship can be described by a 2 or 3 compartment mammillary model with elimination from the central (blood) compartment.[12] For example after a bolus dose;

$$Cp(t) = dose.\sum_{i=1}^{n} A_i.e^{-\lambda_i t}$$

where A_i, λ_i are the parameters of the pharmacokinetic model and n = 2 or 3. *Cp(t)* could also be expressed as a function of the dose, the volumes of distribution in the 3 compartments (V_1, V_2, V_3), the distribution clearances (from blood to each of the peripheral compartments, CL_2 and CL_3) and the elimination clearance from the central compartment (CL_1). For neuromuscular blocking agents, most of the published models have only 2 compartments. The lag time between the plasma concentration and effect could be expressed by a mathematical function called convolution product:[13]

$$Ce\ (t) = Cp\ (t) \otimes k_{e0}.e^{-k_{e0}t} = \int_0^t Cp\ (u).k_{e0}.e^{-k_{e0}(t-u)}du$$

When Cp is stable (steady state), Ce = Cp.

Finally, it is classically assumed that the effect, ***E***, is related to the effect site concentration *Ce* by a sigmoidal Hill model [12], where E_0 is the effect without NMBA (no blockade, $T_1/T_{initial} = 1$ after TOF).

$$E = E_0 - \frac{E_{max}.Ce^{\gamma}}{IC_{50}^{\gamma} + Ce^{\gamma}}$$

E_{max} is the effect induced by a high dose of the drug (100% blockade after TOF), IC_{50} is the concentration of NMBA inducing 50% of blockade and γ is a slope coefficient. The whole PK/PD model including the 3 equations displayed above characterises the average dose-effect relationship for a neuromuscular blocking agent in a population. It could be used in both ways; to predict the effect when the dose given has been a *priori* chosen, or to calculate the dose required to achieve a desired effect (target effect).

The second way to use the PK/PD model "against the current" is known in intravenous anaesthesia as target controlled infusion (TCI). For sedative or analgesic agents, the target is usually the plasma or effect site concentration because quantitative measures of effect are still debated. For neuromuscular blocking agents the measured effect is generally accepted to be directly used as a target, avoiding anaesthesiologists to learn the corresponding concentrations. The anaesthesiologist just needs to enter the drug and the chosen level of blockade in the TCI software that has included a previously published PK/PD model of the neuromuscular blocking agent.[14-16] The software first calculates the dose of the neuromuscular blocking agent to achieve the target blockade according to the model. Then, it regularly checks (every 5-60 sec) the difference between the target and the predicted effect and adjusts the dose in order to minimise this difference. The most famous of these software programs probably is Stanpump*, that can provide target controlled infusion by targeting the percentage of neuromuscular blockade for pancuronium, vecuronium, atracurium and rocuronium.

Adjustment of the model to the individual response: the Bayesian approach

The basic TCI device works clinically pretty well with no measure of effect at all. However, when the level of neuromuscular blockade is measured, it may be different from the blockade predicted by the PK/PD model. This discrepancy may be due to pharmacokinetic differences between the patient and the population used to determine the model, or due to factors that modify the relationship between the neuromuscular blocking agent dose and the effect in this particular patient.

Improving the accuracy of the model is possible by combining the information given by a population model with one or few values of effect measured in the patient (figure 2).[17] It could be done manually (open-loop) or automatically (closed-loop). This approach is called Bayesian, because of Bayes theory which said that the probability of an event (e.g. having the true PK/PD relationship in a particular patient) depends on the probability of a general event A (e.g. know-

---

* written by Dr Steven Shafer, Stanford University, CA; and available at http://pkpd.icon.palo-alto.med.va.gov

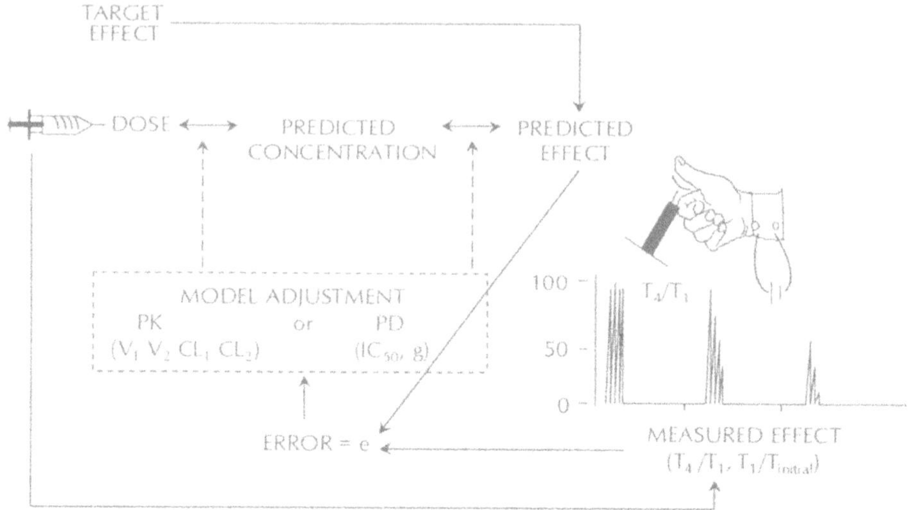

Figure 2
The organisation of a PK/PD model based target controlled infusion device for the administration of neuromuscular blocking agents with adjustment of the PK/PD model to individual responses by means of the Bayesian appraoch.

ing the population PK/PD model) and on the probability of a singular event B, knowing that the general event was true *(P(B/A)*.

$$P(A \text{ and } B) = P(A) \times P(B/A)$$

Correcting the model by adding a measured value makes *P(B/A)* = 1 (assuming there is no error on the measure). This maximises *P(A and B)* i.e. the probability of having the good model in the patient studied. A Bayesian approach has been proposed in numerous studies to adjust the pharmacokinetic model as for example with antineoplasic agents[18, 19] or antibiotics.[20, 21] In anaesthesia, Bayesian regression has been applied to adjust the pharmacokinetic model of alfentanil[22], midazolam[23] and lidocaine[24] by adjusting a population model with individual data. With neuromuscular blocking agents only 2 clinical studies have been performed adjusting respectively, the pharmacokinetics and pharmacodynamics of the model. Both were randomised, but the small number of patients (n = 21 and 22, respectively) may explain why the benefit of adjustment was only partly statistically significant. The first study[25] describes a rocuronium TCI device using Stanpump software with a 50% blockade target maintained for 30-90 min. This study compared the performance of an open-loop TCI device with Bayesian regression on the pharmacokinetic parameters, with a standard TCI device using a published pharmacokinetic model.[16] The errors (displayed graphically by predicted - target values) decreased, especially during the recovery, and the delay to complete recovery decreased significantly in the adapted group (16 versus 25 min). This result was obtained by introducing 1-9 data point per patient into the algorithm.

The second study compared a closed-loop TCI of vecuronium adapting the pharmacodynamic model with manual adjustments by boluses in order to maintain 90% blockade.[26] The level of blockade was more stable over time and the neuromuscular blocking agent consumption was significantly reduced by more than 50% in the feedback-controlled group. In other words, both studies show a better control of neuromuscular blockade using a Bayesian approach, but further clinical studies would be necessary to quantify this. Before performing such studies, one important question needs to be answered first. Which group of parameters needs to be included in the regression: the pharmacokinetic parameters, the pharmacodynamic parameters, or both?

Future development and rational strategy of adjustment

Bayesian adjustment of a pharmacokinetic or pharmacodynamic model is supposed to shift the model from the average values as determined in a large population to the true parameter values corresponding to those of a particular patient at a particular moment of time. This "instantaneous model" may be different from the published average model either because the patient is different from the average (interindividual variability, usually around 30%) or because the model of this patient is changing over time (intraindividual variability, usually below 10%). To decide on which parameters need to be adapted, the factors involved in both components of the variability should be known.

Factors influencing the pharmacokinetic model

Several factors such as age, renal or liver disease could delay the elimination of neuromuscular agents, either by reducing the clearance[27-29] or by increasing the volume of distribution.[30-35] These changes were more or less marked among the different neuromuscular blocking agents, probably due to their different ways of elimination.[36-40] In obese patients, absolute values for volumes and clearances were similar, i.e. the values related the body weight were smaller[41, 42] In other words, a dose calculated upon the real weight in mg/kg induces a higher concentration and a longer blockade in obese patients. In contrast, burns and interactions with other drugs (that may be administered or stopped during the neuromuscular blocking agent infusion) seem to affect the pharmacokinetics of neuromuscular blocking agents hardly.[15, 32, 34]

Factors influencing the pharmacodynamic model

The sensitivity to neuromuscular blocking agents is increased in burned patients[15], in the presence of volatile anaesthetic agents[32,43], after administration of suxamethonium[44] and during hypothermia. Conversely, age[30,33], renal[36,37] or liver disease, and alcohol consumption[45] seem to have little influence, except may be on k_{e0} and onset.[31]

In summary, we may conclude that most of the factors influencing the pharmacokinetic model parameters are related to demographic factors or to a preoperative pathological state, but appear to be constant over the duration of a the neuromuscular blocking agent infusion. Consequently, in general it does make sense to adjust the pharmacokinetic model in order to decrease the interindividual variability. However, in some situations as hypothermia, burns or associated volatile anaesthesia, Bayesian adjustment on the pharmacodynamic model should be considered, because those factors are known to influence mainly the pharmacodynamic model.

Compared to the direct closed-loop systems described above, the use of a PK/PD model to adjust computer-controlled infusion of neuromuscular blocking agents theoretically requires fewer measurements done during an initial period of adjustment. Then, the model is supposed to be roughly adjusted to a patient (at least regarding interindividual variability) and a loss of the signal may not result in dramatic diverging. On the other hand, the algorithm used is more complex, the calculation times are longer and the mathematical modelling of the dose-effect relationship is based on several hypothesis considering the number of compartments, the way of elimination, or the shape of the concentration effect relationship, that may not be true. If, for example, the elimination is not only from the blood compartment but occurs also in tissue or organs[46], an appropriate model should be used. If a neuromuscular blocking agent (as vecuronium, for example) has an active metabolite[47], the effect should be expressed as a function of both the parent compound and the metabolite, and the concentration of both compounds should be known to follow different pharmacokinetic models. Finally, if a deep neuromuscular blockade is achieved (no response to TOF, responses only to PTC), the pharmacodynamic model established with responses to the TOF becomes useless to maintain this level of blockade, while the response to PTC is useless to adjust the model in the presence of only a moderate level of neuromuscular blockade (abdominal closure, prediction of recovery).

Conclusion

Compared to anaesthetic drugs, neuromuscular blocking agents are easier to study and to titrate to effect because the level of blockade can be assessed by well-defined, quantitative measures performed on specific peripheral muscles. These measures can be used as parameters for a direct closed-loop system based on the same tools as non-medical industry processes. They can also be combined with a pharmacokinetic-pharmacodynamic model to adjust the model to a patient, according to Bayesian principles. Adjusting the pharmacokinetic model is likely to decrease mainly the variability between patients, whereas adjusting the pharmacodynamic model may decrease intraindividual variability over the infusion period. The clinical consequences of such sophisticated drug infusion adjustment on safety and economical factors still need to be demonstrated. However, because both the measures of effect and the pharmacokinetic/dynamic models are available for neuromuscular blocking agents, these drugs have a unique theoretical interest to test, choose and optimize the tools that may be used in the near future for any type of computer-controlled infusion.

References

1. Viby-Mogensen J: Neuromuscular Monitoring, Anesthesia. Edited by Miller RD. New York, Churchill Livingstone, 1994,
2. Donati F, Meistelman C, Plaud B: Vecuronium neuromuscular blockade at the diaphragm, the orbicularis oculi, and adductor pollicis muscles. Anesthesiology 73: 870-875, 1990

3. Donati F, Plaud B, Meistelman C: Vecuronium neuromuscular blockade at the adductor muscles of the larynx and adductor pollicis. Anesthesiology 74:833-837, 1991
4. Mason DG, Linkens DA, Abbod MF, Edwards ND, Reilly CS: Automated delivery of muscle relaxants using fuzzy logic control. IEEE engineering in medicine and biology 678-686, 1994
5. Ross JJ, Mason DG, Linkens DA, Edwards ND: Self-learning fuzzy logic control of neuromuscular block. Br J Anaesth 78:412-415, 1997
6. Mason DG, Edwards ND, Linkens DA, Reilly CS: Performance assessment of a fuzzy logic controller for atracurium-induced neuromuscular block. Br J Anaesth 76(3): 396-400, 1996
7. Webster NR, Cohen AT: Closed-loop administration of atracurium : steady-state neuromuscular blockade during surgery using a computer-controlled closed-loop atracurium infusion. Anaesth 42:1085-1091, 1987
8. McLeod AD, Asbury AJ, Gray WM, Linkens DA: Automatic control of neuromuscular block with atracurium. Br J Anaesth 63:31-35, 1989
9. O'Hara DA, Derbyshire GJ, Overdyk FJ, Bogen DK, Marshall BE: Closed-loop infusion of atracurium with four different anesthetic techniques. Anesthesiology 74: 258-263, 1991
10. Assef SJ, Lennon RL, Burke MJ, Behrens TL: A versatile, computer-controlled, closed-loop system for continuous infusion of muscle relaxants. Mayo Clin Proc 68:1074-1080, 1993
11. Stinson LW, Murray MJ, Jones KA, Assef SJ, Burke MJ, Behrens TL, Lennon RL: A computer-controlled closed-loop infusion system for infusing muscle relaxants : its use during motor-evoked potential monitoring. J Cardiothor Vasc Anesth 8:40-44, 1994
12. Hull CJ: Models with more than one compartment, Pharmacokinetics for anaesthesia. Edited by Hull CJ. Oxford, Butterworth-Heinemann, 1991, pp 170-186
13. Sheiner L, Stanski DR, Vozeh S, Miller RD, Ham J: Simultaneous modeling of pharmacokinetics and pharmacodynamics: application to d-tubocurarine. Clin Pharmacol Ther 25:358-371, 1979
14. Rupp SM, Castagnoli KP, Fisher DM, Miller RD: Pancuronium and vecuronium pharmacocinetics and pharmacodynamics in younger and elderly subjects. Anesthesiology 67:45-49, 1987
15. Marathe PH, Dwersteg JF, Pavlin EG, Haschke RH, Heimbach DM, Slattery JT: Effect of thermal injury on the pharmacokinetics and pharmacodynamics of atracurium in humans. Anesthesiology 70:752-755, 1989
16. Plaud B, Proost JH, Pharm D, Wierda MKH, Barre J, Debaene B, Meistelman C: Pharmacokinetics and pharmacodynamics of rocuronium at the vocal cords and the adductor pollicis in humans. Clin.Pharmacol.Ther. 58:185-191, 1995
17. Jelliffe RW, Schumitzky A, Bayard D, Milman M, Van Guilder M, Wang X, Jiang F, Barbaut X, Maire P: Model-based, goal-oriented, individualised drug therapy. Linkage of population modelling, new 'multiple model' dosage design, bayesian feedback and individualised target goals. Clin Pharmacokinet. 34:57-77, 1998
18. Pignon T, Lacarelle B, Duffaud F, Guillet P, Catalin J, Durand A, Favre R: Dosage adjustment of high-dose methotrexate using bayesian estimation : a comparative study of two different concentrations at the end of 8-h infusions. Ther Drug Monit 17:471-478, 1995
19. Bressolle F, Bologna C, Edno L, Bernard JC, Gomeni R, Sany J, Combe B: A limited sampling method to estimate methotrexate pharmacokinetics in patients with

rheumatoid arthritis using a Bayesian approach and the population data modeling program P-PHARM. Eur J Clin Pharmacol 49:285-292, 1996
20. Bruno R, Iliadis MC, Lacarelle B, Cosson V, Mandema JW, Le Roux Y, Montay G, Durand A, Ballereau M, Alasia M: Evaluation of Bayesian estimation in comparison to NONMEM for population pharmacokinetic data analysis: application to pefloxacin in intensive care unit patients. J Pharmacokinet Biopharm 20:653-669, 1992
21. Cropp CD, Davis GA, Ensom MH: Evaluation of aminoglycoside pharmacokinetics in postpartum patients using Bayesian forecasting. Ther Drug Monit 20:68-72, 1998
22. Maitre PO, Stanski DR: Bayesian forecasting improves the prediction of intraoperative plasma concentrations of alfentanil. Anesthesiology 69:652-659, 1988
23. Maitre PO, Bührer M, Thomson D, Stanski DR: A three-step approach combining bayesian regression and NONMEM population analysis : application to midazolam. J Pharmacokinet Biopharm 19:377-384, 1991
24. Vozeh S, Steiner C: Estimates of the population pharmacokinetic parameters and performance of Bayesian feedback: a sensitivity analysis. J Pharmacokinet Biopharm 15:511-528, 1987
25. Devys JM, Billard V, Barreau-Pouhaer L, Mavoungou P, Meistelman C, Debaene B: Administration des curares pour chirurgie plastique : apports de l'adaptation bayésienne. Ann.Fr.Anesth.Reanim. 15:R2791996(Abstract)
26. Ebeling BJ, Muller W, Tonner P, Olkkola KT, Stoekel H: Adaptative feedback-controlled infusion versus repetitive injections of vecuronium in patients during isoflurane anesthesia. Journal of Clinical Anesthesia 3:181-185, 1991
27. Lien CA, Matteo RS, Ornstein E, Schwartz AE, Diaz J: Distribution, elimination, and action of vecuronium in the elderly. Anesth.Analg. 73:39-42, 1991
28. Lynam DP, Cronnelly R, Castagnoli KP, Canfell PC, Caldwell J, Arden J, Miller RD: The pharmacodynamics and pharmacokinetics of vecuronium in patients anesthetized with isoflurane with normal renal function or with renal failure. Anesthesiology 69:227-231, 1988
29. Devlin JC, Head-Rapson AG, Parker CJR, Hunter JM: Pharmacodynamics of mivacurium chloride in patients with hepatic cirrhosis. Br J Anaesth 71:227-231, 1993
30. Kitts JB, Fisher DM, Canfell PC, Spellman MJ, Caldwell JE, Heier T, Fahey MR, Miller RD: Pharmacokinetics and pharmacodynamics of atracurium in the elderly. Anesthesiology 72:272-275, 1990
31. Sorooshian SS, Stafford MA, Eastwood NB, Boyd AH, Hull CJ, Wright PM: Pharmacokinetics and pharmacodynamics of cisatracurium in young and elderly adult patients. Anesthesiology 84:1083-1091, 1996
32. Swerdlow BN, Holley FO: Intravenous anaesthetic agents : pharmacokinetic-pharmacodynamic relationship. Clinical Pharmacokinetics 12:79-110, 1987
33. Fisher DM, Canfell PC, Spellman MJ, Miller RD: Pharmacokinetics and pharmacodynamics of atracurium in infants and children. Anesthesiology 73:33-37, 1990
34. Szenohradszky J, Fisher DM, Segredo V, Caldwell JE, Bragg P, Sharma ML, Gruenke LD, Miller RD: Pharmacokinetics of rocuronium bromide (ORG 9426) in patients with normal renal function or patients undergoing cadaver renal transplantation. Anesthesiology 77:899-904, 1992
35. Wierda JM, Meretoja OA, Taivavainen T, Proost JH: Pharmacokinetics and pharmacokinetic-dynamic modelling of rocuronium in infants and children. Br J Anaesth 78:690-695, 1997
36. Fahey MR, Rupp SM, Fisher DM, Miller RD, Sharma M, Canfell C, Castagnoli K, Hennis PJ: The pharmacokinetics and pharmacodynamics of atracurium in patients with and without renal failure. Anesthesiology 61:699-702, 1984

37. deBros FM, Lai A, Scott R, deBros J, Batson AG, Goudsouzian N, Ali HH, Cosimi AB, Savarese JJ: Pharmacokinetics and pharmacodynamics of atracurium during isoflurane anesthesia in normal and anephric patients. Anesth Analg 65:743-746, 1986
38. Bion JF, Bowden MI, Chow B, Honisberger L, Weatherley BC: Atracurium infusions in patients with fulminant hepatic failure awaiting liver transplantation. Intensive Care Med. 19 Suppl 2:S94-8, 1993
39. Servin FS, Lavaut E, Kleef U, Desmonts JM: Repeated doses of rocuronium bromide administered to cirrhotic and control patients receiving isoflurane. Anesthesiology 84:1092-1100, 1996
40. Fisher DM, Ramsay MAE, Hein T, Marcel RJ, Sharma M, Ramsay KJ, Miller RD: Pharmacokinetics of rocuronium during the three stages of liver transplantation. Anesthesiology 86:1306-1316, 1997
41. Varin F, Ducharme J, Theoret Y, Besner JG, Bevan DR, Donati F: Influence of extreme obesity on the body disposition and neuromuscular blocking effect of atracurium. Clin Pharmacol Ther 48:18-25, 1990
42. Schwartz AE, Matteo RS, Ornstein E, Halevy JD, Diaz J: Pharmacokinetics and pharmacodynamics of vecuronium in the obese surgical patient. Anesth.Analg. 74: 515-518, 1992
43. Stanski DR, Ham J, Miller RD, Sheiner L: Time-dependant increase in sensitivity to d-tubocurarine during enflurane anesthesia in man. Anesthesiology 52:483-487, 1980
44. Donati F, Gill SS, Bevan DR, Ducharme J, Theoret Y, Varin F: Pharmacokinetics and pharmacodynamics of atracurium with and without previous suxamethonium administration [see comments]. Br J Anaesth 66:557-561, 1991
45. Arden JR, Lynam DP, Castagnoli KP, Canfell PC, Cannon JC, Miller RD: Vecuronium in alcoholic liver disease: a pharmacokinetic and pharmacodynamic analysis. Anesthesiology 68:771-776, 1988
46. Fisher DM, Canfell PC, Fahey MR, Rosen JI, Rupp SM, Sheiner LB, Miller RD: Elimination of atracurium in humans: contribution of Hofmann elimination and ester hydrolysis versus organ-based elimination. Anesthesiology 65:6-12, 1986
47. Caldwell JE, Szenohradszky J, Segredo V, Wright PMC: The Pharmacodynamics and Pharmacokinetics of the Metabolite 3- Desacetylvecuronium (ORG 7268) and its Parent Compound, Vecuronium, in Human Volunteers. J.Pharmacol.Exp.Ther. 270: 1216-1216, 1994

NEW NEUROMUSCULAR BLOCKING AGENTS AND FAST-TRACKING ANAESTHESIA

Hermann Mellinghoff and Christoph Diefenbach

Köln, Germany

Introduction

The choice of anaesthetics with a rapid and predictable recovery is essential for a rapid turnover of patients in the operating theatre. "Fast-tracking" after surgery is a concept which was initially developed for patients undergoing cardiac surgery in an attempt to decrease the time from the end of surgery to the extubation of the trachea.[1, 2] An important effect of this concept was the reduction of the time these patients spend in the intensive care unit, postanaesthesia care unit or similar postsurgical wards. Today, "fast-tracking" after ambulatory surgery may also be used to describe the procedure in which patients who meet the discharge criteria in the operating theatre bypass the postanaesthesia care unit.[3]

A muscle relaxant well suited for "fast-tracking" should produce a rapid onset, a short duration of action and it's offset period should allow equally rapid recovery from neuromuscular block. The following considerations are based on a more conservative definition of "fast-tracking", i.e. the attempt to minimise or at least to reliably predict the time patients spend between the end of surgery and their transfer to a ward or step-down unit. The different parts of the time course of neuromuscular block following the injection of a muscle relaxant will be discussed with their relevance to the choice of appropriate drugs for fast-tracking.

The onset of action of neuromuscular block

Decreased neuromuscular blocking potency as well as a rapid clearance seems to be responsible for a more rapid onset of action of muscle relaxants. Bowman has shown in studies in cats that the onset times after the injection of muscle relaxants decreased with increasing molar potency.[4] This relationship was confirmed by iontophoretic experiments by Law Min[5] and by recent clinical research by Kopman and his group [6]. The onset time of succinylcholine also appears to be compatible with this onset - potency relationship. Consistent with these findings rapacuronium (ED95 of 1.0 mg/kg active moiety[8]) has a more rapid onset of action than any of the other available muscle relaxants and, when injected in doses of 1.5-2.5 mg/kg, appears to have an onset of action compatible with that of succinylcholine.

Muscle relaxants are given during induction of anaesthesia to facilitate tracheal intubation. While a rapid onset of action has become an expected phenomenon, at least in part, due to the rapid onset of neuromuscular block of succinylcholine, it is apparently a more important issue in the United States than in other countries.[9] It is well accepted, that the time from injection of a muscle relaxant to its maximum effect is in the order of less than one minute (succinylcholine) to up to three minutes (cisatracurium[11]). This implies that even when the choice of the muscle relaxant for "fast-tracking" is based on a rapid onset of action, the time saved is minimal. Furthermore, Plaud has shown, that onset of neuromuscular block produced by muscle relaxants is faster at the laryngeal muscles than at the adductor pollicis muscles[13,14] and that therefore the clinician is not forced to wait for complete abolition of the peripheral twitch response.

The duration of action of muscle relaxants

With muscle relaxants of ultra-short (succinylcholine), short (mivacurium), short to intermediate (rapacuronium), intermediate (atracurium, vecuronium, cisatracurium and rocuronium) and long duration of action (pancuronium), the anaesthesiologist has a wide array of drugs at his disposal. It is obvious, that the choice of a muscle relaxant depends on the estimated duration of the surgical procedure. Preference should be given to muscle relaxants with a short or intermediate duration of action because they can easily be adapted to a varying duration of surgery.

The recovery from neuromuscular block

Recovery from neuromuscular block is assumed to be complete when any effect of a muscle relaxant has disappeared. As Waud[15] has shown, more than 70% of the acetylcholine receptors can be occupied by muscle relaxants before any reduction of the twitch response to nerve stimulation can be measured. Hence, when no further effect of the twitch response to nerve stimulation after the injection of muscle relaxants can be measured, these drugs may not have completely disappeared from the organism.

For a long time, a train-of-four (TOF) fade ratio of > 0.70 following nerve stimulation has been regarded as a reliable indicator of acceptable clinical recovery, since it had been shown that clinically detectable muscle weakness was associated with a smaller TOF ratio.[16, 17] Once that ratio was greater than 0.70, muscle strength was assumed to have returned to a near-normal state, as indicated by sensitive clinical tests, such as head-lift.[18, 19] In 1979, Viby-Mogensen, using a TOF-ratio of 0.70 as a reference value, investigated the incidence of residual neuromuscular block in recovery rooms following d-tubocurarine or pancuronium.[20] He showed that in patients having been exposed to these muscle relaxants, the incidence of residual paralysis was 42%. Approximately ten years later, Bevan showed that the use of muscle relaxants with intermediate duration of action greatly reduced this incidence of residual neuromuscular block.[21] Also, Kong and Cooper[22] examined postoperative morbidity following atracurium, vecuronium and alcuronium and found that only after administration of alcuronium, patients had signs of muscle weakness for three hours and more despite mandatory reversal. However, neither these reports nor the shorter duration of action of modern muscle relaxants (mivacurium, cisatracurium, rocuronium) have led to the disappearance of residual paralysis: even recent reports demonstrate that residual neuromuscular block is still common in the postsurgical unit.[23, 24]

Even small doses of muscle relaxants have clinically relevant effects as demonstrated by an investigation by Howardy-Hansen.[25] Although the measured TOF-ratio was 0.89 and more, 95% of all volunteers complained of "heavy eyelids" and approximately one third of the subjects had difficulties in swallowing. Similar findings were reported as well for the intermediate-acting relaxants atracurium and vecuronium.[26, 27] Then, in 1997, Kopman et al. presented results in volunteers that indicated that a TOF-ratio of 0.70 could no longer be regarded as an indicator for adequate neuromuscular function.[28] The authors reported that, even at TOF-ratios of 0.90, visual disturbances were present in all subjects. Diplopia and inability to follow moving objects, in this study associated with a TOF-ratio < 0.90, even persisted when the TOF-ratio had fully recovered. Although, the 5-sec head lift, regarded as a reliable clinical sign of full recovery from neuromuscular block[19], could be performed in every subject when the TOF-ratio was > 0.70, grip strength was still significantly reduced. Furthermore, when the TOF-ratio was < 0.75, "all subjects were uncomfortable".[28] In that study, masseter muscle strength was found to be more reliable than head-lift or leg-lift in detecting a small residual neuromuscular block.

Small doses of muscle relaxants also influence ventilation through other mechanisms. Gal[29] reported that with partial paralysis after a small dose of d-tubocurarine, no decrease in ventilation could be detected. Although tidal volumes decreased with increasing paralysis, appropriate resting minute ventilation was maintained by an increased respiratory frequency. As a result, a partially paralysed patient remains normocapnic despite weak peripheral skeletal muscles. This was confirmed by the findings, that the ventilatory response to CO_2 is not significantly reduced under partial paralysis [29], hence the "respiratory sparing" of muscle relaxants. On the other hand, Eriksson has demonstrated in a number of studies[30-32], that in partially paralysed patients, ventilatory regulation is impaired during hypoxia. This effect, confirmed for atracurium, vecuronium and pancuronium, is explained with muscle relaxants interfering with signal transmission in the carotid bodies.[33] It was also shown, that the injection of small doses of vecuronium depresses phrenic nerve activity during hypoxia.[34]

The effect of muscle relaxants is known not to be identical in different muscle groups. In two studies, it was demonstrated that pharyngeal muscles, important for the maintenance of a patent airway, are more sensitive than peripheral muscles to the effects of small doses (0.02 mg/kg) of pancuronium[35] or intubating doses of mivacurium.[36] In another study, it was shown that upper airway function is impaired even after small doses of vecuronium (0.02 mg/kg), as indicated by the greater sensitivity of geniohyoid muscles than the diaphragm to vecuronium.[37] And at TOF-ratios of 0.90 or less, partial paralysis by vecuronium may cause dysfunction of pharyngeal muscles and an increased risk for aspiration.[38] A common feature of these different studies is that peripheral muscles are less sensitive to the effects of muscle relaxants than muscles of the pharynx. This means that any muscle weakness detected in peripheral muscles is almost certainly correlated with problems in maintaining a patent airway and difficulties in swallowing. Extubation of the trachea should therefore not be attempted before complete recovery of neuromuscular transmission.

In another attempt to quantify the effects of a small dose of muscle relaxants, Mahajan has found that after 0.01 mg/kg vecuronium, a dose used as a priming dose, all patients developed ptosis, several had diplopia or were unable to swallow.[39] Furthermore, in eight of ten patients, the SpO_2 decreased significantly.[39]

The effect of small doses of muscle relaxants can be regarded as indicative for the residual effect of doses used in clinical practice. Hence, the findings of these studies suggest that the administration of muscle relaxants influences outcome of patients having undergone surgery. However, only a recently published prospective study by Berg et al.[40] confirmed this relationship. In that study, 693 patients were evaluated with regard to potential causes for postoperative pulmonary complications. The first finding of that study was that, postoperatively, a residual neuromuscular block (TOF-ratio < 0.70) could be detected in 17% of all patients after pancuronium and in 4% of all patients following atracurium or vecuronium, thus confirming earlier findings (see above). A residual block following pancuronium was identified to be a major risk factor for the development of pulmonary complications in the week following surgery, in particular when combined with long-lasting abdominal surgery and in old age.

In view of the studies described above and in the context of a changing clinical practice of anaesthesia (in particular ambulatory anaesthesia), the historical criteria and clinical "gold standards" to exclude residual neuromuscular paralysis (TOF-ratio > 0.70; head-lift or leg-lift) do no longer seem to equal adequate recovery of neuromuscular function. As a consequence, almost complete recovery of neuromuscular transmission (TOF-ratio > 0.90) is to be recommended as a standard criterion before a patient can be discharged from post-operative surveillance. Brull, in a recent editorial[41], has pointed out, that residual paralysis may persist for up to one hour, even after mivacurium-induced block, and that such residual muscle weakness is likely to persist for much longer even after intermediate-acting muscle relaxants, such as atracurium, vecuronium, cisatracurium and rocuronium.

Reversal of neuromuscular block

Ballantyne has shown in a recent study, that the use of long-acting muscle relaxants was associated with prolonged postoperative recovery.[72] Despite routine reversal with neostigmine or glycopyrrulate, in that study, recovery after atracurium was 104 minutes, 18 min faster than after vecuronium (122 min), while recovery after pancuronium was 172 min. Although neuromuscular transmission was not measured in the postoperative phase, this study emphasises the potential clinical relevance of residual neuromuscular block. Even after the administration of mivacurium, Bevan found a high incidence of residual block when the block had not been antagonised at the end of surgery.[24] Consequently, even after short-acting muscle relaxants spontaneous recovery can be slow enough to make residual block visible in the recovery room. Accordingly, pharmacological reversal of neuromuscular block should be based on the findings of neuromuscular monitoring and considered whenever necessary, even after the use of a short-acting relaxant. On the other hand, these facts stress the importance of the choice of a short- or intermediate-acting muscle relaxant for fast-tracking anaesthesia concepts.

Profiles of recently developed non-depolarising muscle relaxants

In the context of fast-tracking anaesthesia, the administration of long-acting muscle relaxants is not appropriate. Therefore, only the recent developments of intermediate and short-acting muscle relaxants will be presented. These new compounds can be classified into two chemical groups: muscle relaxants of the aminosteroidal type (rocuronium and rapacuronium) and those of the benzylisoquinolinium type (mivacurium and cisatracurium).

1. Aminosteroidal compounds

Rocuronium (ED_{95} 0.30 mg/kg[7]) has a time course of action similar to that of vecuronium, with the exception that its onset of action is faster.[42] After an intubating dose of 0.6 mg/kg rocuronium, the volume of distribution is about 0.2 L/kg, the clearance 3 $ml.kg^{-1}.min^{-1}$ and the terminal elimination half-life of rocuronium ($t_{½ß}$) 1.5 h.[43-45] The protein binding of rocuronium is 25%.[46] Rocuronium is assumed to be predominantly eliminated unchanged via the bile, and only to a lesser extent in the urine.[47-49] The recovery interval between 25% and 75% recovery from neuromuscular block (RI25-75) is reported to be between 9 and 19 min.[44, 50] Following repeated injections of rocuronium, the recovery interval is slightly prolonged[51-53], but, after a continuous infusion, Shanks and his group have measured a prolonged recovery interval of 20 to 30 minutes.[54]

Rapacuronium (ED_{95} 1.0 mg/kg active moiety[55]) is a new aminosteroidal muscle relaxant. The volume of distribution after 1.5 mg/kg rapacuronium is 450 ml/kg, the plasma clearance 6-9 $ml.kg^{-1}.min^{-1}$ and the terminal elimination half-life ($t_{½ß}$) 170-190 min.[56] Protein binding is reported to be 62%.[46] Twenty percent of a dose of rapacuronium is excreted in the urine as the parent compound or the metabolite. In patients with renal failure, a reduction in clearance has been found. This suggests that renal elimination is an important factor with respect to the clearance of the drug.[56] After 1.5 mg/kg rapacuronium, the onset of action is almost as rapid as that of succinylcholine, although with a greater variation.[57] Following rapid sequence induction, clinically acceptable intubating conditions after rapacuronium are achieved less frequently than after succinylcholine.[56] This may be explained by a less profound, although equally rapid, neuromuscular blocking effect at the vocal cords than at the adductor pollicis muscles.[58] The duration of action of a single dose of 1.5 mg/kg rapacuronium has been reported to be 14 min.[59] The recovery interval 25%-75% after that dose was 9 minutes [60] and the time from injection to a TOF-ratio > 0.70 was 30 minutes [59]. In another study, spontaneous recovery after three repeat doses or a 30 minute infusion of rapacuronium was 70 min.[61] That time was reduced to 9-10 minutes after the administration of neostigmine.[61] The 3-desacetyl metabolite of rapacuronium (Org9488) has neuromuscular blocking activity with an

ED_{95} of 0.5 mg/kg when assuming identical potency ratios in cats and humans.[8] This activity may become apparent after prolonged maintenance of relaxation with rapacuronium. The lower clearance of the metabolite, which is eliminated via the kidney[55], will gradually prolong the recovery from neuromuscular block after an infusion of rapacuronium.[8]

2. *Benzylisoquinolinium compounds*

Mivacurium is the first short-acting non-depolarising muscle relaxant (ED_{95} 0.08 mg/kg[62]). The rapid hydrolysis by plasma cholinesterase (in vitro at a rate of 80% of that of succinylcholine[10]) is responsible for its short duration of action. Mivacurium is a mixture of three stereoisomers. The only long-acting isomer (cis-cis) accounts for only 4% of the marketed drug. The volume of distribution of the remaining isomers is 0.3 l/kg, clearance during an infusion was 65-110 $ml.kg^{-1}.min^{-1}$ and the elimination half-lives of the two cis-trans and trans-trans isomers is 2 min.[60] Following 0.2 mg/kg mivacurium, complete neuromuscular block is attained at 2.5 min.[63] The clinical duration after that dose is 15-20 min.[10] The onset of mivacurium can be improved using a divided dose technique.[12] Within 90 sec after administration of equipotent doses (3^*ED_{95}), mivacurium 0.25mg/kg provided equal intubation conditions compared to rocuronium 0.9 mg/kg while the clinical duration of block (time to 25% T_1 recovery) was significantly shorter: 17 min for mivacurium versus 43 min for rocuronium. A study on the time course characteristics of neuromuscular block of up to 10 consecutive doses of mivacurium 0.6^*ED_{95} showed a very consistent and short duration of block of 9 min for each dose, confirming the lack of accumulation of this drug.[62] Recovery after discontinuation of an infusion was found in a recent study to be rapid and predictable: the recovery interval 25%-75% was 6 min and the time from discontinuation of the infusion to a TOF-ratio of 0.90 was 20 min.[64]

Cisatracurium (ED_{95} 0.05 mg/kg[65]) is the cis-cis isomer of atracurium. Clearance is 5 $ml.kg^{-1}.min^{-1}$ with Hofmann degradation accounting for 77% of that clearance.[66] The volume of distribution was found to be 0.15 L/kg and the elimination half-life is 22 min.[67] An important finding was that the pharmacokinetics are independent of the dose given.[67] Following intubation doses of 0.1 to 0.4 mg/kg, onset of action (time to 90% T_1 suppression) is attained at 3 to 1.5 min producing a clinical duration of block of 45 to 91 min respectively.[11, 65] The recovery interval (RI25-75) of cisatracurium following a continuous infusion of 2-4 h, is 15-18 min[11, 65] which is comparable to the recovery interval of a single bolus dose of 0.1-0.4 mg/kg.[65] These studies provide evidence that the neuromuscular blocking effect of cisatracurium is not cumulative. A comparative study in young patients (26 ± 6.4 yr) showed no difference in recovery profiles (RI25-75 and time interval 25% T_1 recovery to TOF ratio ≥ 0.75) between equipotent bolus doses of cisatracurium and rocuronium.[69] Another study compared the time course characteristics of neuromuscular block of cisatracurium and vecuronium administered as multiple bolus doses; the study population was stratified for young (18-64 years) and elderly (≥ 65 years) patients.[70] Spontaneous recovery time, defined as the time interval 25% T_1 recovery to TOF ratio ≥ 0.8, was faster for cisatracurium than vecuronium (28 versus 38 min). More interestingly, an age-related increase in clinical duration of neuromuscular block and spontaneous recovery time was found for vecuronium, whereas these values were similar between the young and elderly patients who received cisatracurium. The findings of this last study are consistent with a previous investigation that demonstrated a prolonged spontaneous recovery from neuromuscular block after multiple doses of vecuronium but not atracurium.[71]

Another advantage of cisatracurium is that this drug does not induce a dose dependent histamine release. Furthermore, even a dose as high as 8*ED_{95} shows a haemodynamic stable profile.[68] In summary, cisatracurium combines the cardiovascular stability, previously known from vecuronium, with pharmacological properties such as organ-independent elimination and predictable recovery, previously known from atracurium.

Conclusion

The different pharmacology of the two groups of muscle relaxants is reflected in different pharmacodynamic profiles: the aminosteroidal muscle relaxants rocuronium and rapacuronium have a low potency providing a fast onset of action. However, the pharmacology of these drugs may contribute to prolonged recovery time after administration of multiple doses or continuous infusion; in the group of the benzylisoquinolinium muscle relaxants, rapid metabolism of mivacurium (with the rare exception of patients with pseudocholinesterase deficiency) and Hofmann degradation of cisatracurium both lead to inactive compounds, providing both mivacurium and cisatracurium with predictable and fast recovery, even after administration in multiple repeat doses or continuous infusion.

Recent studies stress the importance of an almost complete recovery of neuromuscular transmission to achieve full neuromuscular function after the administration of muscle relaxants. This is particularly important when muscle relaxants are used in the context of new fast-tracking anaesthesia concepts. Discharge of patients from the recovery area is only possible when no effect of muscle relaxants impairs any muscle function of the patient. These rules almost exclude the use of a long-acting muscle relaxant for fast-tracking anaesthesia, and even influences the choice among the intermediate- and short-acting muscle relaxants. In general, the anaesthesiologist should know in detail the pharmacological properties of a chosen muscle relaxant, and restrict this choice to the muscle relaxant with a sufficiently short duration of action and a rapid and predictable recovery profile for fast-tracking anaesthesia.

References

1. Cheng DCH, Karski J, Peniston C, Ravendran G, Asokumar B, Carroll J, David T, Sandler A. Early tracheal extubation after coronary artery bypass graft surgery reduces costs and improves resource use. A prospective, randomized, controlled trial. Anesthesiol 1996; 85: 1300-10.
2. Mora CT, Dudek C, Torjman MC, White PF. The effects of anesthetic technique on the hemodynamic response and recovery profile in coronary revascularization patients. Anesth Analg 1995; 81: 900-10.
3. Lubarsky DA. Fast-track in the postanesthesia care unit: unlimited possibilities? J Clin Anesth 1996; 8: 70-2.
4. Bowman WC, Rodger IW, Houston J, Marshall, RJ, McIndewar, I. Structure:action relationships among some desacetoxy analogues of pancuronium and vecuronium in the anesthetized cat. Anesthesiol 1988; 69: 57-62.
5. Law Min JC, Bekavac I, Glavinovic MI, Donati F, Bevan DR. Iontophoretic study of speed of action of various muscle relaxants. Anesthesiol 1992; 77: 351-6.
6. Kopman AF, Klewicka MM, Kopman DJ, Neuman GG. Molar potency is predictive of the speed of onset of neuromuscular block for agents of intermediate, short, and ultrashort duration. Anesthesiol 1999; 90: 425-31.
7. Mellinghoff H, Diefenbach C, Bischoff A, Grond S, Buzello, W. Dose-response relationship of rocuronium bromide during intravenous anaesthesia. Eur J Anaesthesiol Suppl 1994; 9: 20-4.
8. Van den Broek L, Wierda JMKH, Smeulers NJ, Proost, JH. Pharmacodynamics and pharmacokinetics of an infusion of Org 9487, a new short-acting steroidal neuromuscular blocking agent. Br J Anaesth 1994; 73: 331-5.

9. Savarese JJ. Some considerations on the new muscle relaxants. Anesth Analg 1998; (Suppl.): 119-27.
10. Savarese JJ, Ali HH, Basta SJ, Embree PB, Scott RPF, Sunder N, Weakly JN, Wastila WB, El Sayad HA. The clinical neuromuscular pharmacology of mivacurium chloride (BW B1090U). A short-acting nondepolarizing ester neuromuscular blocking drug. Anesthesiol 1988; 68: 723-32.
11. Mellinghoff H, Radbruch L, Diefenbach C, Buzello W. A comparison of cisatracurium and atracurium: Onset of neuromuscular block after bolus injection and recovery after subsequent infusion. Anesth Analg 1996; 83: 1072-75.
12. Pino RM, Ali HH, Denman BT, Barrett PS, Schwartz A. A comparison of the intubation conditions between mivacurium and rocuronium during balanced anesthesia. Anesthesiol 1998; 88: 673-8.
13. Plaud B, Proost JH, Wierda JMKH, Barre J, Debaene B, Meistelman, C. Pharmacokinetics and pharmacodynamics of rocuronium at the vocal cords and the adductor pollicis in humans. Clin Pharm Ther 1995; 58: 185-91.
14. Plaud B, Debaene B, Lequeau F, Meistelman C, Donati F. Mivacurium neuromuscular block at the adductor muscles of the larynx and adductor pollicis in humans. Anesthesiol 1996; 85: 77-81.
15. Waud BE, Waud DR. The relation between tetanic fade and receptor occlusion in the presence of competitive neuromuscular block. Anesthesiol 1971; 35: 456-64.
16. Ali HH, Utting JE, Gray TC. Quantitative assessment of residual antidepolarizing block. I. Br J Anaesth 1971; 43: 473-7.
17. Ali HH, Utting JE, Gray TC. Quantitative assessment of residual antidepolarizing block. II. Br J Anaesth 1971; 43: 478-85.
18. Brand JB, Cullen DJ, Wilson NE, Ali HH. Spontaneous recovery from nondepolarizing neuromuscular blockade: correlation between clinical and evoked responses. Anesth Analg 1977; 56: 55-8.
19. Miller RD. How should residual neuromuscular blockade be detected? Anesthesiol 1989; 70: 379-80.
20. Viby Mogensen J, Jorgensen BC, Ording H. Residual curarization in the recovery room. Anesthesiol 1979; 50: 539-41.
21. Bevan DR, Smith CE, Donati F. Postoperative neuromuscular blockade: A comparison between atracurium, vecuronium, and pancuronium. Anesthesiol 1988; 69: 272-6.
22. Kong KL, Cooper GM. Recovery of neuromuscular function and postoperative morbidity following blockade by atracurium, alcuronium and vecuronium. Anaesthesia 1988; 43: 450-3.
23. Fawcett WJ, Dash A, Francis GA, Liban JB, Cashman JN. Recovery from neuromuscular blockade: residual curarisation following atracurium or vecuronium by bolus dosing or infusions. Acta Anaesthesiol Scand 1995; 39: 288-93.
24. Bevan DR, Kahwaji R, Ansermino JM, Reimer E, Smith MF, O'Connor GA, Bevan JC. Residual block after mivacurium with or without edrophonium reversal in adults and children. Anesthesiol 1996; 84: 362-7.
25. Howardy Hansen P, Jorgensen BC, Ording H, Viby Mogensen J. Pretreatment with non-depolarizing muscle relaxants: the influence on neuromuscular transmission and pulmonary function. Acta Anaesthesiol Scand 1980; 24: 419-22.
26. Engbaek J, Howardy-Hansen P, Ording H, Viby-Mogensen J. Precurarization with vecuronium and pancuronium in awake, healthy volunteers: the influence on neuromuscular transmission and pulmonary function. Acta Anaesthesiol Scand 1985 Jan; 29: 117-20.

27. Howardy-Hansen P, Moeller J, Hansen B. Pretreatment with atracurium: the influence on neuromuscular transmission and pulmonary function. Acta Anaesthesiol Scand 1987; 31: 642-4.
28. Kopman AF, Yee PS, Neuman GG. Relationship of the train-of-four fade ratio to clinical signs and symptoms of residual paralysis in awake volunteers. Anesthesiol 1997; 86: 765-71.
29. Gal TJ, Smith TC. Partial paralysis with d-tubocurarine and the ventilatory response to CO2: An example of respiratory sparing? Anesthesiol 1976; 45: 22-8.
30. Eriksson LI, Lennmarken C, Wyon N, Johnson, A. Attenuated ventilatory response to hypoxaemia at vecuronium-induced partial neuromuscular block. Acta Anaesthesiol Scand 1992; 36: 710-5.
31. Eriksson LI, Sato M, Severinghaus, JW. Effect of a vecuronium-induced partial neuromuscular block on hypoxic ventilatory response. Anesthesiol 1993; 78: 693-9.
32. Eriksson LI. Reduced hypoxic chemosensitivity in partially paralysed man. A new property of muscle relaxants? Acta Anaesthesiol Scand 1996; 40: 520-3.
33. Wyon N, Joensen H, Yamamoto Y, Lindahl SGE, Eriksson LI. Carotid body chemoreceptor function is impaired by vecuronium during hypoxia. Anesthesiol 1998; 89: 1471-9.
34. Wyon N, Eriksson LI, Yamamoto Y, Lindahl SGE. Vecuronium-induced depression of phrenic nerve activity during hypoxia in the rabbit. Anesth Analg 1996; 82: 1252-6.
35. Isono S, Ide T, Kochi T, Mizuguchi T, Nishino T. Effects of partial paralysis on the swallowing reflex in conscious humans. Anesthesiol 1991; 75: 980-4.
36. d'Honneur G, Slavov V, Merle JC, Kirov K, Rimaniol JM, Sperry L, Duvaldestin, P. Comparison of the effects of mivacurium on the diaphragm and geniohyoid muscles. Br J Anaesth 1996; 77: 716-9.
37. Isono S, Kochi T, Ide T, Sugimori K, Mizuguchi T, Nishino T. Differential Effects of Vecuronium on Diaphragm and Geniohyoid Muscle in Anaesthetized Dogs. Br J Anaesth 1992; 68: 239-43.
38. Eriksson LI, Sundman E, Olsson R, Nilsson L, Witt H, Ekberg O, Kuylenstiema, R. Functional assessment of the pharynx at rest and during swallowing in partially paralyzed humans: Simultaneous videomanometry and mechanomyography of awake human volunteers. Anesthesiol 1997; 87: 1035-43.
39. Mahajan RP, Hennessy N, Aitkenhead, AR: Effect of Priming Dose of Vecuronium on Lung Function in Elderly Patients. Anesth Analg 1993; 77: 1198-1202.
40. Berg H, Viby Mogensen J, Roed J, Mortensen CR, Engbaek J, Skovgaard LT, Krintel, JJ. Residual neuromuscular block is a risk factor for postoperative pulmonary complications - A prospective, randomised, and blinded study of postoperative pulmonary complications after atracurium, vecuronium and pancuronium. Acta Anaesthesiol Scand 1997; 41: 1095-103.
41. Brull SJ. Indicators of recovery of neuromuscular function: Time for change? Anesthesiol 1997; 86: 755-7.
42. Booth MG, Marsh B, Bryden FM, Robertson EN, Baird, WL. A comparison of the pharmacodynamics of rocuronium and vecuronium during halothane anaesthesia. Anaesthesia 1992; 47: 832-4.
43. Szenohradszky J, Fisher DM, Segredo V, Caldwell JE, Bragg P, Sharma ML, Gruenke L D, Miller RD. Pharmacokinetics of rocuronium bromide (ORG 9426) in patients with normal renal function or patients undergoing cadaver renal transplantation. Anesthesiol 1992; 77: 899-904.
44. Cooper RA, Maddineni VR, Mirakhur RK, Wierda JM, Brady M, Fitzpatrick KT. Time course of neuromuscular effects and pharmacokinetics of rocuronium bromide

(Org 9426) during isoflurane anaesthesia in patients with and without renal failure. Br J Anaesth 1993; 71: 222-6.
45. Khalil M, Dhonneur G, Duvaldestin P, Slavov V, Dehys C, Gomeni R. Pharmacokinetics and pharmacodynamics of rocuronium in patients with cirrhosis. Anesthesiol 1994; 80: 1241-7.
46. Wierda JM, Proost JH. Structure-pharmacodynamic-pharmacokinetic relationships of steroidal neuromuscular blocking agents. Eur J Anaesthesiol Suppl 1995; 11: 45-54
47. Alvarez Gomez JA, Estelles ME, Fabregat J, Perez F, Brugger AJ. Pharmacokinetics and pharmacodynamics of rocuronium bromide in adult patients. Eur J Anaesthesiol Suppl 1994; 9: 53-6.
48. van den Broek L, Wierda JM, Smeulers NJ, van Santen GJ, Leclercq MG, Hennis PJ. Clinical pharmacology of rocuronium (Org 9426): study of the time course of action, dose requirement, reversibility, and pharmacokinetics. J Clin Anesth 1994; 6: 288-96.
49. Wierda JM, Kleef UW, Lambalk LM, Kloppenburg WD, Agoston S. The pharmacodynamics and pharmacokinetics of Org 9426, a new non-depolarizing neuromuscular blocking agent, in patients anaesthetized with nitrous oxide, halothane and fentanyl. Can J Anaesth 1991; 38: 430-5.
50. Huizinga AC, van den Brom RH, Wierda JM, Hommes FD, Hennis PJ. Intubating conditions and onset of neuromuscular block of rocuronium (Org 9426); a comparison with suxamethonium. Acta Anaesthesiol Scand 1992; 36: 463-8.
51. Khuenl-Brady KS, Pühringer F, Koller J, Mitterschiffthaler, G. Evaluation of the time course of action of maintenance doses of rocuronium (ORG 9426) under halothane anaesthesia. Acta Anaesthesiol Scand 1993; 37: 137-9.
52. Lambalk LM, De Wit AP, Wierda JM, Hennis PJ, Agoston S. Dose-response relationship and time course of action of Org 9426. A new muscle relaxant of intermediate duration evaluated under various anaesthetic techniques. Anaesthesia 1991; 46: 907-11.
53. Quill TJ, Begin M, Glass PS, Ginsberg B, Gorback MS. Clinical responses to ORG 9426 during isoflurane anesthesia. Anesth Analg 1991; 72: 203-6.
54. Shanks CA, Fragen RJ, Ling D. Continuous intravenous infusion of rocuronium (ORG 9426) in patients receiving balanced, enflurane, or isoflurane anesthesia. Anesthesiol 1993; 78: 649-51.
55. Schiere S, Proost JH, Schuringa M, Wierda JMKH. Pharmacokinetics and pharmacokinetic-dynamic relationship between rapacuronium (Org 9487) and its 3-desacetyl metabolite (Org 9488). Anesth Analg 1999; 88: 640-7.
56. Szenohradszky J, Caldwell JE, Wright PMC, Brown R, Lau M, Luks AM, Fisher, DM. Influence of renal failure on the pharmacokinetics and neuromuscular effects of a single dose of rapacuronium bromide. Anesthesiol 1999; 90: 24-35.
57. Wierda JMKH, van den Broek L, Proost JH, Verbaan BW, Hennis PJ. Time Course of Action and Endotracheal Intubating Conditions of Org-9487, a New Short-Acting Steroidal Muscle Relaxant - A Comparison with Succinylcholine. Anesth Analg 1993; 77: 579-84.
58. Debaene B, Lieutaud T, Billard V, Meistelman C. ORG 9487 neuromuscular block at the adductor pollicis and the laryngeal adductor muscles in humans. Anesthesiol 1997; 86: 1300-5.
59. Kahwaji R, Bevan DR, Bikhazi G, Shanks CA, Fragen RJ, Dyck JB, Angst MS, Matteo R. Dose-ranging study in younger adult and elderly patients of ORG 9487, a new, rapid-onset, short-duration muscle relaxant. Anesth Analg 1997; 84: 1011-8.
60. Lien CA, Schmith VD, Embree PB, Belmont MR, Wargin WA, Savarese JJ. The pharmacokinetics and pharmacodynamics of the stereoisomers of mivacurium in

patients receiving nitrous oxide/opioid/barbiturate anesthesia. Anesthesiol 1994; 80: 1296-1302.
61. McCourt KC, Mirakhur RK, Lowry DW, Carroll MT, Sparr HJ. Spontaneous or neostigmine-induced recovery after maintenance of neuromuscular block with Org 9487 (Rapacuronium) or rocuronium following an initial dose of Org 9487. Br J Anaesth 1999; 82: 755-6.
62. Diefenbach C, Mellinghoff H, Lynch J, Buzello W. Mivacurium: dose-response relationship and administration by repeated injection or infusion. Anesth Analg 1992; 74: 420-3.
63. Maddineni VR, Mirakhur RK, Mccoy EP, Fee JPH, Clarke RSJ. Neuromuscular Effects and Intubating Conditions Following Mivacurium - A Comparison with Suxamethonium. Anaesthesia 1993; 48: 940-5.
64. Lien CA, Belmont MR, Abalos A, Hass D, Savarese JJ. The nature of spontaneous recovery from mivacurium-induced neuromuscular block. Anesth Analg 1999; 88: 648-653.
65. Belmont MR, Lien CA, Quessy S, Aboudonia MM, Abalos A, Eppich L, Savarese JJ. The clinical neuromuscular pharmacology of 51W89 in patients with receiving nitrous oxide/opioid/barbiturate anesthesia. Anesthesiol 1995; 82: 1139-45.
66. Kisor DF, Schmith VD, Wargin WA, Lien CA, Ornstein E, Cook DR. Importance of the organ-independent elimination of cisatracurium. Anesth Analg 1996; 83: 1065-71.
67. Lien CA, Schmith VD, Belmont MR, Abalos A, Kisor DF, Savarese JJ. Pharmacokinetics of cisatracurium in patients receiving nitrous oxide/opioid/barbiturate anesthesia. Anesthesiol 1996; 84: 300-8.
68. Lien CA, Belmont MR, Abalos A, Eppich L, Quessy S, Aboudonia MM, Savarese JJ. The cardiovascular effects and histamine-releasing properties of 51W89 in patients receiving nitrous oxide/opioid/barbiturate anesthesia. Anesthesiol 1995; 82: 1131-8.
69. Naguib M, Samarkandi AH, Ammar A, Elfaqih SR, AlZahrani S, Turkistani A. Comparative clinical pharmacology of rocuronium, cisatracurium, and their combination. Anesthesiol 1998; 89: 1116-24.
70. Eriksson LI, Pühringer F, Engbaek J, Heier T, Viby-Mogensen J. A double-blind comparison of the pharmacodynamic and safety profiles of cisatracurium and vecuronium. Br J Anaesth 1999; 82: in press.
71. Diefenbach C, Mellinghoff H, Grond S, Buzello W. Atracurium and vecuronium: repeated bolus injection versus infusion. Anesth Analg 1992; 74: 519-22.
72. Ballantyne JC, Chang YC. The impact of choice of muscle relaxant on postoperative recovery time: A retrospective study. Anesth Analg 1997; 85: 476-82.

NEUROMUSCULAR BLOCKING AGENTS IN THE ELDERLY

Frederique Servin

Paris, France

Introduction

Drug dosing schemes of anaesthetic agents in elderly patients are often a challenge for the clinician, and neuromuscular blocking agents (NMBA) are no exception to this rule. Only a good insight in the pharmacokinetic and pharmacodynamic changes in the elderly may allow a rational use of these agents in elderly patients.

Clinical findings

Onset of action

The onset of action of NMBAs is usually prolonged in the elderly, whatever the study drug (vecuronium[1], rocuronium[2], pipecuronium[3], succinylcholine[1], cis-atracurium[4,5] and doxacurium[6]). In studies where no difference in NMBA onset times has been found between elderly and younger patients (vecuronium[7], rocuronium[8], mivacurium[9]), the initial dose was 2 to 3 times the ED95, thus precluding an accurate measurement of the time to maximal effect.

Maintenance doses and continuous infusion

The duration of action of maintenance doses of rocuronium[2] and vecuronium[10] is significantly prolonged in the elderly, whereas that of atracurium doses[10] is not. The maintenance infusion rate of mivacurium required to ensure adequate muscle relaxation is lower in elderly patients[9,11,12]. Hart et al[13] have demonstrated a strong influence of pseudocholinesterase activity on the mivacurium infusion rates required to maintain 50% or 90% twitch depression. Similarly in Goudsouzian's study, the lowest infusion rate was observed in patients with low pseudocholinesterase activity[12].

Recovery

Recovery for muscle relaxation is usually delayed in elderly patients. Thus, the recovery index from 25% to 75% recovery of twitch height is increased by 60% (39 to 62 min) for pancuronium[14], 230% (15 to 49 min) for vecuronium[15], 62% (13 to 21 min) for rocuronium[8], 42% (5.5 to 7.8 min) for mivacurium[9]; and the time to reach 25% recovery of twitch height is delayed in the elderly for doxacurium by 43% (68 to 97 min)[6]. On the contrary, recovery from muscle relaxation is not modified by ageing for atracurium[10], cisatracurium[4], and pipecuronium[3].

Pharmacokinetic changes

As a result of the ageing process a number of changes occur such as deterioration in renal and hepatic function, alteration in body composition with a decrease in lean body mass and in total body water. As a consequence, the pharmacokinetics of muscle relaxants is modified in elderly patients.

Steroid compounds

The muscle relaxants with a steroid structure (pancuronium, vecuronium, rocuronium, pipecuronium, and rapacuronium) are mainly eliminated by the liver through metabolism and biliary excretion, and partially excreted in the urine. Their large molecules are highly ionised regardless of pH, which limits their distribution to the extracellular compartment. As a consequence, their volume of distribution can be expected to remain unchanged or to slightly decrease with ageing. Indeed, pancuronium and pipecuronium distribution volumes remain unchanged whereas vecuronium and rocuronium have significantly reduced distribution volumes in the elderly (table 1).

Pancuronium is predominantly (30 to 70 %) excreted unchanged in the urine, and approximately 20% of the drug undergoes deacetylation. Glomerular filtration rate is reduced in the elderly, and as a consequence, so is the clear-

Table 1
Volume of distribution of NMBAs (L/kg) (mean ± SD)

Agent	Younger patients	Elderly patients
Pancuronium		
V_{DAUC}[14]	0.28 ± 0.06	0.32 ± 0.10
Vss[16]	0.21 ± 0.08	0.22 ± 0.04
Vecuronium		
Vss[16]	0.24 ± 0.04	0.18 ± 0.03 *
Rocuronium		
V_{DAUC}[8]	0.55 ± 0.28	0.40 ± 0.12 *
Pipecuronium		
Vss[3]	0.31 ± 0.07	0.39 ± 0.13
Atracurium		
Vss[18]	0.10 ± 0.02	0.19 ± 0.06 *
Mivacurium[25]		
Trans-trans	0.23 ± 0.11	0.20 ± 0.10
Cis-trans	0.52 ± 0.32	0.24 ± 0.16 *
Cis-cis	0.25 ± 0.11	0.35 ± 0.19
Cisatracurium		
Vss[4]	0.11 ± 0.01	0.13 ± 0.01 *
Doxacurium		
Vss[6]	0.15 ± 0.04	0.22 ± 0.08 *

* $p<0.05$

Table 2
Elimination clearance of NMBAs ($ml.kg^{-1}.min^{-1}$) (mean ± SD)

Agent	Younger patients	Elderly patients
Pancuronium[14]	1.8 ± 0.4	1.2 ± 0.4 *
[16]	1.5 ± 0.5	1.2 ± 0.3
Vecuronium[16]	5.2 ± 0.8	3.7 ± 1.0 *
Rocuronium[8]	5.0 ± 1.5	3.7 ± 1.0 *
Pipecuronium[3]	2.5 ± 0.7	2.4 ± 1.0
Atracurium[18]	5.3 ± 0.9	6.5 ± 1.1
Mivacurium[25]		
Cis-trans	74 ± 39	39 ± 17 *
Trans-trans	45 ± 22	27 ± 10 *
Cis-cis	4.2 ± 1.2	4.5 ± 1.2
Cisatracurium[4]	5.0 ± 0.9	4.6 ± 0.8
Doxacurium[6]	2.2 ± 1.1	2.5 ± 0.7

* $p<0.05$

ance of pancuronium[14] (table 2). Nevertheless, phase I metabolic reactions are not consistently modified by ageing, and when urinary excretion is reduced, it is possible that some enhancement of the metabolic rate of pancuronium exists, explaining why in some studies no difference in pancuronium clearance was found between younger adults and elderly patients[16]. If this is the case, a greater proportion of active metabolite might be produced in the elderly.

Vecuronium is scarcely metabolised, with 40% excreted unchanged in the bile and 30% in the urine. A limited amount of the drug (30%) is deacetylated in the liver with one active metabolite. As both liver blood flow and glomerular filtration rate are reduced in the elderly, vecuronium clearance is reduced by approximately 30% in this population[16].

The elimination of rocuronium is very similar to that of vecuronium with approximately 75% eliminated in the bile and 10% in the urine. A little rocuronium undergoes deacetylation, and no significantly active metabolites are produced. Rocuronium clearance is also reduced by 30% in the elderly[8].

In conclusion, pharmacokinetic parameters for steroid NMBAs are significantly but moderately modified by ageing, with a trend towards reduction in both clearance (around 30%) and distribution volumes (around 25%). These modifications have been proposed to explain prolonged duration of action, but this prolongation (at least 60%) appears important when compared to the kinetic changes.

Benzylisoquinoliniums

The currently available benzylisoquinoliniums include atracurium, mivacurium, cisatracurium and doxacurium. Atracurium and mivacurium are mixtures of stereoisomers with varying potencies and pharmacokinetics. Cisatracurium is one of the ten isomers of atracurium.

Atracurium is a mixture of ten isomers, one of them being cisatracurium. No study has yet considered the pharmacokinetics of the different atracurium isomers in young and elderly patients, and the published data have all taken atracurium as if it was a single compound, which is not accurate, but much less complex. Mivacurium is a mixture of three isomers, two of them (cis-trans and trans-trans), potent and metabolised by plasma pseudocholinesterases represent more than 90% of the mivacurium dose. The less potent cis-cis isomer represents less than 10% of the dose, and participates only marginally to mivacurium relaxant action[12].

Like steroid NMBAs, benzylisoquinoliniums are big molecules that do not travel through lipophilic barriers easily. Their distribution volumes are therefore in the same order of magnitude compared to that of the steroid compounds (table 1). Distribution volumes of benzylisoquinoliniums are slightly enhanced in elderly patients (table 1). This may be due to a potential decrease in plasma protein binding in this population, these compounds being more extensively protein bound than the steroids.

Biodisposition of benzylisoquinolinium compounds is very varied. Some of them (doxacurium) are not metabolised at all but are excreted mainly in the urine and marginally in the bile. Atracurium and cisatracurium undergo spontaneous degradation through Hofmann elimination and ester hydrolysis. This process accounts for about 83% of cisatracurium elimination clearance, but only for about 40% of the elimination clearance of atracurium[17]. The part of the atracurium that does not undergo Hofmann elimination is probably metabolised mainly in the liver. If the elimination clearance of atracurium is not modified by ageing, its organ clearance is reduced, but this reduction is counterbalanced by an enhancement of non-organ clearance[18]. The main mivacurium isomers are metabolised by plasma pseudocholinesterases and the cis-cis isomer has a much lower clearance. Maddineni, in a letter to the British Journal of Anaesthesia[19], reported a decrease in pseudocholinesterase activity in elderly patients when compared to younger ones, though the activity remained in the normal range. This observation, which has not been confirmed by a full manuscript, might contribute to the reduced trans-trans and cis-trans isomers clearances (table 2).

Effect site concentration

Muscle blood flow has been suggested as a factor that influences delivery of drugs to the end plate[20]. Regional blood flows, including muscle blood flow, are reduced in elderly people[21]. There might therefore exist a more important concentration gradient between the effect site and the plasma in elderly patients, illustrated by a lower exit rate constant (ke0) in the aged. The slow onset and longer duration of action of most NMBAs in elderly patients, poorly explained by the scarce changes in elimination kinetics might correspond to this phenomenon. When cisatracurium was studied, the time to maximum block was more rapid in young patients compared with elderly ones, owing to a reduction in ke0 with age[5].

Pharmacodynamics

So far, all the clinical changes in NMBA behaviour in elderly patients have been explained by pharmacokinetic but not pharmacodynamic alterations[22]. Plasma concentrations corresponding to a fixed degree of paralysis are not modified by ageing (pancuronium[14], Conversely, the concentration response relationships remain usually unchanged[2-6,8,14,16,18,23,24], suggesting that the ageing process has no influence on the pharmacodynamic component of NMBAs behaviour.

Conclusion

The analysis of the currently available literature shows that muscle relaxant action is usually slower and longer in elderly patients, but ageing does not modify the sensitivity to those compounds. For some compounds, there is a discrepancy between the clinical profile and the pharmacokinetic changes that might at least partially be explained by a slower transfer rate to the effect site. The duration of action of atracurium and cisatracurium is not modified by ageing and may therefore be the drugs of choice in this patient population. These agents may therefore be the drugs of choice in this patient population.

References

1. Koscielniak-Nielsen Z J, Bevan J C, Popovic V, et al.Onset of maximum neuromuscular block following succinylcholine or vecuronium in four age groups. Anesthesiology 1993 ; 79 : 229-34.
2. Bevan D R, Fiset P, Balendran P, et al.Pharmacodynamic behaviour of rocuronium in the elderly. Can J Anaesth 1993 ; 40 : 127-32.
3. Ornstein E, Matteo R S, Schwartz A E, et al.Pharmacokinetics and pharmacodynamics of pipecuronium bromide (Arduan) in elderly surgical patients. Anesth Analg 1992 ; 74 : 841-4.
4. Ornstein E w, Lien C A, Matteo R S, et al.Pharmacodynamics and pharmacokinetics of cisatracurium in geriatric surgical patients. Anesthesiology 1996 ; 84 : 520-5.

5. Sorooshian S S, Stafford M A, Eastwood N B, et al.Pharmacokinetics and pharmacodynamics of cisatracurium in young and elderly adult patients. Anesthesiology 1996; 84 : 1083-91.
6. Dresner D L, Basta S J, Ali H H, et al.Pharmacokinetics and pharmacodynamics of doxacurium in young and elderly patients during isoflurane anesthesia. Anesth Analg 1990 ; 71 : 498-502.
7. McCarthy G, Elliott P, Mirakhur R K, et al.Onset and duration of action of vecuronium in the elderly: comparison with adults. Acta Anaesthesiol Scand 1992 ; 36 : 383-6.
8. Matteo R S, Ornstein E, Schwartz A E, et al.Pharmacokinetics and pharmacodynamics of rocuronium (Org 9426) in elderly surgical patients. Anesth Analg 1993 ; 77 : 1193-7.
9. Maddineni V R, Mirakhur R K, McCoy E P, et al.Neuromuscular and haemodynamic effects of mivacurium in elderly and young adult patients. Br J Anaesth 1994 ; 73 : 608-12.
10. Slavov V, Khalil M, Merle J C, et al.Comparison of duration of neuromuscular blocking effect of atracurium and vecuronium in young and elderly patients. Br J Anaesth 1995 ; 74 : 709-11.
11. Dahaba A A, Rehak P H and List W F.A comparison of mivacurium infusion requirements between young and elderly adult patients. Eur J Anaesthesiol 1996 ; 13: 43-8.
12. Goudsouzian N, Chakravorti S, Denman W, et al.Prolonged mivacurium infusion in young and elderly adults. Can J Anaesth 1997 ; 44 : 955-62.
13. Hart P S, McCarthy G J, Brown R, et al.The effect of plasma cholinesterase activity on mivacurium infusion rates. Anesth Analg 1995 ; 80 : 760-3.
14. Duvaldestin P, Saada J, Berger J L, et al.Pharmacokinetics, pharmacodynamics, and dose-response relationships of pancuronium in control and elderly subjects. Anesthesiology 1982 ; 56 : 36-40.
15. Lien C A, Matteo R S, Ornstein E, et al.Distribution, elimination, and action of vecuronium in the elderly. Anesth Analg 1991 ; 73 : 39-42.
16. Rupp S M, Castagnoli K P, Fisher D M, et al.Pancuronium and vecuronium pharmacokinetics and pharmacodynamics in younger and elderly adults. Anesthesiology 1987 ; 67 : 45-9.
17. Fisher D M, Canfell P C, Fahey M R, et al.Elimination of atracurium in humans: contribution of Hafmann elimination and ester hydrolysis versus organ-based elimination. Anesthesiology 1986 ; 65 : 6-12.
18. Kitts J B, Fisher D M, Canfell P C, et al.Pharmacokinetics and pharmacodynamics of atracurium in the elderly. Anesthesiology 1990 ; 72 : 272-5.
19. Maddineni V R, Mirakhur R K and McCoy E P.Plasma cholinesterase activity in elderly and young adults [letter]. Br J Anaesth 1994 ; 72 : 497.
20. Donati F.Onset of action of relaxants. Can J Anaesth 1988 ; 35 : pS52-8.
21. Fleg J.Alterations in cardiovascular structure and function with advancing age. Am J Cardiol 1986 ; 57 : 33c-44c.
22. Parker C J, Hunter J M and Snowdon S L.Effect of age, gender and anaesthetic technique on the pharmacodynamics of atracurium. Br J Anaesth 1993 ; 70 : 38-41.
23. Bell P F, Mirakhur R K and Clarke R S.Dose-response studies of atracurium, vecuronium and pancuronium in the elderly. Anaesthesia 1989 ; 44 : 925-7.
24. D'Hollander A A, Nevelsteen M, Barvais L, et al.Effect of age on the establishement of muscle paralysis induced in anesthetized adult subjects by ORG NC45. Acta Anaesth Scand 1983 ; 27 : 108-110.
25. Servin F, Lavaut E, Peytavin G, et al. A pharmacokinetic and dynamic study of mivacurium infusion in elderly patients. Anesthesiology 1997 ; 87 : A855.

THE USE OF NEUROMUSCULAR BLOCKING AGENTS IN THE ICU

Karin S. Khünl-Brady

Innsbruck, Austria

Introduction

The rapid development in the field of intensive care medicine, particularly during the past 20 years, is characterised by spectacular advances in monitoring techniques that, however, are not paralleled by the development of equally advanced pharmacotherapeutic concepts for the use of drugs in the intensive care unit (ICU). This holds true for sedatives and analgesic drugs but specially for neuromuscular blocking agents. The frequency of use of sedatives and analgesics in various hospitals and the choice of the individual neuromuscular blocking agents are extremely variable and hardly based on anything more than empiricism dominated by local standards and the physician's personal preferences.[1]

In Europe approximately 0% to 25% of ventilated patients require a muscle relaxant during a period of their stay in the ICU. Until recently, this seemed to be the opposite in the United States; almost every ventilated patient received a muscle relaxant for a variable length of time.[2] According to one of the first surveys on primary muscle relaxants used in the ICU in the United States, including anaesthesiologists with a special certificate of competence in critical care, 52%, 28%, and 3% of the responders indicated vecuronium, pancuronium, and atracurium as compounds of their first choice, respectively.[3] The current choice of agent differs from the above as more and more muscle relaxants become available for use in the ICU.[4] Although the usefulness and safety of neuromuscular relaxants in surgical anaesthesia is widely accepted, detailed data in critically ill patients are scarce. More importantly, only the surgical application of muscle relaxants is supported by adequate animal pharmacology and toxicology. Yet in the ICU muscle relaxants are commonly employed for weeks without monitoring in doses exceeding those used in the operating room. The selection and dosing of muscle relaxants in the ICU do not seem to be of great concern because it is erroneously believed that these compounds can do no harm as long as the patient is ventilated.

Problems associated with the use of neuromuscular blocking agents

Critical illness polyneuropathy

This syndrome was first described by Zochodne and Bolton in 1987.[5] The clinical signs impose as muscle weakness with concomitant problems of weaning patients from the ventilator, especially after sepsis and multiple organ failure. Histological and electrophysiological signs consist of axon degeneration with (in most cases) normal nerve conduction velocity. Neurological changes are usually followed by myopathy, so the term "polyneuromyopathy" was created.[6] The aetiology of the critical illness polyneuropathy is still unclear, however, today it is considered to be a part of the systemic inflammatory response syndrome (SIRDS) of patients with multiple organ failure and/or septic syndrome. It is important to notice that in most cases neuromuscular blocking agents have not been involved at all.

Prolonged paralysis

During the past years, the number of reports on complications associated with the long-term use of neuromuscular blocking agents has increased considerably. The most frequently reported adverse events include muscle weakness with peripheral paresis, disuse muscular atrophy, occasionally with histological alterations consistent with pharmacological denervation, tetraplegia and areflexia, prolonged residual paralysis due to neuromuscular blockade, polyneuropathy and myopathy requiring ventilatory support for up to four months after termination of the administration of the muscle relaxant. The above complications have been described with the use of all available neuromuscular blocking drugs. The frequency of these case reports is not associated with a particular agent, but reflects mainly the frequency of their use. With a few exceptions, in most of the reported cases, no adequate neurologic differential diagnosis was carried out to distinguish between critically illness polyneuropathy, myopathy, or compromised neuromuscular transmission. In none of these reports is there any information on parenteral or enteral nutrition and daily carbohydrate intake. Clinical studies, however, indicate that impairment of carbohydrate metabolism may be an essential cause of polyneuropathy that might be confused with the various neuromuscular complications observed after long-term administration of neuromuscular blocking agents in the ICU.[7]

Most likely, the combination of the underlying disease and subsequent complications, concurrent administration of other drugs (antibiotics, but specially corticosteroids), alterations in the pharmacokinetics of the muscle relaxant, but also in the function of the neuromuscular transmission secondary to "pharmacological denervation" and, more importantly, absolute or relative overdoses of the paralysing agents will, to a variable extent, contribute to the complex causes of the reported neuromuscular complication. The use of excessive doses or irrational combinations of neuromuscular blocking agents is probably the most likely cause of prolonged paralysis in critically ill patients. These complications are even more likely to occur with the concomitant use of high dose corticosteroids and the lack of neuromuscular monitoring.[1, 8]

Tolerance development

Not only prolonged paralysis, but also tolerance development to muscle relaxants has been reported.[9-11] The continuous blockade of the acetylcholine receptors, leads to an upregulation of the number of receptors (much like that one observed during chronic therapy with ß- receptor blocking agent) and contributes to the increase in muscle relaxant requirements. Although the above changes occur in all ICU patients studied, tolerance development to neuromuscular blocking agents occurs only in some. It was shown that the number of acetylcholine receptors strongly correlated with the amount of muscle relaxant needed in patients developing tolerance to different neuromuscular blocking agents during long-term administration.[11]

Prevention of problems

Limited familiarity of the ICU staff with the pharmacology of muscle relaxants and the omission of monitoring of the neuromuscular blockade are probably the most important factors contributing to the injudicious use of muscle relaxants in the ICU setting.

Education

The medical staff of the ICU consists of anaesthesiologists, surgeons, specialists in internal medicine, paediatricians, and other healthcare professionals. However, only the anaesthesiologist is truly familiar with the use of neuromuscular blocking agents. Until recently, little or no information on optimal clinical dosing regimens for neuromuscular blocking agents in the ICU was available. Even standard textbooks on critical care medicine advise either doses that are used in surgical anaesthesia or provide only vague information on the pharmacological properties and erroneous dose recommendations for the use of neuromuscular blocking agents in the ICU.[12, 13] Therefore, it is not surprising that physicians and nurses in the ICU often equate neuromuscular blocking effects with sedation and analgesia, being insufficiently aware of the need for continuous sedation when muscle relaxants are used. There is obviously a need for an educational program for ICU physicians and nurses focused on the pharmacology and biodisposition of analgesics, sedatives, and neuromuscular blocking agents. Lately, this is increasingly done in newer editions of ICU text books and journals of intensive care nurses.[14, 15]

Monitoring

Critically ill patients have little in common with most surgical patients. Consequently, not only the drug use should be adapted for the specific requirements and tolerance of the critically ill, but also the monitoring techniques and criteria. For the assessment of the neuromuscular blockade, a peripheral nerve stimulator, used in the train-of-four (TOF) mode, seems to be a suitable satisfactory method. However, it remains an open question whether and how the confounding pathological conditions in the critically ill might affect neuromuscular transmission. In a recent report, two patients with diabetic polyneuropathy were described in whom, on repeated occasions, monitoring of neuromuscular blockade was impossible owing to failure of electric stimuli up to 100 mA to evoke twitch contraction of the adductor pollicis muscle.[16] This applies also for patients with sepsis, peripheral oedema and severe vasoconstriction. Conceivably, the TOF ratio may not be associated with the same level of neuromuscular blockade in surgical patients as in patients in the ICU, that often suffer from concurrent sepsis and critical illness polyneuropathy. Also a newly developed accelerographic monitor (TOF guard®), which was used in several studies in the ICU, may not give reliable results of TOF ratios in the critically ill patient.[17] Nevertheless, the peripheral nerve stimulator is the best available tool to be used for monitoring of the neuromuscular transmission during long-term administration of muscle relaxants in the ICU. It can be used (preferably) at the ulnar nerve at the wrist inducing contractions of the adductor muscle of the thumb, or at the posterior tibial nerve at the medial malleolus, inducing movements of the first toe. Visual and tactile assessment of the evoked responses is easy and reliable enough to protect the patient from inadvertent overdosing of the muscle relaxant.[1] During intermittent bolus administration, maintenance doses should not be given before the second response of the TOF becomes detectable by visual or tactile assessment. If the drug is administered by intravenous infusion, at least the first twitch of the TOF should be clearly detectable. In this way, 80% to 90% neuromuscular blockade can be maintained throughout. More importantly, adherence to the above principles will prevent absolute or relative overdosing and, most likely, greatly diminish most of the neuromuscular complications described after long-term use of muscle relaxants. It was shown in a prospective randomised study that patients under neuromuscular monitoring do not only require significantly less drug for adequate relaxation, but they also recovered faster from neuromuscular block and showed less neuromuscular complications.[8] In addition, monitoring may also alleviate the socio-economic consequences of prolonged paralysis, necessitating artificial ventilation and full nursing care for weeks, which might pose additional health risks and stress to the patient together with considerably increases in hospital costs.

Indications for the use of muscle relaxants in the ICU

Intubation

If muscle relaxation is only required for intubation, a short acting nondepolarizing drug with no side effects is preferably administered together with adequate analgesia and sedation. Succinylcholine is strictly contraindicated in the critically ill patient. Vecuronium or, because of its faster onset of action, rocuronium might by the drug of choice for intubation if the patient is supposed to resume spontaneous ventilation after the placement of the tracheal tube.

Continuous mechanical ventilation

Owing to the forced application of ventilatory techniques that augment spontaneous breathing activities, the continuous (prolonged) administration of neuromuscular blocking agents is very limited. However, in a particular number of ICU patients, the application of controlled mechanical ventilation for a given time period is necessary to achieve stable cardiopulmonary conditions including patients with adult respiratory distress syndrome (ARDS), chronic obstructive pulmonary disease (COPD) in critical condition, tetanus or severe brain trauma with elevation of intracranial pressure. In these patients, the temporary or continuous administration of neuromuscular blocking agents can be mandatory because of difficulties in the adaptation period (initialisation of continuous mechanical ventilation), fighting against the ventilator (risk of barotrauma, intracranial pressure rise), and the danger of exhausting work of breathing (status asthmaticus, neurologic diseases).

For the above purposes, a long-acting agent could be satisfactory when used as intermittent bolus doses, or a compound of intermediate duration of action can be administered as intravenous infusion. Which drug however, administered whichever way, the effects of muscle relaxants should be monitored and the dose altered accordingly to the patient's individual requirements.

Choice of agents and usefulness in the ICU

The classifications of the time course of the neuromuscular blocking agents is usually based on the clinical duration, which is defined as the time from the administration of the muscle relaxant to the recovery of the twitch response to 25% of its control value. In clinical practice of anaesthesia for surgical procedures, pancuronium became a standard for long-acting muscle relaxants, whereas atracurium and vecuronium were classified as agents with intermediate duration of action. Besides the time course profile, the side effects of the various agents are also an important factor in the choice of a particular compound. It is generally known that the administration of pancuronium is associ-

Table 1
Mean dose requirements of different muscle relaxants.

Vecuronium	adults[19, 27]	4 - 7 mg/h (range 2-13 mg/h)
	adults[8, 20]	0.04-1.03 $mg.kg^{-1}.h^{-1}$
	renal failure[20]	0.5 - 5 mg/h
	children [22,23]	0.1 - 0.14 $mg.kg^{-1}.h^{-1}$
	neonates/infants[22,23]	0.05 - 0.1 $mg.kg^{-1}.h^{-1}$
Rocuronium	adults[24]	30 mg/h (bolus) - 45 mg/h (infusion)
	children[10]	0.3 - 2.2 $mg.kg^{-1}.min^{-1}$
Atracurium	adults[31, 26]	0.47-1.0 $mg.kg^{-1}.h^{-1}$
	children[25]	1.6 $mg.kg^{-1}.h^{-1}$
Cisatracurium	adults[27]	11 mg/h (0.17-0.37 $mg.kg^{-1}.h^{-1}$)
	adults[31]	0.19 $mg.kg^{-1}.h^{-1}$
Mivacurium	no data available	
Pancuronium	adults[28, 29]	2.2 - 3.1 mg/h (range 1.4 - 5.4 mg/h)
	children[30]	0.03 - 0.22 $mg.kg^{-1}.h^{-1}$
Pipecuronium	adults[28]	2.89 mg/h (range 1.8 - 4.3 mg/h)
Doxacurium	adults[29]	1 mg/h

ated with an increase in the heart rate that is not inherent to pipecuronium. Atracurium frequently causes hypotension and tachycardia secondary to histamine release, whereas vecuronium is the most commonly chosen muscle relaxant because of its paucity of haemodynamic and other side effects. A task force recruited from members of the American College of Critical Care and the Society of Critical Care Medicine recently recommended pancuronium as first choice muscle relaxant followed by vecuronium as second choice if the patient is cardiovascular unstable.[17]

A summary of the currently available dose finding studies for neuromuscular blocking agents in ICU patients can be found in table 1. All values (if not indicated otherwise) are mean values from different studies, in some cases the range is shown as well to stress the interindividual variation in dose requirements of the critically ill.

Pharmacokinetic aspects and breakdown products

Critically ill patients requiring prolonged administration of muscle relaxants may be at additional risk for alterations in the expected pharmacokinetics and pharmacodynamics of these agents. Concurrent administration of other drugs and certain disease states may alter the normal response of the neuromuscular junction to acetylcholine or change the body's ability to distribute and eliminate a drug or its metabolites. In the ICU setting the breakdown products of neuromuscular blocking agents may play an important clinical role. The biotransformation pattern of vecuronium[32], pancuronium[32], and atracurium[33] is generally known; however, little or no information is available on the rate of formation, maximum concentrations and elimination pattern of their metabolites after long-term administration of the parent compound to critically ill patients. Breakdown products should be considered as different pharmacological entities with the same or different pharmacological effect and pharmacokinetic profile as the parent compound from which they are formed. Pancuronium, pipecuronium and vecuronium undergo the same type of desacetylation reaction to yield 3-desacetyl 17-desacetyl and 3,17-desacetyl metabolites. All 3 breakdown products of these compounds are active neuromuscular blocking agents. The 3-desacetyl derivatives are considered to be the main metabolite because they are the only breakdown products ever demonstrated in appreciable quantities in body fluids in humans. In human volunteers, the potency of 3-desacetyl vecuronium is about 80% that of its parent compound, with 25% of the administered drug being excreted in the urine.[34] This might indicate that the above breakdown product contributes to the effect of vecuronium and might play a role in prolonged paralysis after long term administration of high doses of vecuronium.[35]

One of the advantages of rocuronium over vecuronium is the lack of detectable levels of metabolites, because this compound is already desacetylated at the 3-position. Therefore accumulation of a metabolite of rocuronium is unlikely to contribute to prolonged paralysis and neuromuscular effects of the parent compound.

Atracurium is a bisquaternary benzylisoquinolinium compound, inactivated partly by Hofmann elimination.[33] The Hofmann elimination reaction yields as breakdown products laudanosine and a quaternary monoacrylate, the products of the ester hydrolysis are a quaternary alcohol and a quaternary acid. The latter two metabolites undergo further conversion by Hofmann elimination into laudanosine, which is the ultimate breakdown product of atracurium. Laudanosine is a central nervous system stimulant that has been shown, together with some glycine antagonists, to cause strychnine like convulsions.[36] Based on the existing experimental evidence so far, it is unlikely that laudanosine concentrations might reach convulsive levels after clinical doses of atracurium. However, the terminal half-life of laudanosine is considerably prolonged, up to 20 times or even longer than that of atracurium, in patients with hepatic or renal disease.[37] Therefore, during and after long-term intravenous infusion of atracurium and cisatracurium, aiming at maintaining a stable neuromuscular block, the concentrations of laudanosine will inevitably accumulate.[38] Although cisatracurium undergoes the same metabolism (i.e. its end product yields laudanosine), the expected plasma levels of this metabolite are much lower than after atracurium, because due to its higher potency, a smaller dose (in mg/kg) is needed.[39] Therefore, accumulation of laudanosine probably is of no importance after the long term use of cisatracurium.

Conclusion

Neuromuscular blocking agents, together with sedatives and analgesic drugs, provide the pharmacological basis for controlled ventilation that can be life-saving in critically ill patients. During the last few years, an increasing number of reports focused attention on the possible role of neuromuscular blocking agents in muscle weakness, prolonged paralysis, and other neuromuscular dysfunction after their long-term use in critically ill patients. The impact of critically illness polyneuropathy as part of the systemic inflammatory response of septic patients remains to be elucidated in this context. Of the various mechanisms suggested, the use of absolute or relative overdoses and the combination of neuromuscular blocking agents with high dose corticosteroids are probably the most likely explanations for the above complications. The most prominent reasons for the use of excessive doses seem to be the limited familiarity of the ICU staff with the pharmacological properties of this class of agents and the omission of monitoring of the neuromuscular transmission during their long-term administration. Consequently, pharmacological misconceptions among health care professionals may be corrected by a suitable educational program and the use of a peripheral nerve stimulator for monitoring of the neuromuscular blockade must be made mandatory whenever muscle relaxants are used in the ICU. The dose ranges of muscle relaxants reported above can only serve as guidelines for initiation of the administration of muscle relaxation with the strong recommendation for individual dose adjustments needed because of the wide variation of dose requirements in critically ill patients.

References

1. Agoston S, Khuenl-Brady KS, M. Seyr et al. The use of neuromuscular blocking agents in the intensive care unit In: Partridge B., W. B. Saunders (Eds.): Anesthesiology Clinics of North America. (1994) 345-359
2. Jones RM, Payne JP. Recent Developments in Muscle Relaxation: Atracurium in Perspective. International Congress and Symposium Series No. 131, Royal Society of Medicine Services Ltd., New York 1988
3. Klessig H. T., H. J. Geiger, M. J. Murray et al: A national survey on the practical patterns of anesthesiologists/intensivists in the use of muscle relaxants. Crit Care Med 20 (1992) 1341-1345
4. Murray MJ, Strickland RA, Weiler C. The use of neuromuscular blocking drugs in the ICU: A US perspective. Int Care Med 19 (1993) S40-S 44
5. Zochodne DW, Bolton CF, Wells GA et al. Critical illness polyneuropathy. A complication of sepsis and multiple organ failure. Brain 110 (1987) 819- 841
6. Lee C. Intensive care unit neuromuscular syndrome ? Anesthesiology 83 (1995) 237-240
7. Waldhausen E, Keser G: Lähmungen durch Kohlenhydrate unter Intensivtherapie. Anaesthesist 40 (1991) 332-338
8. Rudis MI, Sikora CA, Angus E et al. A prospective, randomized, controlled evaluation of peripheral nerve stimulation versus standard clinical dosing of neuromuscular blocking agents in critically ill patients. Crit Care Med 25 (1997) 575-583
9. Coursin DB., Klasek G, Goelzer SL. Increased requirements for continuously infused vecuronium in critically ill patients. Anesth Analg 69 (1989) 518-521
10. Tobias JD. Continuous infusion of rocuronium in a paediatric intensive care unit. Can J Anaesth. 43 (1996) 353-357
11. Dodson BA, Kelly BJ, Braswell LM. Cohen NH. Changes in acetylcholine receptor number in muscles from critically ill patients receiving muscle relaxants; an investigation of the molecular mechanism of prolonged paralysis Crit Care Med 23 (1995) 815-821
12. Kaplan RE : Postanaesthetic problems In: Civetta JM , Taylor RW Kirbv RR (Eds) Critical Care. Philadelphia, IB Lippincott, pp 157-160, 1988
13. Luce JM. Neuromuscular blockade. In: Luce J. M., D. J. Person (Eds.): Critical Care Medicine. Philadelphia, WB Saunders, 1988, 474
14. Shoemaker WS, Ayres S, Grenvik A, et al (eds): Textbook of Critical Care .Medicine. Philadelphia, LB Saunders, 1994
15. Miller JN. Comprehensive review: Neuromuscular blocking agents in critical care. Crit Care Nurs 18 (1995) 60-73

16. Knüttgen D, Bremench J, Rings J, et al. Relaxometrie bei diabetischer Polyneuropatie. Anaesthesist 41(1992) 559-563
17. Loan PH, Paxton LD, Mirakhur RK et al. The TOF-Guard neuromuscular transmission monitor. Anaesthesia 50 (1995) 699-702
18. Shapiro BA, Warren J Egol A et al. Practice parameters for sustained neuromuscular blockade in the adult critically ill patient: An executive summary. Crit Care Med 23 (1995) 1601-1605
19. Sparr HJ, Khuenl-Brady KS, Pühringer F et al. Long-term use of aminosteroidal neuromuscular blocking drugs in the intensive care unit. Int Care Med 20 (1994) S125
20. Darrah WC, Johnston JR, Mirakhur RK: Vecuronium infusions for prolonged muscle relaxation in the intensive care unit. Crit Care Med 17 (1989) 1297-1300
21. Smith CL, Hunter JM, Jones RS. Vecuronium infusions in patients with renal failure in an ICU. Anaesthesia 42 (1987) 387-393
22. Hodges UM. Vecuronium infusion requirements in paediatric patients in intensive care units: the use of acceleromyography. Br J Anaesth 76 (1996) 23-28
23. Fitzpatrick KT, Black GW, Ceran PM et al. Continuous vecuronium infusion for prolonged muscle relaxation in children. Can J Anaesth 38 (1991) 169-174
24. Sparr HJ, Wierda JMKH Proost JH et al. Pharmacodynamics and pharmacokinetics of rocuronium in intensive care patients. Br J Anaesth 78 (1998) 267-273
25. Kushimo OT, Darowski MJ, Morris P et al. Dose requirements of atracurium in paediatric intensive care patients. Br J Anaesth 67 (1991) 781-783
26. Griffiths RB, Hunter JM, Jones RS. Atracurium infusions in patients with renal failure in an ICU. Anaesthesia 41 (1986) 375-381
27. Prielipp RC, Coursin DB, Scuderi PE et al. Comparison of the infusion requirements and recovery profiles of vecuronium and cisatracurium (51W89) in intensive care unit patients. Anesth Analg 81 (1995) 3-12
28. Khuenl-Brady KS, Reitstätter B, Schlager A et al: Long term administration of pancuronium and pipecuronium in the intensive care unit. Anesth Analg 78 (1994) 1082-1086
29. Murray MJ, Coursin DB, Scuderi PE et al. Double-blind, randomized, multicenter study of doxacurium vs. pancuronium in intensive care unit patients who require neuromuscular-blocking agents. Crit. Care Med. 23 (1995) 450-458
30. Tobias JD, Lynch A, McDuffee A, Garrett JS. Pancuronium infusion for neuromuscular block in children in the pediatric intensive care unit. Anesth. Analg 81 (1995) 13-16
31. Boyd AH, Eastwood NB, Parker CJ et al. Comparison of the pharmacodynamics and pharmacokinetics of an infusion of cis-atracurium (51 W89) or atracurium in critically ill patients undergoing mechanical ventilation in an intensive therapy unit. Br J Anaesth 76 (1996) 382-388
32. Marshall IG, Gibb AJ, Durant NN. Neuromuscular and vagal blocking actions of pancuronium bromide, its metabolites, and vecuronium (Org NC 45) and its potential metabolites in the anaesthetized cat. Br J Anaesth 55 (1983) 703-714
33. Stenlake JB, Waigh RD, Urwin J et al. Atracurium conception and inception. Br J Anaesth 55 (1983) 98-108
34. Caldwell CE, Szenohradszky J, Segredo V et al. The pharmacodynamics and pharmacokinetics of the metabolite 3-desacetylvecuronium (Org 7268) and its parent compound, vecuronium, in human volunteers. J Pharm Exper Therap 270 (1994) 1216-1222
35. Segredo V, Caldwell JE, Matthay MA et al: Persistent paralysis in critically ill patients after long-term administration of vecuronium. N Engl J Med 327 (1992) 524-428

36. Pong SF, Graham LT Jr. A relatively simple screening test for gaba or glycine antagonists using rat electroretinography. Arch Int Pharmacodyn Ther 220 (1976) 275-279
37. Fahey MR, Rupp SM, Canfell C et al. Effect of renal failure on laudanosine excretion in man. Br J Anaesth 57 (1985) 1049-1051
38. Parker CJR, Jones JE, Hunter JM. Disposition of infusions of atracurium and its metabolite, laudanosine, in patients in renal and respiratory failure in an ICU. Br J Anaesth 61 (1988) 531-540
39. Smith CE, Van Mierst MM, Parker CJR, Hunter JM. The pharmacokinetics of 51W89 administered by constant infusion: a comparison with atracurium Br J Anaesth 75 (1995) 275P-276P

NEUROMUSCULAR BLOCKING AGENTS AND NEUROMUSCULAR DISEASES

Benoît Plaud and François Donati

Villejuif, France and Montréal, Québec, Canada

Introduction

Acquired neuromuscular diseases or congenital disorders either affect the neuromuscular transmission or the muscle itself. When the neuromuscular transmission is involved, two pathophysiological mechanisms must be distinguished: the abnormality of the nicotinic receptor at the endplate (myasthenia gravis, upregulation of the receptor) and the abnormality of acetylcholine release (Lambert-Eaton myasthenic syndrome, iatrogenic myasthenic syndrome). In both situations pharmacodynamic properties of neuromuscular blocking agents (NMBA) are profoundly affected.[1-7]

Myasthenia gravis

Myasthenia gravis is an autoimmune disorder of neuromuscular transmission. The presence of antibodies against the acetylcholine receptor at the neuromuscular junction results in a reduction of the number of the functional receptors with a decreased safety margin of neuromuscular transmission. Major symptoms are muscle weakness and fatigability, relieved by rest (table 1). Anticholinesterase drugs provide symptomatic improvement in most patients. Myasthenia gravis is frequently associated with abnormalities of the thymus, so thymectomy is the main surgical procedure offered to these patients.[8] Respiratory failure with a need of prolonged ventilation, myasthenic or cholinergic crisis,

Table 1
Osserman and Genakins classifications of myasthenia gravis.[3]

I	Ocular signs and symptoms only
II A	Generalised mild muscle weakness
II B	Generalised moderate weakness, and/or bulbar dysfunction
III	Acute fulminating presentation, and/or respiratory dysfunction
IV	Late severe generalised myasthenia gravis

and swallowing depression are the main perioperative complications.[5,9] The goal of the preoperative management is to optimise clinical status.[10] Preoperative respiratory function tests must be performed since respiratory status is a predictive criterion for postoperative respiratory support. Naguib et al. demonstrated that a model can be used for predicting the need for postoperative mechanical ventilation in myasthenia gravis patients who underwent transcervical-transternal thymectomy.[11] The immunosuppressive therapy (corticosteroids, azathioprine, cyclosporin) must be continued. Preoperative plasmapheresis has been proposed but no direct benefit has been demonstrated.[8,12] Preoperative respiratory physiotherapy is recommended even if respiratory symptoms are not serious. Drugs that depress respiratory function such as benzodiazepines and opioids must be avoided for premedication. The risk for prolonged postoperative ventilation is difficult to predict, but it is advised to plan the eventuality of a stay in intensive care unit. Following transcervical thymectomy, only 7.4 % of patients required prolonged ventilation.[1,13] Anticholinesterase drugs should be stopped a few days before surgery if the clinical status of the patient allows this, because they could increase the effect of succinylcholine and inhibit the effect of nondepolarising NMBAs. Muscle relaxants are not contraindicated in myasthenia gravis but adequate understanding of the response of the myasthenic patient to NMBAs is necessary for their safe administration (table 2).

Concerning depolarising NMBAs a resistance (decreased potency) is observed because the number of available receptors at the endplate is reduced.[2,14] High doses of succinylcholine may be required for rapid sequence tracheal intubation but phase II block is frequent even after a single dose.[15] The sensitivity to, and the duration of action of nondepolarising NMBAs are increased, reducing the intraoperative needs. A reduction of 50 to 75% of the

Table 2
Comparative potency of succinycholine, atracurium and vecuronium in normal and myasthenic patients. A resistance is observed with succinylcholine in myasthenia gravis (higher ED). In contrast sensitivity to non depolarising NMBAs is increased (lower ED).[2,7,14,16,17,30]

	succinylcholine		atracurium		vecuronium	
	normals	myasthenia	normals	myasthenia	normals	myasthenia
	n = 20	n = 10	n = 10	n = 5	n = 10	n = 5
ED_{50} (mg/kg)	0.17	0.33	0.13	0.07	0.019	0.010
ED_{90} (mg/kg)	0.27	0.66	0.21	0.12	0.031	0.017
ED_{95} (mg/kg)	0.31	0.82	0.24	0.14	0.036	0.020

ED_{50}, ED_{90} and ED_{95} : effective dose producing 50, 90 and 95% neuromuscular blockade at the adductor pollicis muscle.

usual dose is common.[16,17] Nondepolarising NMBAs of intermediate duration of action must be chosen.[6] Administration of reduced doses and the use of neuromuscular monitoring allow early extubation in most cases. All the risk factors that predispose to neuromuscular function impairment must be controlled (i.e. hypothermia, hypokalemia, acidosis). The need for anticholinesterase drugs is decreased in the first 48 postoperative hours. These drugs must be restarted carefully and titrated to avoid the risk of cholinergic crisis. During the postoperative period ventilatory function must be monitored carefully because myasthenic patients are at high risk of postoperative respiratory failure. This complication requires mechanical ventilation because it is difficult to distinguish a myasthenic from a cholinergic crisis.

Myasthenic crisis is defined as a respiratory failure with the need of mechanical ventilation and it is the most severe complication of myasthenia gravis. In a retrospective study, Berrouschot et al. showed that the incidence of this complication is about 2.5% with a mortality rate of 13%. In this survey, 17% of the cases of myasthenic crisis occurred after thymectomy.[5] The authors compared 3 therapeutic regimens: continuous intravenous infusion of pyridostigmine, pyridostigmine plus prednisolone, and plasma exchange). None of these treatments demonstrated any advantage. The high incidence of pulmonary infections is related to a poor cough capacity, decreased secretion clearance and defective swallowing.

Myasthenic syndromes

The main causes of myasthenic syndromes are the Lambert-Eaton myasthenic syndrome and iatrogenic myasthenic syndromes. The Lambert-Eaton myasthenic syndrome is characterised by a proximal fatigability, relieved by exercise. It is mainly associated with malignant tumours (pulmonary). The production of anti-calcium voltage dependent channel antibodies implies a presynaptic neuromuscular blockade with abnormal acetylcholine release.[18] Symptoms disappear with treatment of the underlying disease in 50 to 70 % of cases. Their reappearance often precedes a recurrence of the malignant process. Symptomatic treatment is provided by 3,4 diaminopyridine, which promotes release of acetylcholine at the endplate. For the anaesthetic management only case reports are published due to the rare occurrence of this illness.[19] It is recommended to continue the 3,4 diaminopyridine up to the morning of the surgery. The response to succinylcholine seems to be normal but the sensitivity to non-depolarising NMBAs is increased.[19] If muscle relaxants are required, titration beginning with the tenth of the usual dose and careful monitoring of neuromuscular blockade are necessary. Pyridostigmine is not effective and calcium antagonists are contraindicated.

Some drugs are responsible for myasthenic syndromes, such as penicillamine and aminoglycosides. These syndromes regress after stopping the administration of the drug. They can worsen a myasthenia gravis or even induce it.[20] Others drugs that are suspected to be responsible for myasthenic syndromes are the anticonvulsivants (phenytoin sodium, trimethadione), anti-infectives (ciprofloxacine hydrochloride), beta-adrenergic receptor-blocking drugs (propanolol, practolol, timolol), and lithium carbonate.

Muscle disorders

Muscle disorders include several types of neuromuscular dysfunctions: muscle dystrophy (pseudohypertrophic dystrophy or Duchenne muscular dystrophy), myotonic dystrophy (Steinert's disease) and metabolic myotonia.

Table 3
Cause of death in 33 patients with Duchenne muscular dystrophy.[22]

Cause of death	n	Percent of total
Respiratory failure	21	64
Congestive heart failure	4	12
Sudden death	4	12
Acute pneumonia	2	6
Paralytic ileus	1	3
Renal artery thrombosis	1	3

Duchenne muscular dystrophy (DMD) is the most common of childhood muscular dystrophies (3 per 10 000 births). The disease is caused by an X-linked recessive gene and is often undiagnosed until the age of 3 to 5 years. The initial symptoms involve the proximal muscle groups of the pelvis. Kyphoscoliosis may develop and skeletal muscle atrophy predisposes to long bone fractures. Elevated plasma creatinine kinase concentrations result from muscle fibre necrosis. Pulmonary complications and congestive heart failure are the main causes of death which occurs between the ages of 15 and 25 years (table 3).[21,22] Anaesthesia is required for scoliosis correction, tendon releases for contractures or exploratory laparotomies for ileus. These procedures improve the quality of life and must be carried out early in order to limit the operative risk. The preoperative preparation should avoid or limit sedation. Anaesthesiologists must consider impaired cardiac function and the risk of life-threatening cardiac dysrhythmia and avoid depression of cardiac contractility.[23] Up to 25% of the patients may have mitral valve prolapse. Pulmonary and cardiac function have to be evaluated preoperatively (respiratory function tests, echocardiography, Holter) because impaired muscle function limits symptomatology.[24,25] The patients with Duchenne muscular dystrophy must potentially be considered as having a full stomach (weak laryngeal reflexes, long gastric emptying times). Succinylcholine is formally contraindicated because of a risk of lethal hyperkalemia that can simulate malignant hyperthermia. Therefore, all malignant hyperthermia-triggering agents must be avoided.[26] Sensitivity to nondepolarising NMBAs is increased. A study demonstrated a significant increase in the sensitivity to vecuronium for both maximal effect and duration of action.[27] It is the first study comparing neuromuscular sensitivity of nondepolarising NMBAs in DMD and normal patients (eight subjects in each group). There is a significant increase in the sensitivity to the neuromuscular relaxing effect of vecuronium in patients with DMD as compared with normal patients. These results concern both maximal effect and duration of action of neuromuscular block. For example after 0.05 μg/kg of vecuronium (approximately the ED_{95}) the median value of the train-of-four ratio (TOFr) was 0.86 in the control group versus 0.14 in the DMD group. Likewise the recovery of TOFr from 0.1 to 0.25 was slower in the patients with DMD: 36 min versus 6 min in the control group.

Most postoperative complications are respiratory including the need of prolonged ventilation, especially if vital capacity is less than 30 % of predicted and infectious complications. Perioperative chest physiotherapy seems to be effective. If suitable, regional anaesthesia is a good alternative to avoid general anaesthesia and may facilitate chest physiotherapy.

Myotonic dystrophy

Myotonic dystrophy designates a group of hereditary degenerative diseases of skeletal muscles characterised by persistent contracture of skeletal muscles after their stimulation, resulting from abnormal calcium metabolism. Steinert's disease is the most common and serious form of this group (3 to 5 per 100 000 population). It is predominantly seen in adults. There is a progressive involvement of skeletal, cardiac or smooth muscles. The association of mental retardation, frontal baldness and cataract formation is characteristic. The incidence of diabetes mellitus, hypothyroidism, adrenal insufficiency, central sleep apnoea and cholelithiasis is increased. Mitral valve prolapse is present in 20 % of the patients. Cardiac dysrhythmia and conduction defects with pulmonary aspiration are the main causes of death, which occurs by the sixth decade.[4,28] The treatment is symptomatic, and may include phenytoin, quinine or procainamide Preoperative management must consider asymptomatic cardiac and pulmonary dysfunction, especially the risk of conduction blockade. Many complications may occur during anaesthesia.[29] Delayed oesophageal and gastric emptying increase the risk of aspiration but like in DMD succinylcholine is formally contraindicated because of the risk of lethal hyperkalemia. A myotonic crisis can be triggered by succinylcholine, hypothermia, surgical manipulations, electrocautery or drugs (clofibrate, propanolol, neostigmine, potassium).[29] Nondepolarising NMBAs are not effective in these crises. The use of nondepolarising NMBAs, if they are needed, requires monitoring of the neuromuscular blockade. Reversal agents can precipitate skeletal muscle contraction by facilitating

Table 4
Conditions associated with up- and down-regulation of acetylcholine receptors.[15]

Resistance to NMBAs ***Hyperkalaemia with succinylcholine*** Any neurologic motor defect Muscle trauma Thermal trauma Disuse atrophy ICU - prolonged use of relaxants Severe infection	↑ ***nicotinic acetylcholine receptors***
Cerebral palsy Myeloméningocele chronic anticonvulsivants ***Resistance to NMBAs*** ***no Hyperkalaemia***	
Myasthenia gravis Exercise conditioning Organophosphorus poisoning ? ***Sensitivity to NMBAs*** ***Resistance with succinylcholine***	↓ ***nicotinic acetylcholine receptors***

depolarisation of the endplate. Postoperative management in the intensive care unit includes chest physiotherapy and extended observation of cardiac and respiratory functions.

Up-regulation of skeletal muscle acetylcholine receptor

Clinical conditions in which the neuromuscular responses simulate an increased receptor number include denervation, disuse muscle atrophy, thermal and direct muscle trauma, infection, and chronic treatment with antagonists of neuromuscular transmission (table 4).[15] In these conditions, the new acetylcholine receptor (or immature) differs from the normal (or mature) with the substitution of the ε-subunit for the γ-subunit. As a result, the pharmacological effects of NMBAs are profoundly modified. The increased sensitivity to agonists such as succinylcholine may induce a lethal hyperkalemic response. Therefore, succinylcholine is formally contraindicated from 48 h after the injury and until the symptoms disappear. The sensitivity to non depolarising NMBAs is decreased because the number of receptors in the extra-junctional area is increased.[15]

Conclusion

Neuromuscular diseases represent an entity including very various pathologies with different patterns. The perioperative complications (cardiac and respiratory) are serious and potentially life-threatening. Preoperatively, an evaluation of the pulmonary and cardiac systems, which are often involved in these diseases, must be performed. Some anaesthetic agents may lead to specific complications. If muscle relaxants are needed, careful monitoring of neuromuscular blockade is necessary. Succinylcholine is formally contraindicated in muscle disorders and in conditions with up-regulation of acetylcholine receptors.

References

1. Akpolat N, Tilgen H, Gursoy F, Saydam S, Gurel A. Thoracic epidural anaesthesia and analgesia with bupivacaine for transsternal thymectomy for myasthenia gravis. Eur J Anaesthesiol 1997;14:220-3.
2. Baraka A. Neuromuscular response to succinylcholine-vecuronium sequence in three myasthenic patient undergoing thymectomy. Anesth Analg 1991;72:827-30.
3. Baraka A. Anaesthesia and myasthenia gravis. Can J Anaseth 1992;39:476-86.
4. Bégin P, Mathieu J, Almirall J, Grassino A. Relationship between chronic hypercapnia and inspiratory-muscle weakness in myotonic dystrophy. Am J Respir Crit Care Med 1997;156:133-9
5. Berroushot J, Baumann I, Kalischewski P, Sterker M, Schneider D. Therapy of myasthenic crisis. Crit Care Med 1997;25:1228-35.
6. Bevan DR, Bevan J, Donati F. Neuromuscular diseases (pp 414-430). In : Muscles relaxants in clinical anesthesia. Bevan DR, Bevan JC, Donati F eds. Year Book Medical Publishers, Chicago, 1988.
7. Buzello W, Noeldge G, Krieg N, Brobmann GF. Vecuronium for muscle relaxation in patients with myasthenia gravis. Anesthesiology 1986;64:507-9.
8. Drachman DB. Myasthenia gravis. N Engl J Med 1994;330:1797-810.
9. Zulueta JJ, Fanbourg BL. Respiratory dysfunction in myasthenia gravis. Clin Chest Med 1994;15:683-91.
10. Froelich J, Eagle CJ. Anaesthetic management of a patient with myasthenia gravis and tracheal stenosis. Can J Anaesth 1996;43:84-9.
11. Naguib M, Eldawlatly AA, Ashour M, Bamgboye EA. Multivariate determinants of the need for postoperative ventilation in myasthenia gravis. Can J Anaesth 1996;43: 1006-13.
12. Evoli A, Batocchi AP, Tonali P. A practical guide to the recognition and management of myasthenia gravis. Drugs 1996;52:662-70.
13. Mineo TC, Pompeo E, Ambrogi V, Sabato AF, Bernardi G, Casciani CU. Adjuvant pneumomediastinum in thoracoscopic thymectomy for myasthenia gravis. Ann Thorac Surg 1996;62:1210-2.
14. Eisenkraft JB, Book WJ, Mann SM, Papatestas AE, Hubbard M. Resistance to succinylcholine in myasthenia gravis: a dose-response study. Anesthesiology 1988;69: 760-3.

15. Martyn JAJ, White DA, Gronert GA, Jaffe RS, Ward JM. Up and down regulation of skeletal muscle acetylcholine receptors. Anesthesiology 1992;76:822-43.
16. Eisenkraft JB, Book WJ, Papatestas AE. Sensitivity to vecuronium in myasthenia gravis: a dose-response study. Can J Anæsth 1990;37:301-6.
17. Nilsson E, Meretoja OA. Vecuronium dose-response and maintenance requirements in patient with myasthenia gravis. Anesthesiology 1990;73:28-32.
18. Pelucchi A, Ciceri E, Clementi F, Marazzini L, Foresi A, Sher E. Calcium channel autoantibodies in myasthenic syndrome and small cell lung cancer. Am Rev Respir Dis 1993;147:1229-32.
19. Telford RJ, Hollway TE. The myasthenic syndrome: anaesthesia in a patient treated with 3,4 diaminopyridine. Br J Anaesth 1990;64:363-6.
20. Wittbrodt ET. Drugs and myasthenia gravis: an update. Arch Intern Med 1997;157: 399-408.
21. Melacini P, Vianello A, Villanova C, Fanin M, Miorin M, Angelini C, Dalla Volta S. Cardiac and respiratory involvement in advanced stage Duchenne muscular dystrophy. Neuromuscul disord 1996;6:367-76.
22. Yanagisawa A, Miyagawa M, Yotsukura M, Tsuya T, Shirato C, Ishihara T, Aoyagi T, Ishikawa K. The prevalence and prognostic significance of arrhythmias in Duchenne type muscular dystrophy. Am Heart J 1992;124:1244-50.
23. Ducceschi V, Nigro G, Sarubbi B, Comi LI, Politano L, Petretta VR, Nardi S, Briglia N, Santogelo L, Nigro G, Iacono A. Autonomic nervous system imbalance and left ventricular systolic dysfunction as potential candidates for arrhythmogenesis in Becker muscular dystrophy. Int J of Cardiol 1997;59:275-9.
24. Melacini P, Fanin M, Danieli GA, Villanova C, Martinello F, Miorin M, Freda MP, Miorelli M, Mostacciuolo ML, Fasoli G, Angelini C, Dalla Volta S. Myocardial involvement is very frequent among patients affected with subclinical Becker's muscular dystrophy. Circulation 1996;94:3168-75.
25. Quinlivan RM, Lewis P, Marsden P, Dundas R, Robb SA, Baker E, Maisey M. Cardiac function, metabolism and perfusion in Duchenne and Becker muscular dystrophy. Neuromuscul disord 1996;6:237-46.
26. Obata R, Yasumi Y, Suzuki A, Nakajima Y, Sato S. Rhabdomyolysis in association with Duchenne's muscular dystrophy. Can J Anaesth 1999;46:564-6.
27. Ririe DG, Shapiro F, Sethna NF. The response of patients with Duchenne's muscular dystrophy to neuromuscular blockade with vecuronium. Anesthesiology 1998;88: 351-4.
28. Phillips MF, Harper PS. Cardiac disease in myotonic dystrophy. Cardiovasc res 1997;33:13-22.
29. Russel SH, Hirsch NP. Anaesthesia and myotonia. Br J Anaesth 1994;72:210-6.
30. Smith CE, Donati F, Bevan D. Cumulative dose-response curves for atracurium in patients with myasthenia gravis. Can J Anaesth 1989;36:402-6.

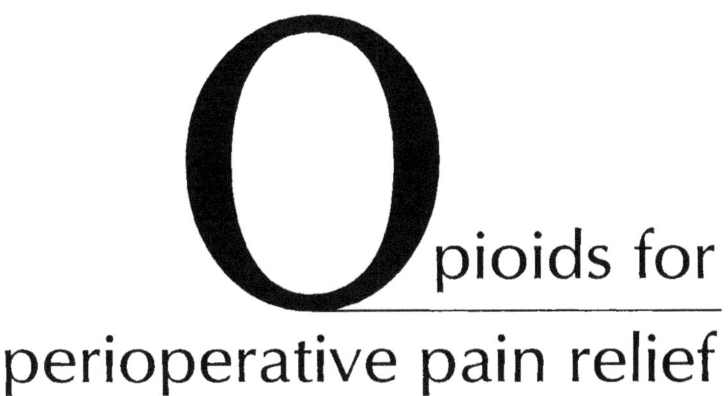
Opioids for
perioperative pain relief

Sites of Respiratory Action of Opioids

Elise Sarton and Albert Dahan

Leiden, The Netherlands

Introduction

Potent opioids are frequently used during diagnostic procedures (monitored anesthesia care), surgery, trauma and in the post-operative period. Apart from their intended effect (i.e., analgesia), these drugs posses life-threatening side effects such as respiratory depression. Depending on potency and dose, respiratory depression is either mild, serious or lethal. High doses of potent intravenous opioids as used during surgery depress ventilation to such an extent that ventilatory support by a ventilator is necessary. However, also at low doses, such as used during monitored anesthesia care, opioids inflict sometimes severe respiratory depression.

Worldwide, morphine, the prototype μ-agonist, is still the first choice in the treatment of postoperative pain. Recent studies in μ-opioid-receptor (MOR) gene (exon 1 and exon 2) knockout mice indicate that, at least for its analgesic effects, morphine acts at the μ-receptor.[1,2] It is of interest to note that μ-opioids such as morphine-6-glucuronide (M6G) and heroin seem to act through receptor mechanisms distinct from the μ-receptor at which morphine acts (i.e., the μ_1-receptor).[2] In contrast to morphine and methadone, heroin and (spinal and supraspinal) M6G still retained their analgesic activity in homozygous exon 1-deficient mice. M6G and morphine were inactive in the exon 2 MOR-1 mutant mice. Although respiratory and analgesic studies in exon 2 MOR-1 mutant mice indicate functional interactions between μ- and δ- but not with κ-opioid receptors,[3] the mechanism by which morphine (and other opioids) interacts with the control of breathing remains poorly understood. Furthermore, important sex differences exist in the analgesic and respiratory effects of morphine and alfentanil.[4-6] While animal studies indicate greater analgesic potency of opioids in male animals, the opposite seems true in humans (Sarton and Dahan, unpublished observation).

Alfentanil, a more selective μ-receptor agonist than morphine, is used in patients during monitored anaesthesia care (i.e., they breathe spontaneously). In this short review we will discuss the influences of morphine and alfentanil on the control of breathing in a cat model and in healthy human volunteers.

Chemical control of breathing

In awake and anaesthetized mammals, an increase in arterial PCO_2 increases ventilation by stimulation of the peripheral and central chemoreceptors. The peripheral chemoreceptors contribute 30%, the central chemoreceptors 70% to the total ventilatory response to carbon dioxide. In the steady-state, ventilation is related in a linear fashion to end-tidal PCO_2 ($P_{ET}CO_2$) above resting $P_{ET}CO_2$ values, which is mathematically expressed as:

$$\text{Ventilation} = (G_P + G_C)\,[P_{ET}CO_2 - B]$$

where G_P is the ventilatory reactivity or sensitivity to CO_2 of the peripheral chemoreceptors, G_C the ventilatory sensitivity to CO_2 of the central chemoreceptors and B the apneic threshold or extrapolated $P_{ET}CO_2$ at zero ventilation. B determines the position of the response curve relative to the x-axis. The peripheral chemoreceptors are located in the carotid bodies which are found at the bifurcation of the carotid arteries in the neck. Neurotransmitters in the carotid bodies include dopamine, acetylcholine, serotonine, NO, CO and opioid peptides. Central chemoreceptors are located in the ventral medulla. Their exact position is unknown. The peripheral chemoreceptors are fast responding receptors, the central chemoreceptors are slow responding receptors (see below). Information from both receptors, together with information from other sites (such as propioceptors, cortex and subcortical areas, hypothalamus, etc) are integrated in the respiratory centers in the brain stem.

Apart from responding to carbon dioxide, the peripheral chemoreceptors react to hypoxia. This causes a brisk increase in ventilation. Glutamate and the *N*-methyl-D-aspartate (NMDA) receptor play a crucial role in the central processing of afferent input from the peripheral chemoreceptors. When hypoxia lasts longer than 3 to 5 min, the central depressant effects of hypoxia cause ventilation to decline. Reduction of oxygen saturation to about 80% will causes an initial increase in ventilation by about 100% followed by a slow decline. Steady-state ventilation will be reached after 15 min and is about 40 to 60% higher than baseline (normoxic) ventilation. The mechanism(s) of the slow decline in ventilation due to sustained hypoxia is unknown but may be related to: (1) An increase in cerebral blood flow due to hypoxia and the resultant wash-out of acid metabolites from the brain stem (this will reduce central respiratory drive); (2) The increase of neurotransmitters and neuromodulators with a net inhibitory effect on ventilation. Candidate neurotransmitters are: γ-aminobutyric acid, dopamine, adenosine, neuronal NO. (3) At deep hypoxic levels, direct depression of respiratory neurones. It is of interest to note that an intact peripheral (i.e., carotid body) response is a necessity for the development of the slow ventilatory decline due to central hypoxia.[7] Furthermore, the larger the peripheral response in terms of minute ventilation the larger the magnitude of the slow decline.[7] The reverse is also true. See for a review of the recent literature reference 7.

The dynamic end-tidal forcing technique (DEF)

The extensive literature on the influences of opioids on respiration shows that various methods of investigation are employed. Invariably all studies indicate that opioid administration causes a reduction in resting ventilation which is accompanied by a rise in end-tidal and arterial PCO_2 and depression of ventilatory responses to carbon dioxide and hypoxia. However, because of the differences in methods used to study the ventilatory changes due to hypoxia and hypercapnia, results of most studies are incomparable. This makes it difficult to investigate the mechanism(s) of respiratory depression caused by opioids.

In our opinion, the dynamic end-tidal forcing (DEF) technique is best suited for drug studies. An extensive description of the DEF technique is given in reference 8. In short, by manipulating the inspired gas concentrations, independent of changes in ventilation or mixed venous return, this technique forces end-tidal carbon dioxide and oxygen to follow a predescribed pattern in time, on a breath-to-breath basis. Carbon dioxide forcing involves steps in $P_{ET}CO_2$ at a background of strict normoxia. Oxygen forcing involves step decreases in $P_{ET}O_2$ against the background of strict isocapnia. Using a mathematical model of the respiratory controller, end-tidal carbon dioxide forcing gives the ventilatory steady-state CO_2 sensitivities of the peripheral and central chemoreflexes and provides valuable information on the dynamics of the receptors involved. This is done by taking into account and identifying the time delays and time constants of the peripheral and central chemoreflex loops which differ by a factor of about 2 and 10, respectively (time delay of the peripheral and central chemoreflex loops are ~6 and ~12 s, time constants are ~10 and ~120 s). DEF of oxygen enables the study of the temporal characteristics of the hypoxic response.

Studies in cats

Using the DEF technique, Berkenbosch et al.[9,10] investigated the effects of i.v. morphine (0.15 mg/kg) in an (α-chloralose-urethan) anaesthetized cat model. Their primary interest was to locate the respiratory site(s) of action of morphine. They considered the following sites: central chemosensitive structure, the peripheral chemoreceptors of the carotid bodies, the integrating centers in the brainstem where information from both group of chemoreceptors is processed and/or the neuromechanical link between brainstem and ventilation (this includes motor neurons, efferent nerves and respiratory muscles). They obtained the following results:

i. Morphine decreased isocapnic normoxic, hyperoxic and hypoxic ventilation by ~60%;
ii. Morphine decreased the overall ventilatory CO_2 sensitivity by 30% and shifted the position of the response curve to the right (shift of about 4 mmHg or 0.5 kPa). Central and peripheral CO_2 sensitivities decreased to the same extent;

iii. Part of the respiratory depression could be antagonized by physostigmine;
iv. Morphine had no effect on the ventilatory increase due to steady-state isocapnic hypoxia.

Note that the steady-state ventilatory response to isocapnic hypoxia is due to two opposing effects: an increase in ventilation due to effects of hypoxia at the peripheral chemoreceptors and a decrease in ventilation due to the depressant effects of central hypoxia (see earlier). While these results indicate that morphine acts at sites within the peripheral and central chemoreflex loop (result 1 and 2), they provide little insight in the interaction of central hypoxia, morphine and ventilation at the μ-receptor. These data do suggest a role for the central cholinergic system in the development of respiratory depression from opioids.

Human studies

Morphine

We compared the effects of i.v. morphine at an analgesic dose (bolus of 100 μg/kg, followed by a continuos infusion of 30 $\mu g.kg^{-1}.h^{-1}$) on hypercapnic and acute (i.e., non-steady-state) and sustained (i.e., steady-state) ventilatory responses in men and women (in both phases of their menstrual cycle) using the DEF technique.[5,6] Hypercapnic ventilatory responses were separated into a peripheral and central component using the DEF technique. A summary of our results is given here:

i. The half-life (t_2) for changes in ventilation and end-tidal PCO_2 ranged between 1 and 5 min in men and women (steady-state obtained after 15 to 20 min, men *versus* women NS, see figure 1 of reference 6).
ii. In men, there was no or little decrease in ventilatory CO_2 sensitivity but a rightward shift of the response curve of 4.2 mmHg or 0.6 kPa (figure 1);
iii. In women, a decrease in CO_2 sensitivity of –30% without a shift of the response curve (men *versus* women $P < 0.05$);
iv. Depression of the acute increase in ventilation due to hypoxia by >50% in women; 0 to 20% depression in men (men *versus* women $P < 0.05$).
v. Sex-related differences were located in the peripheral chemoreflex pathway but not in the central chemoreflex pathway;

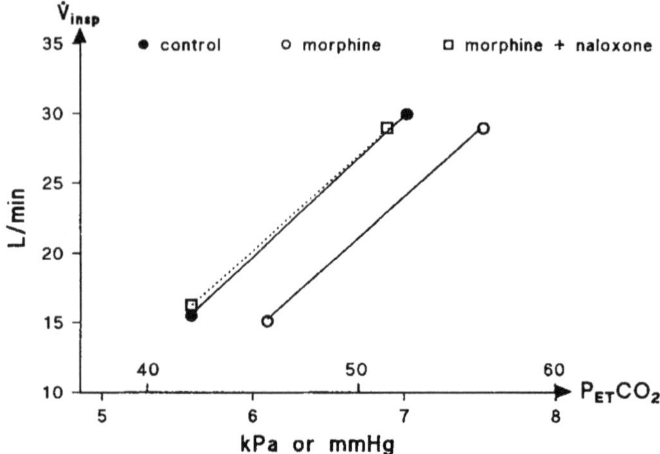

Figure 1
Influence of morphine and naloxone on the ventilatory response to carbon dioxide in a male subject. Morphine shifted the response curve to the right but did not affect the slope. Naloxone after morphine reversed the effects of morphine completely. The parallel shift seen with morphine is typical for men.

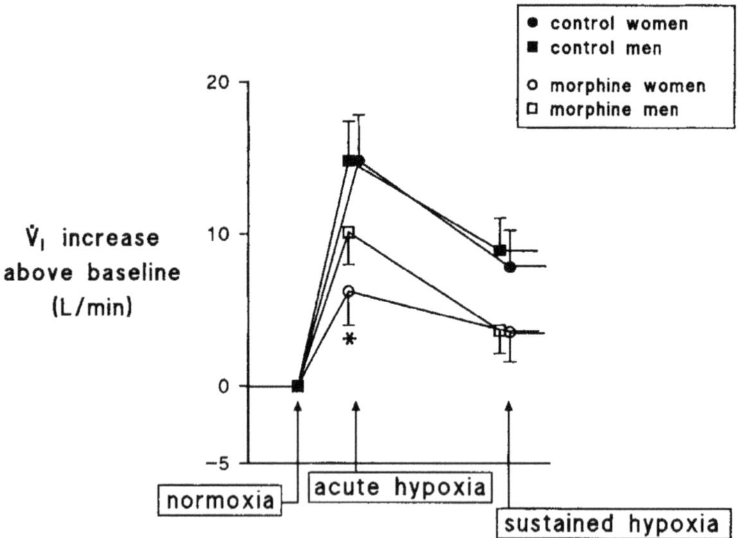

Figure 2
Influence of morphine on the ventilatory response to 3 (acute) and 15 min (sustained) of isocapnic hypoxia. Note the absence of sex differences in the control responses, large differences in the acute response during morphine administration, and the absence of differences in the sustained response during morphine. * $P < 0.05$ morphine women *versus* morphine men. Adapted from reference 6 (with permission).

vi. In women, the phase of the menstrual cycle had no effect on the influences of morphine on hypoxic and hypercapnic ventilatory responses;
vii. Complete reversal of respiratory depression after 5 μg/kg naloxone in men and women (figure 1);
viii. Morphine did not interfere with the development of the secondary decline in ventilation due to central hypoxia (i.e., no interaction of central hypoxia, morphine and ventilation at the μ-receptor). See also figure 2.

Alfentanil

In a pilot study, we examined the influence of alfentanil on the ventilatory response when subjects were awake and when asleep due to inhalation of 0.08% sevoflurane. During the study, the EEG was monitored. One male subject showed little to no effect of 20 to 40 ng/mL alfentanil when awake but showed a reduction in acute ventilation due to hypoxia when asleep with sevoflurane (i.e., he showed an immediate decrease in ventilation upon the introduction of hypoxia, figure 3). This indicates a synergistic interaction between opioids and light non-REM sleep induced by a subanaesthetic concentration of sevoflurane on ventilatory control. A second male subject showed the abolishment of the hypoxic ventilatory response with alfentanil and sevoflurane. Isobolographic analysis of his data indicate an additive effect of the two agents on the ventilatory response to hypoxia.

Conclusions

Individual studies on the mechanisms of respiratory action of opioids in animals and humans provide only limited information. Comparison and combining of study results is needed but is only possible when reliable and comparable techniques are employed. Our studies indicate that opioids act at μ-receptors within the peripheral and central chemoreflex pathways. In this respect anaesthetized cats and awake humans are comparable. In humans, our studies indicate important sex differences. These seem to reside in the peripheral chemoreflex loop but not in the central chemoreflex loop. If these observations are due to sex differences in μ-receptors (involving density, binding affinity, second messenger activation, etc.) or due to interactions with other receptors (such as the NMDA receptor) remains unknown. Our findings are analogous to

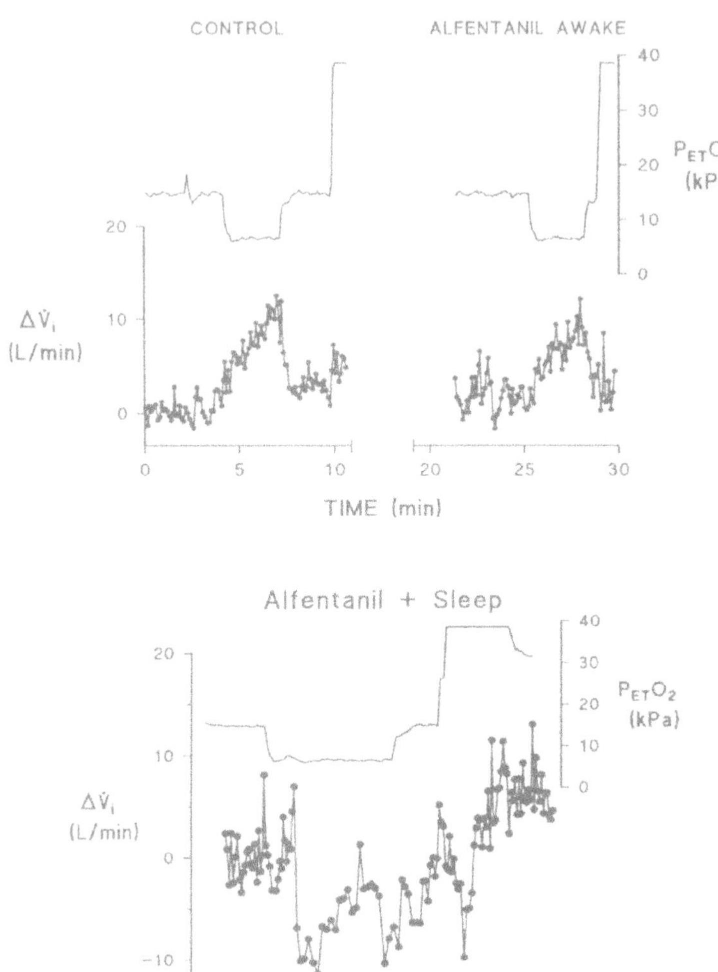

Figure 3
Influence of alfentanil delivered by TCI (target blood conc. 40 ng/mL) on the ventilatory response to acute hypoxia in a male subject. A 2 L/min decrease in the awake alfentanil response compared to control response was observed (top two panels). At the identical alfentanil blood target concentration, the inhalation of 1/20th of a minimum alveolar concentration of sevoflurane which caused light non-REM sleep did not cause an increase in ventilation but a decrease below baseline (bottom panel).

sex-related differences in opioid-mediated analgesia.[4,11] The basis of opioid-related sex differences are biological differences in pharmacodynamics rather than pharmacokinetics. Further studies are warranted to examine sex-dependent and sex-independent factors on opioid- and also anaesthetic-induced respiratory depression and analgesia.

The preliminary alfentanil data support the notion that changes in the central nervous system arousal state has an important influence on the ability to increase ventilatory drive when hypoxic and hypercapnic.[12] This is of clinical importance since frequent and repetitive hypoxic events are associated with monitored anaesthesia care and postoperative analgesia (especially in sleeping patients).

References

1. Matthes HWD, Maldonado R, Simonin F, Valverde O, Slowe S, Kitchen I, Befort K, Dierich A, Le Meur M, Dollé P, Tzavara E, Hanoune J, Roques BP, Kieffer BL. Loss of morphine-induced analgesia, reward effect and withdrawal symptoms in mice lacking the μ-opioid-receptor gene. Nature 1996; 383: 819-23
2. Schuller AGP, King MA, Zhang J, Bolan E, Pan YX, Morgan DJ, Chang A, Czick ME, Unterwald EM, Pasternak GV, Pintar JE. Retention of heroin and morphine-6β-glucuronide analgesia in a new line of mice lacking exon 1 of MOR 1. Nature Neuroscience 1999; 2: 151-6
3. Matthes HWD, Smadja C, Valverde O, Vonesch JL, Foutz AS, Boudinot E, Denavit-Saubié M, Severini C, Negri L, Roques BP, Maldonado R, Kieffer BL. Activity of the δ-opioid receptor is partially reduced, whereas activfity of the κ-receptor is maintained in mice lacking the μ-receptor. J Neuroscience 1998; 18: 7285-95
4. Cicero TJ, Nock B, Meyer ER. Sex-related differences in morphine=s antinociceptive activity: relationship to serum and brain morphine concentrations. J Pharmacol Exper Therap. 1997; 282: 939-44
5. Dahan A, Sarton E, Teppema L, Olievier C. Sex-related differences in the influence of morphine on ventilatory control in humans. Anesthesiology 1998; 88: 903-13
6. Sarton E, Teppema L, Dahan A. Sex-differences in morphine-induced ventilatory depression resides within the peripheral chemoreflex loop. Anesthesiology 1999: 90: 1329-38
7. Dahan A, Ward D, van den Elsen M, Temp J, Berkenbosch A. Influence of reduced carotid body drive during sustained hypoxia in hypoxic depression fo ventilation in man. J Appl Physiol 1996; 81: 565-72
8. Dahan A, DeGoede J, Berkenbosch A, Olievier I. The influence of oxygen on the ventilatory response to carbon dioxide. J Physiol (Lond) 1990; 428: 485-99
9. Berkenbosch A, Olievier C, Wolsink J, DeGoede J, Rupreht J. Effects of morphine and physostigmine on the ventilatory response to carbon dioxide. Anesthesiology 1994; 80: 1303-10
10. Berkenbosch A, Teppema L, Olievier C, Dahan A. The influences of morphine on the ventilatory response to isocapnic hypoxia. Anesthesiology 1997; 86: 1342-9

11. Kest B, Sarton E, Mogil J, Dahan A. Opioid-induced analgesia and respiratory depression: Sex differences. In: Physiology and Pharmacology of Cardio-Respiratory Control, edited by Dahan A, Teppema L, van Beek H. Dordrecht, Kluwer Academic Publishers, 1998, pp 93-100
12. Sarton E, Dahan A, Teppema L, Olofsen E, Berkenbosch A. Acute pain and central nervous system arousal do not restore impaired hypoxic response during sevoflurane sedation. Anesthesiology 1996; 85: 295-303

REMIFENTANIL – A NEW AGE IN ANAESTHESIA?

Johan Raeder

Oslo, Norway

Introduction

A new drug may represent progress, either in terms of an improvement in clinical efficacy, a reduction in side effects, an improvement in the pharmaco-economic profile or in terms of a combination of these. Surgical procedures characterised by significant differences in intra- or interindividual anaesthetic needs, require hypnotic and analgesic agents with a rapid on- and offset. Development of such "on-off" agents may improve the ease of titration, even if their pharmacodynamic characteristics remain unchanged. Does remifentanil really initiate a new age in anaesthesia? The only apparent novelty of remifentanil compared to the other opioids is its remarkable pharmacokinetic profile; the pharmacodynamic characteristics and drug costs are more or less similar. However, because of its pharmacokinetic characteristics, remifentanil may be used in a different way and provide specific clinical effects directly when needed. The safe haemodynamic stability of high dose opioid anaesthesia and the rapid recovery characteristics may also have profound economical implications, when total peri-operative costs are considered.[1] In order to elucidate the way remifentanil may change our way of providing anaesthesia, we need to discuss the pharmacokinetics and pharmacodynamics of remifentanil and the role of opioids in anaesthesia.

Opioids in anaesthesia

Analgesia and hypnosis (and eventually muscular relaxation) are the cornerstones of general anaesthesia. Pure μ-opioid agonists are unique in their ability of providing potent dose-dependant analgesia. A total control of the stress-response may be achieved with these agents. Whereas other anaesthetic drugs, such as inhalational agents, may blunt most of the stress response in the presence of significant haemodynamic depression, opioids may be used in high doses without compromising myocardial contractility.[2] The absence of allergic reactions, malignant hyperthermia or organ toxicity are other features that make opioids attractive. Opioids may also be used as sedative agents during local or regional anaesthesia, providing anxiolysis and additional analgesia with minor hypnotic or amnesic effect, when the dose is carefully titrated. The potent μ-agonist opioids do have well known side effects that may limit their use: respiratory depression, itching, nausea, and vomiting. The sedative action of opioids is complex: even in very high concentrations unconsciousness remains unreliable and mono-opioid anaesthesia has a high risk of awareness. At the same time opioids are known to induce muscular rigidity especially when high doses are rapidly administered.[3] For these reasons, opioids are not suited as sole induction agents. On the other hand, administration of opioids during induction reduces the requirement of hypnotic agents and facilitates endotracheal intubation, even without the use of muscle relaxants.[4] In most patients opioids provide sedation, which may cause a significant delay in the recovery process. The quality of opioid sedation is much less predictable compared to the classic hypnotic agents such as the barbiturates or the benzodiazepines. Some patients may feel dysphoria after opioid administration.[5] The effects of opioids on sleep also include suppression of REM-phase sleep, which may lead to rebound phenomena and disturbed sleep quality for many days after discontinuation of the administration.

Thus, whereas opioids have many unique characteristics that are very useful during general anaesthesia, their use in high doses has been limited by the fear of postoperative side effects. This phenomenon has lead to an anaesthetic strategy in which the opioid dose is often kept as low as possible and is combined with high doses of hypnotic agents, such as propofol or inhalational anaesthetic agents or both.

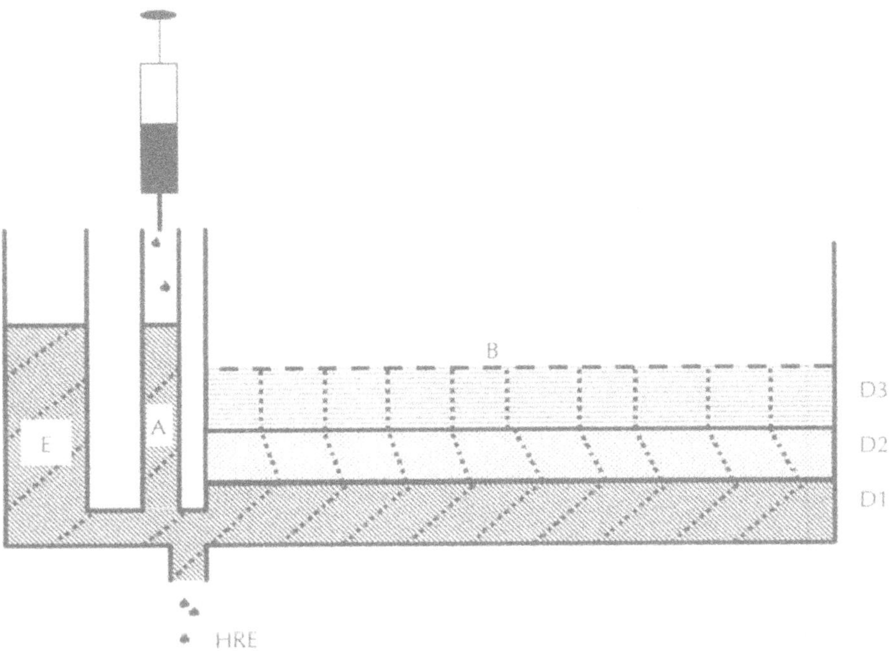

Figure 1
A continuous infusion of a drug is given into the blood compartment (A) which after 6-7 min (propofol) is in equilibrium with the effect compartment (E). During prolonged infusion increasing drug levels (D1-D3) are built up in the rest of the body (B). The longer the infusion, the higher the levels (D1-D3) and the longer it will take for the levels in serum and effect compartment to decrease, due to limited hepatorenal eliminination (HRE).

Opioid pharmacokinetics

Opioids are highly lipid soluble drugs with a rapid transfer across the blood-brain barrier. Differences in intracerebral binding characteristics result in a variable delay in onset of the maximal clinical effect from 1-1.5 (remifentanil and alfentanil) to 4-6 min (fentanyl and sufentanil). The elimination is limited by hepatic degradation to hydrophilic metabolites that are excreted by the kidneys. As a result, with repeated administration or continuous infusion, the opioids increasingly accumulate in the body. This phenomenon gains clinical relevance with increasing infusion duration (figure 1). The context-sensitive half-life is used to describe this process; it is the time required for a 50% reduction in

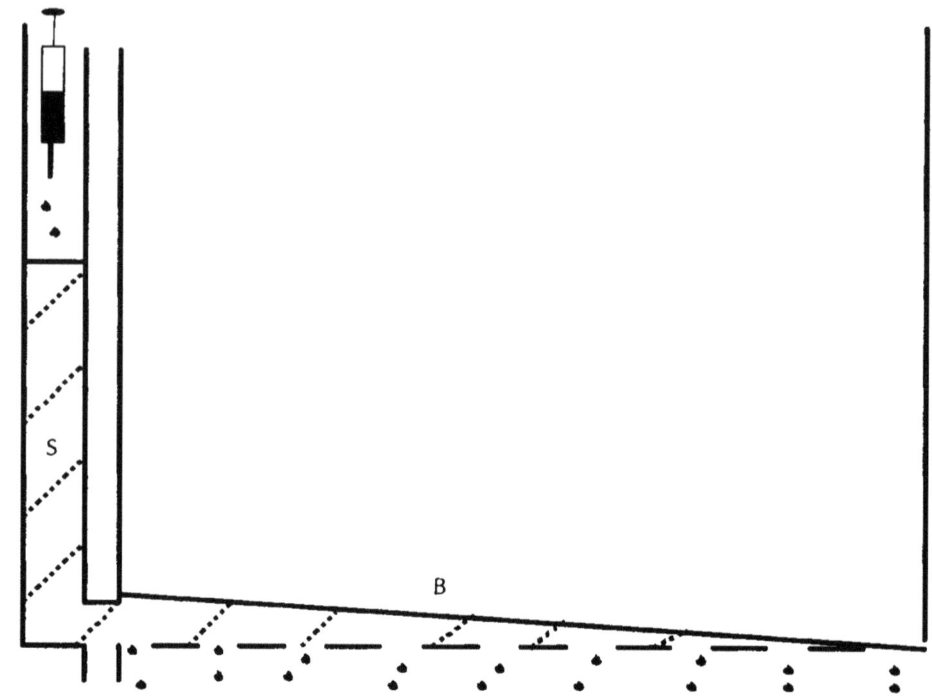

Figure 2
With remifentanil, extensive elimination takes place in serum (S) and in extracellular fluid. As a consequence, the drug will never builds up high levels in the body (B), and elimination will be rapid irrespective of the duration of administration.

the plasma concentration after discontinuation of a continuous infusion. The context-sensitive half-life embodies both the redistribution and the clearance of a drug and is usually positively correlated with the duration of administration.

Remifentanil pharmacokinetics

Remifentanil is metabolised by various types of non-specific esterases throughout the body. The clearance of remifentanil grossly exceeds that of the other opioids fentanyl, alfentanil and sufentanil. There is no known major genetic deficiency in the ability to metabolise remifentanil. The rate of metabolism is not influenced by hepatic[6] or renal failure[7], or by extremes of age[8], but it is slightly decreased (with 20%) by hypothermia during cardiopulmonary bypass.[9]

The clearance of remifentanil is so rapid and extensive, that it prevents the drug from accumulating in the body tissues (figure 2). For this reason the context-sensitive half-life of remifentanil is only 3-5 min, irrespective of the duration of infusion; it is thus context-*in*sensitive.

Lean body-mass is better correlated with the clearance than body-weight and it has been shown that fat tissue is virtually not involved in the distribution of this drug.[10] Remifentanil has a metabolite with a very low intrinsic activity, which may accumulate in renal failure, but for procedures of less than 12 h this metabolite is of no clinical importance.[11] In the elderly, the pharmacokinetics of remifentanil are more predictable than with other opioids.[12] The sensitivity to remifentanil is, just as with the other opioids, enhanced in the elderly. Compared to a 20 year old individual, a 85 year old individual will require a reduction of up to 50% with respect to the bolus dose and of up to 65% with respect to the maintenance infusion rate to establish a similar effect.[13] Although the drug readily passes the placenta no effects on the newborn have been observed when remifentanil is used for Caesarean section.[14]

Remifentanil pharmacodynamics

The pharmacodynamic characteristics of remifentanil do not differ significantly from the other potent µ-agonists, i.e. at equipotent plasma and effect site concentrations, the effects of remifentanil are identical to those of the other opioids. The rapid onset of effect may predispose for the risk of chestwall rigidity, as this complication is most frequently observed with alfentanil and remifentanil.[3] Whereas most anaesthesiologist are familiar with spontaneous laryngeal mask ventilation in patients undergoing minor to intermediate surgical procedures during propofol infusion supplemented with low doses of alfentanil or fentanyl, this seems to demand more skills when using remifentanil. Some studies have addressed this issue[15] and report difficulties in maintaining reliable spontaneous ventilation with remifentanil[16] in excess of 0.08-0.1 $\mu g.kg^{-1}.min^{-1}$. While this infusion rate is sufficient for postoperative analgesia or peri-operative sedation (with loco-regional anaesthesia)[17], it is often inadequate for surgical anaesthesia. While anaesthesia with alfentanil or fentanyl may provide residual analgesia during the initial post-operative period, remifentanil's short duration of action requires administration of long-acting analgesics prior to its discontinuation.[18-21] The incidence of post-operative nausea and vomiting after general anaesthesia with remifentanil has been reported comparable to that of the other opioids[20, 21], although the nausea following sedative doses of remifentanil may be shorter-lived. This raises the question on how drug effects may last even after the drug is cleared from the plasma and effect compartment. Extensive drug binding to the receptor may be one mechanism that may explain this phenomenon. Intracellular processes initiated by drug binding but not necessarily reversed immediately after the drug is dissolved from the receptor, may be another explanation. The latter concept is designated as " the drug footprint theory"; i.e. drug effects are still present after the drug has left. An interesting recent study by Black et al.[22] adds to these concerns. In healthy volunteers, behavioural and physiological impairment was still present one hour after termination of a minor target concentration of 3 ng/ml of remifentanil.[22] On the other hand, a comparative study in patients undergoing day case surgery showed significantly better recovery of psychomotor and psychometric function between 30 and 90 min after anaesthesia with remifentanil compared to alfentanil.[37]

Less is known on the development of acute tolerance to opioids during an anaesthetic procedure. In a study in volunteers, Vinik and Kissin[23] showed a rapid developing tolerance for cold- and pressure-induced pain after a 3-h infusion of remifentanil at an infusion rate of 0.1 $\mu g.kg^{-1}.min^{-1}$. In contrast, a recent study with alfentanil and remifentanil for post-operative pain relief could not prove a rapid development of opioid tolerance (Schraag et al., submitted to Anesth Analg). Similarly, no clinical studies are known that observed an increased need of remifentanil during the course of anaesthesia. The use of remifentanil in the intensive care setting may provide more information on this subject.

Practical implications

Remifentanil may be used in bolus doses during the start of anaesthesia or during maintenance of monitored anaesthesia care or general anaesthesia,[24] However, the ultra-rapid elimination makes remifentanil a drug typically to be given by continuous infusion. An increase in the infusion rate will cause a rapid increase in effect while a decrease in the infusion rate, or even a termination of the infusion, will cause a rapid decrease in effect, irrespective of how long the drug has been given. Following alterations in pump speed, in general, a new steady plasma level is reached after 4 to 5 elimination half-lives, which is within 15-20 min for remifentanil. This period may be shortened by administering bolus injections (dose up) or by infusion cessation (dose down), either done manually or by a target controlled infusion device (TCI).[25] At this moment, target controlled infusion devices for the infusion of remifentanil are only available for scientific purposes. However, such systems may soon become commercially available. When combined with propofol TCI, remifentanil TCI will provide the clinician with a very simple and logic way of providing tailored anaesthetic care. One TCI pump can then be used to infuse remifentanil to provide the analgesic component of anaesthesia, to be adjusted on the basis of haemodynamic indices of stress suppression. The second TCI pump can be used to provide the hypnotic component of anaesthesia with propofol guided, for instance, by the bispectral index (BIS). This concept we allow us to provide adequate anaesthesia for prolonged procedures, followed by a rapid emergence, of within 4-5 min after the end of surgery. The benefits of this TIVA technique compared to an inhalational anaesthetic technique are numerous; an improved control of the stress-response, less cardiovascular depression, no pollution with waste products into the surroundings, the ability to use 100% oxygen when needed, less postoperative nausea and vomiting[1], less confusion or agitation.[26] This technique may also be very useful for specific procedures such as during neurosurgery requiring patients to regain consciousness transiently during the procedure[27], or following neurosurgery when the neurological function of the patient needs to be evaluated as soon as possible, postoperatively.

Practical guidelines

Dosage schemes are usually reported in $\mu g.kg^{-1}.min^{-1}$ (table 1). During steady state conditions, an infusion rate of 0.1 $\mu g.kg^{-1}.min^{-1}$ results in a blood concentration of about 2.5 ng/ml in a healthy, average weight individual.[28] It is of utmost importance that the infusion line is reliable and secure throughout the procedure. In the absence of a sufficient concentration of a hypnotic agent, the rapid offset of remifentanil can result in intra-operative awakening of the patient when the infusion is interrupted. Bolus doses in excess of 1 μg/kg and given

Table 1
Ultiva continuous infusion dose schedule. A loading dose may be administered as a continuous infusion of 1 $\mu g.kg^{-1}.min^{-1}$ over a period of 1.5 min. The average maintenance infusion rate (when combined with propofol or an inhalational agent) is 0.25 $\mu g.kg^{-1}.min^{-1}$ and may be titrated to the patient's individual need between 0.05 and 2.0 $\mu g.kg^{-1}.min^{-1}$.

Loading dose	Maintenance dose
1 $\mu g . kg^{-1} .min^{-1}$ for 1½ minute	**0.25 $\mu g . kg^{-1} .min^{-1}$** (range: 0.05 - 2)

during less than 30 seconds should not be given because of the risk of chestwall rigidity.[3] Furthermore, it is important to have appropriate analgesia established with alternative means when the remifentanil infusion is terminated at the end of the procedure.

Major surgery

For this type of surgery a high-dose opioid anaesthetic technique may be used while still having the option of a rapid emergence, extubation and resumption of spontaneous respiration. High-dose remifentanil anaesthesia has also been used successfully in haemodynamically unstable patients, such as patients with compromised myocardial function[31] or critically ill children.[32] Anaesthesia may be induced with a remifentanil infusion of 0.5 - 1.0 $\mu g.kg^{-1}.min^{-1}$ for 1.5 min, combined with an intermediate dose of a hypnotic agent (e.g. propofol 1.0 - 1.5 mg/kg, or a target concentration of 2.5-3 μg/ml. Bradycardia and hypotension may occur and some authors advocate the use of cholinergic agents routineously.[29, 30] Maintenance of anaesthesia may be accomplished with remifentanil 0.05 - 2.0 $\mu g.kg^{-1}.min^{-1}$ adjusted to the clinical needs of the individual patient and type of surgical procedure, supplemented with 0.3 - 0.5 MAC of an inhalational agent or propofol at a target concentration of 2.5 μg/ml to maintain loss of consciousness. Tapering down the infusion regimen of propofol (or the ET % of an inhalational anaesthetic agent) by the end of the procedure may be considered to speed up recovery. Because spontaneous respiration in the presence of remifentanil occurs at infusion rates below 0.1 $\mu g.kg^{-1}.min^{-1}$, it will take 3-4 times the context-sensitive half-times until the patient breaths spontaneously (approximately 15 min) following the discontinuation of a 1.0 $\mu g.kg^{-1}.min^{-1}$ infusion of remifentanil.

Whenever possible, NSAIDs, paracetamol or local infiltration anaesthesia of the wound should be effective to supplement post-operative analgesia when the patient regains consciousness. If otherwise appropriate, a low dose bupivacaine-opioid infusion through an epidural catheter should be started in due time before the end of surgery. In the absence of epidural analgesia, most major surgery requires (iv) administration of an opioid for postoperative pain relief, prior to the end of surgery. The time of administration of this opioid depends on its onset time; e.g. fentanyl 20-30 μg/kg should be administered intravenously within 5-10 min before the anticipated end of surgery. When morphine is used as postoperative analgesic agent, 0.2 mg/kg should be given, iv, 20-30 min before the end of surgery while a 0.3 mg/kg dose of piritramide, iv, should be administered 10-15 min before the end of surgery.

Intermediate-minor surgery

In our experience, an initial infusion rate of 0.1-0.3 $\mu g.kg^{-1}.min^{-1}$ is appropriate. The patient will become sedated, continue to breathe and receive analgesic protection for the aching of propofol during induction. A propofol bolus dose of 1.0-2.0 mg/kg (or a target concentration of 4.0-5.0 μg/ml) given 2-3 min after the start of the remifentanil infusion, will induce loss of consciousness. The lower dose may be appropriate if the patient has received a proper dose of a premedicant, or receives midazolam 1-2 mg, iv, as part of the induction. Maintenance with remifentanil 0.1-0.3 $\mu g.kg^{-1}.min^{-1}$ is often adequate, combined with inhalational agents and/or propofol at target concentrations of 2.0-3.0 μg/ml. Preferably, non-opioid multimodal analgesia should be present before the emergence of the patients. For procedures with a painful post-operative period, intravenous administration of fentanyl 10-20 μg/kg, 5-10 min before the end of surgery may be useful.

Sedation

Sedation may be accomplished either with remifentanil alone or with remifentanil combined with midazolam or propofol. Unless analgesia is a very important aspect of the procedure, a small dose of midazolam, iv, 1-2 mg, at the start of the procedure may be beneficial in terms of reducing the remifentanil dose, providing better respiration and less nausea and itching in the absence of a prolonged emergence.[33] For sedation and spontaneous ventilation, infusion rates of 0.04 - 0.1 $\mu g.kg^{-1}.min^{-1}$ of remifentanil are sufficient.[34]

Postoperative analgesia

The initial infusion rate for postoperative analgesia is in the order of 0.05-0.15 $\mu g.kg^{-1}.min^{-1}$, individually adjusted.[17] PCA devices for remifentanil have also been used with some success[35], however, due to the very rapid on- and offset of the effect, a continuous infusion at a low rate (i.e. 0.025-0.05 $\mu g.kg^{-1}.min^{-1}$) is necessary.[24]

Conclusions

Remifentanil is a classic μ-agonist with strong analgesic effects. At equipotent concentrations remifentanil exhibits the same pharmacodynamic profile as fentanyl, alfentanil and sufentanil. However, the rapid onset and offset of the effect of remifentanil (even after prolonged infusion and independent of the total dose administered) is totally new and different from the other opioids. This exciting pharmacokinetic profile gives us an improved titration precision that allows us to experience the opioid effects when we need them and to avoid the side effects of residual drug concentrations when the analgesic need is reduced or vanished. These clinical benefits may also result in pharmaco-economical advantages. In the near future, the introduction of reliable delivery systems for remifentanil combined with propofol will provide us with a new concept in intravenous anaesthesia, the double TCI anaesthesia.

References

1. Suttner S, Boldt J, Schmidt C, Piper S, Kumle B: Cost analysis of target-controlled infusion-based anesthesia compared with standard anesthesia regimens. Anesth Analg 1999; 88: 77-82
2. Michelsen LG, Hug CC, Jr.: The pharmacokinetics of remifentanil. [Review] [16 refs]. Journal of Clinical Anesthesia 1996; 8: 679-82
3. Jhaveri R, Joshi P, Batenhorst R, Baughman V, Glass PS: Dose comparison of remifentanil and alfentanil for loss of consciousness. Anesthesiol 1997; 87: 253-9
4. Robinson DN, O'Brien K, Kumar R, Morton NS: Tracheal intubation without neuromuscular blockade in children: a comparison of propofol combined either with alfentanil or remifentanil. Paediatric Anaesthesia 1998; 8: 467-71
5. Raeder JC, Breivik H: - Premedication with midazolam in out-patient general anaesthesia. A comparison with morphine-scopolamine and placebo. Acta Anaesthesiologica Scandinavica 1987 Aug;31(6):509-14
6. Dumont L, Picard V, Marti RA, Tassonyi E: Use of remifentanil in a patient with chronic hepatic failure. British Journal of Anaesthesia 1998; 81: 265-7

7. Hoke JF, Shlugman D, Dershwitz M, Michalowski P, Malthouse-Dufore S, Connors PM, Martel D, Rosow CE, Muir KT, Rubin N, Glass PS: Pharmacokinetics and pharmacodynamics of remifentanil in persons with renal failure compared with healthy volunteers. Anesthesiol 1997; 87: 533-41
8. Minto CF, Schnider TW, Shafer SL: Pharmacokinetics and pharmacodynamics of remifentanil. II. Model application. Anesthesiol 1997; 86: 24-33
9. Russell D, Royston D, Rees PH, Gupta SK, Kenny GN: Effect of temperature and cardiopulmonary bypass on the pharmacokinetics of remifentanil. British Journal of Anaesthesia 1997; 79: 456-9
10. Egan TD, Huizinga B, Gupta SK, Jaarsma RL, Sperry RJ, Yee JB, Muir KT: Remifentanil pharmacokinetics in obese versus lean patients [see comments]. Anesthesiol 1998; 89: 562-73
11. Hogue CWJ, Bowdle TA, O'Leary C, Duncalf D, Miguel R, Pitts M, Streisand J, Kirvassilis G, Jamerson B, McNeal S, Batenhorst R: A multicenter evaluation of total intravenous anesthesia with remifentanil and propofol for elective inpatient surgery. Anesth Analg 1996; 83: 279-85
12. Shafer SL: The role of newer opioids in geriatric anesthesia. [Review] [69 refs]. Acta Anaesthesiologica Belgica 1998; 49: 91-103
13. Minto CF, Schnider TW, Egan TD, Youngs E, Lemmens HJ, Gambus PL, Billard V, Hoke JF, Moore KH, Hermann DJ, Muir KT, Mandema JW, Shafer, SL: Influence of age and gender on the pharmacokinetics and pharmacodynamics of remifentanil. I. Model development. Anesthesiol 1997; 86: 10-23
14. Scott H, Bateman C, Price M: The use of remifentanil in general anaesthesia for caesarean section in a patient with mitral valve disease. Anaesthesia 1998; 53: 695-7
15. Peacock JE, Luntley JB, O'Connor B, Reilly CS, Ogg TW, Watson BJ, Shaikh S: Remifentanil in combination with propofol for spontaneous ventilation anaesthesia. British Journal of Anaesthesia 1998; 80: 509-11
16. Avramov MN, Smith I, White PF: Interactions between midazolam and remifentanil during monitored anesthesia care. Anesthesiol 1996; 85: 1283-9
17. Bowdle TA, Camporesi EM, Maysick L, Hogue CWJ, Miguel RV, Pitts M, Streisand JB: A multicenter evaluation of remifentanil for early postoperative analgesia. Anesth Analg; 83: 1292-7
18. Philip BK, Scuderi PE, Chung F, Conahan TJ, Maurer W, Angel JJ, Kallar, SK, Skinner EP, Jamerson BD: Remifentanil compared with alfentanil for ambulatory surgery using total intravenous anesthesia. The Remifentanil/Alfentanil Outpatient TIVA Group. Anesth Analg 1997; 84: 515-21
19. Kovac AL, Azad SS, Steer P, Witkowski T, Batenhorst R, McNeal S: Remifentanil versus alfentanil in a balanced anesthetic technique for total abdominal hysterectomy. Journal of Clinical Anesthesia 1997; 9: 532- 541
20. Guy J, Hindman BJ, Baker KZ, Borel CO, Maktabi M, Ostapkovich N, Kirchner J, Todd MM, Fogarty-Mack P, Yancy V, Sokoll MD, McAllister A, Roland C, Young WL, Warner DS: Comparison of remifentanil and fentanyl in patients undergoing craniotomy for supratentorial space-occupying lesions [see comments]. Anesthesiol 1997; 86: 514-24
21. Davies G, Kingswood C, Street M: Pharmacokinetics of opioids in renal dysfunction. [Review] [93 refs]. Clinical Pharmacokinetics 1996; 31: 410-22
22. Black ML, Hill JL, Zacny JP: Behavioral and physiological effects of remifentanil and alfentanil in healthy volunteers. Anesthesiol 1999; 90: 718-26
23. Vinik HR, Kissin I: Rapid development of tolerance to analgesia during remifentanil infusion in humans. Anesth Analg 1998; 86: 1307-11

24. Sa RM, Inagaki Y, White PF: Remifentanil administration during monitored anesthesia care: are intermittent boluses an effective alternative to a continuous infusion? Anesth Analg 1999; 88: 518-22
25. Milne SE, Kenny GN: Future applications for TCI systems. [Review] [27 refs]. Anaesthesia 1998; 53 Suppl 1: 56-60
26. Grundmann U, Uth M, Eichner A, Wilhelm W, Larsen R: Total intravenous anaesthesia with propofol and remifentanil in paediatric patients: a comparison with a desflurane-nitrous oxide inhalation anaesthesia. Acta Anaesthesiologica Scandinavica 1998; 42: 845-50
27. Johnson KB, Egan TD: Remifentanil and propofol combination for awake craniotomy: case report with pharmacokinetic simulations [published erratum appears in J Neurosurg Anesthesiol 1998 Apr;10(2):69]. Journal of Neurosurgical Anesthesiology 1998; 10: 25-9
28. Vuyk J: Pharmacokinetic and pharmacodynamic interactions between opioids and propofol. [Review] [13 refs]. Journal of Clinical Anesthesia 1997; 9: 23S-26S
29. Thompson JP, Hall AP, Russell J, Cagney B, Rowbotham DJ: Effect of remifentanil on the haemodynamic response to orotracheal intubation. British Journal of Anaesthesia 1998; 80: 467-9
30. DeSouza G, Lewis MC, TerRiet MF: Severe bradycardia after remifentanil [letter]. Anesthesiol 1997; 87: 1019-20
31. Lehmann A, Boldt J, Zeitler C, Thaler E, Werling C: Total intravenous anesthesia with remifentanil and propofol for implantation of cardioverter-defibrillators in patients with severely reduced left ventricular function. Journal of Cardiothoracic & Vascular Anesthesia 1999; 13: 15-9
32. Eck JB, Lynn AM: Use of remifentanil in infants. Paediatric Anaesthesia 1998; 8: 437-9
33. Gold MI, Watkins WD, Sung YF, Yarmush J, Chung F, Uy NT, Maurer W, Clarke MY, Jamerson BD: Remifentanil versus remifentanil/midazolam for ambulatory surgery during monitored anesthesia care [see comments]. Anesthesiol 1997; 87: 51-7
34. Lauwers M, Camu F, Breivik H, Hagelberg A, Rosen M, Sneyd R, Horn A, Noronha D, Shaikh S: The safety and effectiveness of remifentanil as an adjunct sedative for regional anesthesia. Anesth Analg 1999; 88: 134-40
35. Schraag S, Kenny GN, Mohl U, Georgieff M: Patient-maintained remifentanil target-controlled infusion for the transition to early postoperative analgesia. British Journal of Anaesthesia 1998; 81: 365-8
36. Baker KZ, Ostapkovich N, Sisti MB, Warner DS, Young WL: Intact cerebral blood flow reactivity during remifentanil/nitrous oxide anesthesia. Journal of Neurosurgical Anesthesiology 1997; 9:134-40
37. Cartwright DP, Kvalsvik O, Cassuto J, Jansen JP, Wall C, Remy B, Knape JT, Noronha D, Upadhyaya BK: A randomized, blind comparison of remifentanil and alfentanil during anesthesia for outpatient surgery Anesth Analg. 1997; 85(5): 1014-9

MONITORED ANAESTHESIA CARE WITH REMIFENTANIL

J. Robert Sneyd and Aileen Craig

Plymouth, United Kingdom

Introduction

Monitored Anaesthesia Care (MAC) refers to the provision of sedation and/or analgesia during diagnostic and therapeutic procedures in the presence or absence of regional anaesthesia. Monitored anaesthesia care has developed as a key component of modern ambulatory surgery and offers patients the benefits of regional anaesthesia with sufficient sedation to permit the patient to tolerate the procedure. Sedation is not the exclusive province of the anaesthetist. Sedative techniques are practised by other clinicians using a wide variety of agents. Used appropriately, monitored anaesthesia care extends the repertoire of surgical procedures that can be considered for ambulatory patients and may also permit day surgery in patient groups who would traditionally be considered unsuitable for outpatient general anaesthesia. Monitored anaesthesia care spans the continuum between conscious sedation and general anaesthesia. It is recognised that in such cases, the level of sedation may vary widely during a single case and the potential jeopardy to the cardiovascular and respiratory systems justifies the continuous presence of an anaesthetist and the deployment of additional monitoring techniques.

Intravenous anaesthetics and MAC

Currently, a range of drugs is used for monitored anaesthesia care. The opioids, benzodiazepines and propofol are used most frequently. Although anaesthetists are familiar with managing the airway in anaesthetised or heavily sedated patients, these skills are not invariably possessed by other professional groups and the inappropriate use of sedatives has caused some well publicised disasters[1,2]. In the UK, working parties of the Royal College of Anaesthetists, Royal College of Radiologists and Royal College of Surgeons of England have published guidelines for sedation by non-anaesthetists[3,4] and offer advice on selection of patients, use of monitoring and appropriate staffing. The use of sedative "cocktails" is common practice, with benzodiazepine-opioid combinations as most frequent applied mixture. The Royal College of Surgeons recognises the interaction between these agents and states that *"Failure to modify dosage of these drugs, when used in combination, may lead to life-threatening complications."* The continued use of these combinations reflects the clinical experience that most surgical procedures, including those performed in the presence of regional anaesthesia, include elements of patient discomfort. In the presence of this type of discomfort an opioid may enhance the tolerability of the patient for such stimulation. Most countries' Medical Practitioners have unrestricted (or minimally restricted) rights to prescribe the drugs of their choice. Nevertheless, there is general recognition that certain agents are reserved, by custom, rather than by legislation, for anaesthetists or others with additional training in anaesthesia. Specifically, the intravenous induction agents and the opioids; fentanyl, alfentanil, sufentanil and remifentanil are seldom used by non-anaesthetists who usually restrict themselves to using benzodiazepines, morphine and/or pethidine (meperidine).

Remifentanil for MAC

The rapid onset of the clinical effect of remifentanil (i.e. its rapid access to the "effect site"[5]) and prompt elimination by extra-hepatic metabolism makes remifentanil attractive for monitored anaesthesia care. These characteristics offer the clinician a rapid response of the sedative level of the patient to bolus doses or changes in the infusion rate. Before this technique is generally adopted we should ask three questions. Is remifentanil effective for monitored anaesthesia care? Is it safe? How does it compare with the use of propofol and midazolam? When a new technique is introduced, it is customary to commence clinical investigations with simple efficacy studies in which the agent is compared with a placebo. Ethical considerations dictate that all participants in such a study should receive sedation adequate for their clinical needs and this inevitably inflicts some compromise on study design. Lauwers et al.[6] compared remifentanil with a saline placebo in 160 patients undergoing hip replacement in the presence of a spinal blockade (n = 61) or hand surgery in the presence of a brachial plexus blockade (n = 93). Patients received a sedative infusion, of 0.04, 0.07 or 0.1.μg.kg^{-1} min^{-1} remifentanil or placebo, which was subsequently titrated to effect. Midazolam was given by intermittent bolus injection if adequate sedation could not be produced by titration of the remifentanil or placebo infusion within the restrictions of the protocol. Treatment effects were similar in the hand and hip surgery groups and the ED_{50} for sedation was estimated as 0.043 μg.kg^{-1}.min^{-1}. The ED_{90} was not determined because the estimate was outside the studied dose range i.e. greater that 1 μg.kg^{-1}.min^{-1}. Thirteen patients were withdrawn because of adverse events with 8 having respiratory depression or oxygen desaturation (SpO_2 < 90%). Many patients did require supplementation with midazolam with those patients receiving the highest dose of remifentanil being least likely to require midazolam. Nevertheless, midazolam was still required in 18% of patients receiving the highest dose of remifentanil (0.1 μg. kg^{-1}.min^{-1}). In this study, regional anaesthesia was described as "incomplete" in many patients (30 - 35% of those undergoing hand surgery and a smaller proportion of those undergoing hip surgery) and the analgesia offered by the titrated remifentanil infusions was considered a valuable supplement. Nausea and respiratory depression were significantly more common during the infusion phase of the study however, this disappeared during the post-operative period. This finding suggests that the typical μ-opioid effects were limited to the period of infusion. Two studies have examined the interaction between midazolam and remifentanil for monitored anaesthesia care. Gold et al.[7] studied 159 patients undergoing outpatient surgery who received either a bolus dose of remifentanil of 1 μg/kg in 1 min, followed by an infusion of 0.1 μg.kg^{-1}.min^{-1} or an alternative regimen with half the dose of remifentanil i.e. 0.5 μg/kg in 1 min, followed by an infusion of 0.05 μg.kg^{-1}.min^{-1} in the presence of an additional intravenous midazolam bolus of 1 or 2 mg. The addition of midazolam did not influence the efficacy of sedation, which was satisfactory in both groups; however, its use permitted a lower infusion rate of remifentanil with a reduction in anxiety and nausea. The authors concluded that the remifentanil-midazolam technique represented a significant improvement on the use of remifentanil alone. Avramov et al.[8] studied 81 women scheduled for elective breast biopsy. Patients received an intravenous bolus of either saline or midazolam 2, 4 or 8 mg, followed by an infusion of remifentanil of 0.1 $\mu g.kg^{-1}.min^{-1}$ that was changed to patient responses and the desired level of sedation. Midazolam produced a dose dependant increase in the degree of sedation and the authors concluded that the regimen of intravenous midazolam, 2 mg, followed by an infusion of remifentanil of 0.05 - 0.1 $\mu g.kg^{-1}.min^{-1}$ was the optimal combination. In addition to the co-administration with midazolam, remifentanil has been critically compared to propofol in two studies. Lauwers et al.[9] randomised 28 patients to remifentanil 0.1 $\mu g.kg^{-1}.min^{-1}$ or propofol 50 $\mu g.kg^{-1}.min^{-1}$ and reported that remifentanil provided a smoother haemodynamic profile than propofol. However, it caused significantly more respiratory depression and oxygen desaturation. Both agents were easily titrated to effect and recovery times were similar. Smith et al.[10] studied 44 females undergoing breast biopsy and all received intravenous midazolam, 2 mg, followed either by propofol 75 $\mu g.kg^{-1}.min^{-1}$ or remifentanil 0.1 $\mu g.kg^{-1}.min^{-1}$ with subsequent titration to the desired level of sedation. Those patients receiving propofol were significantly more sedated than the patients receiving remifentanil. In the presence of remifentanil respiratory depression and oxygen desaturation occurred more often. Recovery times were faster after propofol infusion despite the high initial infusion rate.

How should we administer remifentanil for monitored anaesthesia care? As illustrated by the studies above, intravenous administration of midazolam, 2 mg, as a single intravenous bolus dose before the start of sedation appears to be advantageous. All previous studies have reported administration of remifentanil by infusion. Sa Rego et al.[11] studied 45 patients undergoing extracorporeal shock wave lithotripsy with all patients receiving intravenous midazolam, 2 mg, followed by a propofol infusion of 50 $\mu g.kg^{-1}.min^{-1}$. Analgesia during the period of shock waves was provided by remifentanil given either as an infusion, a bolus injection or a combination of infusion and bolus injection. Additional remifentanil was given by titration of the infusion rate or by administering additional bolus injections. These authors reported that the use of intermittent bolus doses (12.5 - 25 μg) alone or in combination with an infusion (0.05 $\mu g.kg^{-1}.min^{-1}$) were satisfactory alternatives to a variable rate infusion. Although, in this study, the bolus injections of remifentanil were given by the anaesthetists, the data suggest that a patient controlled system with a suitable lock-out period may be worthy of further investigation. Bolus injections may be particularly advantageous in controlling painful stimuli because plasma and effect site concentrations of remifentanil will rise rapidly after a bolus dose, whereas, a simple infusion rate increase will require several minutes to achieve a new steady state concentration. In the future, target controlled infusion of remifentanil may be considered in similar situations and may be advantageous to the above described dosing techniques. Remifentanil is undoubtedly efficacious as an agent for monitored anaesthesia care and is licensed to be used in this indication in many countries. Sedation is not the primary action of opioids and could reasonably be described as a side effect. It may be argued that using a drug for a side effect is poor pharmacology and that the well known dose related respiratory depression induced by all μ-opioid receptor agonists makes conscious sedation of spontaneously breathing patients by means of an opioid infusion an intrinsically unsafe technique. These concerns are theoretically valid and are partially supported by the clinical experience reported above with several authors describing respiratory depression in patients sedated with remifentanil. Furthermore, the use of pulse oximetry to confirm adequate respiration during remifentanil sedation has been criticised[1,2] and the published studies may therefore underestimate the magnitude of this problem. Serious consideration should be given to using a benzodiazepine or propofol as the hypnotic component of a monitored anaesthesia technique with opioids reserved for provision of analgesia if the regional anaesthetic technique is insufficient. Remifentanil may be relatively expensive in comparison to propofol and midazolam. However, drug acquisition costs form only a small portion of the total costs of a surgical episode and additional costs of a specific technique may, in certain circumstances, be offset by savings generated by swift patient recovery. There are few formal health economic evaluations in day surgery and there is currently no evidence that the use of remifentanil for monitored anaesthesia care offers overall economic benefits. The advantages and disadvantages of the agents propofol, midazolam and remifentanil for monitored anaesthesia care

Table 1
Summaries of comparative studies of remifentanil for monitored anaesthesia care (MAC)

Mingus 1998[13] Orthopaedic and urogenital surgery. Remifentanil (n=72) 0.09 $\mu g.kg^{-1}.min^{-1}$ (mean infusion rate) versus propofol (n=35) 53.8 $\mu g.kg^{-1}.min^{-1}$ **Efficacy**: fewer remifentanil patients had pain and less were over-sedated. **Safety**: remifentanil was associated with more respiratory depression and short-term nausea

Lauwers 1998[9] TURP and hand surgery. Remifentanil (n=14) 0.075 $\mu g.kg^{-1}.min^{-1}$ ('appropriate infusion rate') versus propofol (n=14) 50 $\mu g.kg^{-1}.min^{-1}$. **Efficacy:** remifentanil had less haemodynamic depression, similar scores for comfort and sedation in both groups. **Safety**: more respiratory depression and nausea with remifentanil.

Smith 1997[10] Breast biopsy. Remifentanil (n=22) 0.095 $\mu g.kg^{-1}.min^{-1}$ (mean infusion rate) versus propofol (n=22) 50.6 $\mu g.kg^{-1}.min^{-1}$. **Efficacy:** Both agents provided acceptable sedation, longer time to home readiness with remifentanil. **Safety**: Remifentanil was associated with more respiratory depression.

Lauwers 1999[6] Hand and hip surgery. Remifentanil (n=117) ED_{50} = 0.043 $\mu g.kg^{-1}.min^{-1}$ versus placebo (n=37). **Efficacy:** satisfactory sedation in most patients given remifentanil. **Safety**: nausea, pruritis, respiratory depression with remifentanil.

Table 2
Comparison of propofol, midazolam and remifentanil when used for monitored anaesthesia care (MAC)

	Propofol	Midazolam	Remifentanil
Onset of sedation	rapid	moderate	rapid
Recovery	rapid	slow	rapid
Pain on injection	yes	no	no
Water soluble	no	yes	yes
Supports rapid bacterial growth	yes	no	no
Haemodynamic depression	moderate	minimal	minimal
Respiratory depression	minimal	minimal	significant
Cost	moderate	low	moderate
Specific reversal agent	none	flumazenil	naloxone

are summarised in table 2. Remifentanil is a potent and efficacious analgesic and has performed well when used to provide the analgesic component of a 'balanced' sedative technique[11]. In view of the reservations about respiratory depression we must look critically at proposals to make general use of this agent in monitored anaesthesia care.

As summarised above, remifentanil works best when combined with another agent, usually a small dose of midazolam. If it is not an ideal single agent for monitored anaesthesia care then consideration should be given to reserving this opioid for what opioids do best i.e. relieve pain. Administration of remifentanil at doses likely to provide adequate sedation in most patients, i.e. 0.1 $\mu g.kg^{-1}.min^{-1}$, may cause unacceptable respiratory depression in a significant minority.

Conclusion

In conclusion, monitored anaesthesia care with remifentanil is an effective technique which has worked well in clinical trials. Its role in the large number of patients who routinely undergo this technique has not yet been convincingly demonstrated. So far, remifentanil appears a useful agent as an adjunct analgesic in patients whose primary sedative is a benzodiazepine or propofol.

References

1. Jastak JT, Peskin RM. Major morbidity or mortality from office anesthetic procedures: a closed-claim analysis of 13 cases. *Anesthesia Progress* 1991;38(2):39-44.
2. Krippaehne JA, Montgomery MT. Morbidity and mortality from pharmacosedation and general anesthesia in the dental office. *Journal Of Oral And Maxillofacial Surgery* 1992;50(7):691-8; discussion 698-9.
3. Sedation and anaesthesia in radiology: Joint working party of The Royal College of Anaesthetists and the Royal College of Radiologists, 1992.
4. Guidelines for sedation by non-anaesthetists: Royal College of Surgeons of England, 1993.
5. Egan TD, Minto CF, Hermann DJ, Barr J, Muir KT, Shafer SL. Remifentanil versus alfentanil: comparative pharmacokinetics and pharmacodynamics in healthy adult male volunteers. *Anesthesiology* 1996;84(4):821-33.
6. Lauwers M, Camu F, Breivik H, Hagelberg A, Rosen M, Sneyd R, et al. The safety and effectiveness of remifentanil as an adjunct sedative for regional anesthesia. *Anesthesia And Analgesia* 1999;88(1):134-40.
7. Gold MI, Watkins WD, Sung YF, Yarmush J, Chung F, Uy NT, et al. Remifentanil versus remifentanil/midazolam for ambulatory surgery during monitored anesthesia care. *Anesthesiology* 1997;87(1):51-7.
8. Avramov MN, Smith I, White PF. Interactions between midazolam and remifentanil during monitored anesthesia care. *Anesthesiology* 1996;85(6):1283-9.
9. Lauwers MH, Vanlersberghe C, Camu F. Comparison of remifentanil and propofol infusions for sedation during regional anesthesia. *Reg Anesth Pain Med* 1998;23(1):64-70.

10. Smith I, Avramov MN, White PF. A comparison of propofol and remifentanil during monitored anesthesia care. *J Clin Anesth* 1997;9(2):148-54.
11. Sa Rego MM, Inagaki Y, White PF. Remifentanil administration during monitored anesthesia care: are intermittent boluses an effective alternative to a continuous infusion? *Anesthesia and Analgesia* 1999;88:518-522.
12. Ramsay MAE, A. M, Hein HAT, Cancemi E. Use of remifentanil in patients breathing spontaneously during monitored anesthesia care and in the management of acute postoperative care. *Anesthesiology* 1998;88(4):1124-1125.
13. Mingus ML, Monk TG, Gold MI, Jenkins W, Roland C. Remifentanil versus propofol as adjuncts to regional anesthesia. Remifentanil 3010 Study Group. *J Clin Anesth* 1998;10(1):46-53.

REMIFENTANIL ANAESTHESIA AND POSTOPERATIVE PAIN MANAGEMENT

Stefan Schraag

Ulm, Germany

Introduction

Remifentanil, one of the latest developments among the fentanyl congeners, is a novel, short-acting μ-receptor opioid agonist, which has been introduced into clinical anaesthetic practice in most European countries and the United States within the last three years. It is the hydrochloride salt of 3-[4-methoxycarbonyl-4-[(1-oxopropyl) phenylamino]-1-piperidine] propanoic acid methyl ester. Incorporation of the methyl ester into the *N*-acyl moiety is the structural basis of the vulnerability of remifentanil to metabolism. The unique metabolism, based on organ independent ester hydrolysis in blood and tissue, results in a favourable pharmacokinetic profile with a rapid offset of drug effect, and thus the need for a continuous infusion to administer the drug. This essential feature is expressed as a context-sensitive half-time of about 3-4 min, regardless the duration of infusion[1].

These pharmacokinetic properties should confer ease of titration to changing intraoperative surgical stimulation and facilitate "real-time" management of intraoperative stressful conditions. Therefore, a large variety of anaesthetic techniques in today's clinical practice contain remifentanil as the analgesic component. As it has been shown to provide superior haemodynamics and faster time to extubation, remifentanil contributes to an improved overall effectiveness in anaesthesia services[2].

A major disadvantage of remifentanil, however, is the appropriate transition to postoperative pain control. Although the quick offset of action is beneficial with regard to recovery and respiratory control, this fact simultaneously leads to inadequate analgesia in the immediate postoperative phase[3], which may adversely affect patient's recovery and outcome. This manuscript gives a detailed discussion of the available options for the transition to adequate pain control after anaesthesia with remifentanil.

Analgesia and patient outcome

Adequate analgesia after major surgery is a relevant determinant of patient outcome [4]. For example Mangano and co-workers[5] examined whether the use of intense analgesia in the stressful perioperative period could decrease post-operative ischaemia after cardiac surgery. A total of 106 patients undergoing myocardial revascularisation received either morphine (low intensity group) or sufentanil (high intensity group) for intraoperative and postoperative analgesia up to 18 hours post-bypass, supplemented with benzodiazepines. The high intensity group had significantly less severe and less incidence of ischaemic events in the postoperative period.

Analgesic strategies

Since remifentanil was introduced into clinical practice, there has been a variety of suggested solutions to overcome the problem of immediate postoperative pain control, which becomes evident significantly earlier compared with other opioids, like alfentanil or sufentanil[6] (figure 1). An attractive means of providing longer lasting high quality analgesia with minimal side effects is the use of local anaesthetics. Especially in minor and body surface surgery the application of a local block is easy and highly efficient. Larger surgical interventions, such as total hip replacement, thoracic surgery or laparotomies often require a spinal or epidural block. Unfortunately, for various reasons the combination of general with regional anaesthesia may be limited to a small percentage of patients presenting for major surgery.

Presently, the most popular technique used to provide analgesia following remifentanil anaesthesia is the administration of longer acting analgesics, either as an intraoperative supplement or as a supplement prior to the end of surgery.

This strategy has been reported successfully both for opioids, such as morphine, piritramide and fentanyl, and for non-steroidal analgesics, like ketorolac, diclofenac or metamizol. A combination of both appears to act synergistic and thus optimise the analgesic effect. However, the crucial point with this technique remains the optimal timing of the drug administration and the anticipated dose requirements in the individual patient. Giving too much may result in an inadvertent and prolonged respiratory depression deleting the benefits of remifentanil´s recovery profile, whereas underdosing automatically leads to a patient with painful emergence from anaesthesia. Another technique of covering the problem of immediate postoperative analgesia is to continue the remifentanil infusion, at least until the patient can be adequately assessed in the recovery room, and subsequently administer a longer acting analgesic in accordance with the individual requirements.

Clinical trials

The challenge of postoperative pain management following remifentanil-based anaesthesia has also been addressed by some controlled clinical studies, published within the last three years. Minkowitz et al.[7] evaluated the effect of two loading doses of morphine (0.12 and 0.20 mg/kg) and compared the 24 hours morphine requirements, as administered with a patient-controlled infusion device, after remifentanil or fentanyl as the intraoperative analgesic components during urogenital surgery. Both morphine doses were comparably effective for an adequate analgesic transition and the overall analgesic requirements were similar between remifentanil and fentanyl regimens. Albrecht et al.[8] undertook a prospective, controlled and blinded study in 80 ASA 1-3 patients after midazolam premedication undergoing major abdominal surgery. All patients received propofol-remifentanil based anaesthesia. Twenty minutes before the anticipated end of surgery they were allocated into four groups to receive intravenously, either fentanyl 0.15 mg, morphine 15 mg, buprenorphine 0.3 mg or piritramide 15 mg. Additional analgesia was provided by PCA piritramide. All four groups showed a comparable recovery profile, but the majority of patients required a second bolus of the study drug. The best analgesia profile was seen in the patients receiving piritramide.

To overcome the disadvantage of immediate painful conditions after termination of a remifentanil infusion, several studies examined the feasibility of a manual controlled remifentanil infusion. Bowdle et al.[9] compared different infusion rates (0.05-0.15 $\mu g.kg^{-1}.min^{-1}$) and the effect of incremental bolus doses in a multi-centre study. They found adequate analgesia in 78% of patients within 30 minutes, but adverse respiratory effects were a notable problem, which affected 29% of patients, including 7% with apnoea. It is quite astonishing, that the same authors report in a subsequent study[10], when a postoperative remifentanil infusion was studied for the first 30 minutes after abdominal surgery before further transition to either morphine PCA or epidural analgesia, that no respiratory problems occurred. However, this particular study enrolled only 22 patients and the design had to be modified after treating 13 patients, because of inadequate pain control. This assumes a systematic underdosing and thus may explain the lack of respiratory events. In another multi-centre study comparing remifentanil with alfentanil for major abdominal surgery, Schüttler et al.[11] titrated a manual remifentanil infusion beginning with 0.1 $\mu g.kg^{-1}.min^{-1}$. They found that rapid changes in remifentanil blood concentration by bolus administrations or increases of the infusion rate, although effective with regard to analgesia, resulted in a high frequency of muscle rigidity, respiratory depression and apnoea. An editorial comment to this paper states, that using remifentanil in the manner described is unacceptable[12]. Similar results were recently reported by Yarmush et al[13]. They conducted a double blind comparison of manually controlled remifentanil infusion (median infusion rate: 0.125 $\mu g.kg^{-1}.min^{-1}$) with morphine boluses during the first 25 min after the end of surgery. Transient respiratory depression, apnoea or both (14%) were the most frequent adverse effects in the remifentanil group.

A randomised, double-blind study by Sá Rêgo et al.[14] was designed to evaluate the analgesic effectiveness and respiratory stability of remifentanil when administered as intermittent bolus injections, a variable-rate infusion, or a combination of a constant basal infusion supplemented with intermittent boluses during monitored anaesthesia care and propofol sedation. Although the authors found that both intermittent bolus injections of remifentanil (25 µg) and a continuous infusion (0.05 $\mu g.kg^{-1}.min^{-1}$) supplemented with boluses (12.5 µg) may be more effective than a variable-rate infusion, the overall incidence of respiratory adverse events were high in all groups with at least one period of apnoea

Table 1
Postoperative remifentanil manual infusion. Studies on analgesic efficiency and repiratory side effects (numbers in brackets refer to references in the text).

Author	n	Infusion rates ($\mu g.kg^{-1}.min^{-1}$)	Adequate pain control (%)	Respiratory adverse events* (%)	Apnoea (%)
Bowdle [9]	157	0.05 - 0.15	64	29	7
Bowdle [10]	22	0.04 - 0.26	86	0	0
Schüttler [11]	116	0.05 - 0.10	71	21	11
Yarmush [13]	72	0.05 - 0.23	58	14	4
Sá Rêgo [14]	30	0.10	n.a.**	30	25-28

* Respiratory adverse events are reported with slightly different definitions in the respective paper. But the majority of events required interventions, such as additional oxygen, assisted ventilation, adjustment of remifentanil infusion rate or reversal of opioid effect by naloxone.
** During propofol sedation.

in 25-30 % of the patients. A summary of studies evaluating postoperative remifentanil infusions is given in table 1.

Remifentanil and respiratory depression

The relationship between remifentanil induced ventilatory suppression and its predicted effect-site concentration is more or less linear[15]. In fact, the equilibration time $T_{1/2}k_{eo}$ for respiratory effects is almost double the 1.6 min reported for the onset of EEG spectral-edge effects. This suggests that one must wait at least 2-3 min to assess the respiratory effects of a bolus dose. The effect of a change in the manual infusion scheme will therefore be apparent only after a time interval that can vary between 10 and 15 min.

When remifentanil infusion rates of 0.025-0.1 $\mu g.kg^{-1}.min^{-1}$ were administered in combination with propofol (6 $mg.kg^{-1}.h^{-1}$) as part of a total intravenous anaesthesia technique, Peacock et al.[16] found that infusion rates $\leq$ 0.05 $\mu g.kg^{-1}.min^{-1}$ were associated with adequate spontaneous ventilation. In contrast, Murdoch et al.[17] reported some difficulties with adequate ventilation during remifentanil infusion. They examined 20 unpremedicated patients undergoing day case surgery during remifentanil-propofol anaesthesia. After induction and insertion of a laryngeal mask, anaesthesia was maintained with

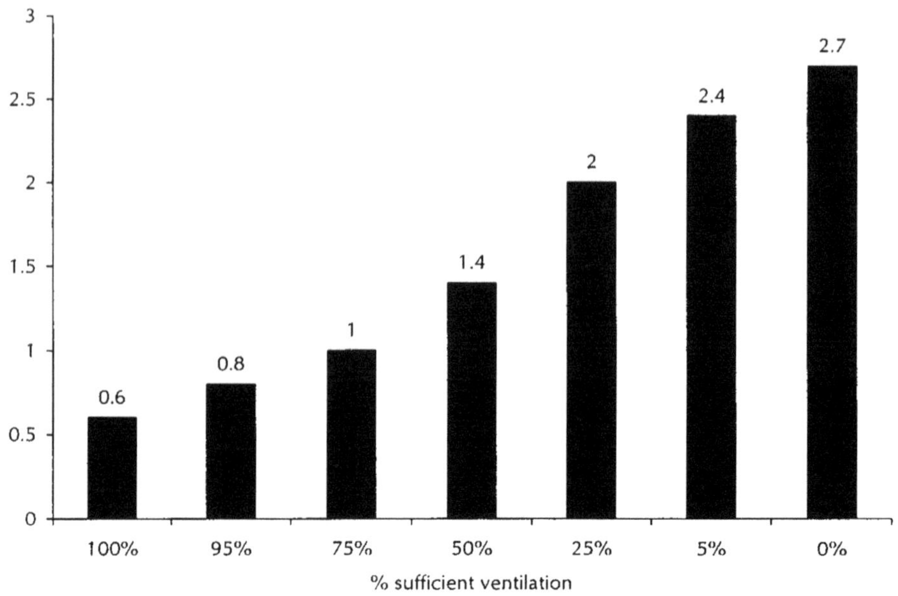

Figure 1
Remifentanil target concentrations and the percentage of adequate spontaneous ventilation during propofol anaesthesia. Adequate ventilation is defined as an end tidal CO_2 partial pressure of 6.5-7.0 kPa and an oxygen saturation (SaO_2) of 94% or higher achieved for a period of at least five minutes (n=25).

propofol TCI at a constant level of 4.5 µg/ml. After ensuring spontaneous ventilation, remifentanil, administered by a target-controlled infusion device, was increased and decreased in increments of 0.2 ng ml^{-1} until adequate spontaneous ventilation, defined as an ET-CO_2 of 6.5-7.0 kPa, was achieved for a period of at least 5 min. Success rate was only 60% and the median remifentanil target concentration during the periods of respiratory stability was 1.6 ng ml^{-1}. This corresponded to a median infusion rate of 0.05 $\mu g.kg^{-1}.min^{-1}$ (range 0.019-0.107 $\mu g.kg^{-1}.min^{-1}$). An essential finding in this study was the large variability of over 4.7 fold around the median. Similar results were obtained by us in a series of 25 patients, where we tried to determine the remifentanil threshold for adequate ventilation during propofol anaesthesia (figure 1).

However, one must keep in mind that possible interactions between remifentanil and propofol on respiration pattern during anaesthesia may account for

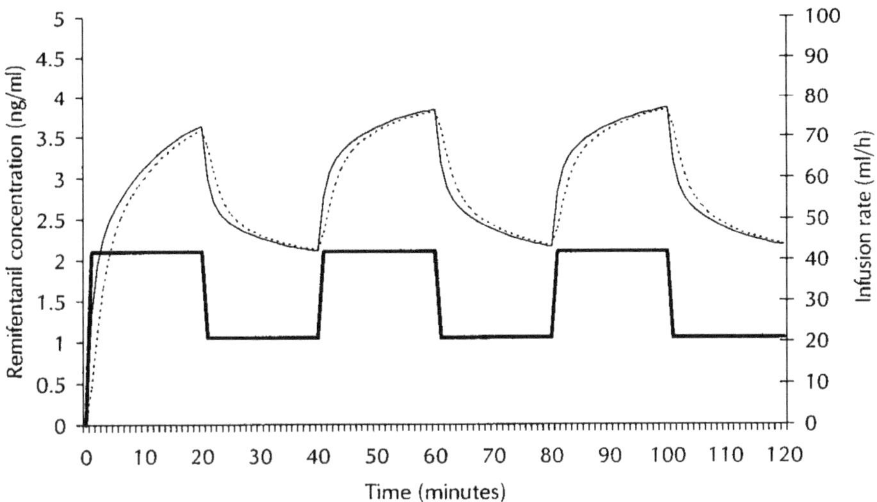

Figure 2
Time course of remifentanil blood concentration (solid line) and calculated effect site concentration (dashed line) during repeated changes between two different infusion rates every 20 minutes (0.2 μg.kg^{-1}.min^{-1} versus 0.1 μg.kg^{-1}.min^{-1}).

the less good results compared with postoperative remifentanil infusions in awake patients

Target controlled infusion (TCI) with remifentanil

A couple of studies have now been published showing that remifentanil is a suitable intraoperative alternative to the other fentanyl congeners[6, 11]. But, as expressed by a wide variation of infusion rates these studies also show still an uncertainty about the appropriate dosing guidelines necessary to blunt different noxious stimulation using remifentanil by manual infusion. Why target controlled infusion of remifentanil? Intravenous anaesthetic drugs that possess a rapid equilibration with the effect compartment like propofol, alfentanil or remifentanil offer the opportunity for titrating the anaesthetic or analgesic effect close to the drug's blood concentration. In this respect pharmacokinetic model based TCI-propofol and TCI-alfentanil have been successfully used to confer ease of titration of the anaesthetic and analgesic effect, respectively[18, 19]. In contrast, a manual infusion of remifentanil will require a considerable time span to achieve steady state blood concentrations. Furthermore, every manual adjustment of the infusion rate will again result in a sluggish equilibration to the new steady state condition (figure 2). Even intermittent bolus administrations of this rapid metabolised drug will not result in a more rapid equilibrium. Furthermore, the effect of a manual application of remifentanil, based on the currently available dosing recommendations, is highly variable and dependent on the condition of the individual patient. For example, the same infusion regime applied to an obese old patient will result in more than double the blood concentration of remifentanil compared to a young lean patient. A target controlled infusion of remifentanil, which compensates for the distribution and elimination by adjusting the infusion rate on the basis of a pharmacokinetic model makes individual titration of the drug to the effect more predictable. Although small boluses are given when using TCI-remifentanil, these have not been associated with side effects like bradycardia and hypotension seen with uncontrolled manual boluses. Recent developments the pharmacokinetic models used in TCI- remifentanil also include parameters such as age, weight, height (lean body mass) and body surface area as covariates[20].

Transition to postoperative analgesia with a patient-maintained remifentanil TCI

We developed a target controlled infusion of remifentanil to ensure individually predictive and adequate intraoperative drug delivery without overshoot and overdosing, which seemed to be common in the early reports using remifentanil as the "forgiving opioid"[21]. The logical consequence to overcome the problem with postoperative pain control was to continue TCI Remifentanil into the early postoperative phase, as serious side effects, mainly respiratory depression, have been reported with manual infusions[9]. We studied 30 male patients in the early postoperative period to assess the efficacy, safety and feasibility of a patient-demand, target-controlled infusion remifentanil[22]. All patients received the same TCI based propofol-remifentanil anaesthetic for elective orthopaedic surgery. After discontinuation of propofol at the end of surgery, the remifentanil infusion was progressively reduced by decrements of 0.1 ng/ml until the patients were breathing spontaneously. After extubation and transfer to the post anaesthesia care unit (PACU), they were given control of a handset, which was connected to the TCI controller, and were able to increase the target remifentanil blood level by increments of 0.2 ng/ml with a 2 min lockout interval. If there were no demands within a 30-min period, the TCI controller reduced the target concentration by 0.2 ng/ml. Every 3 min pain scores, sedation level, respiration rate, oxygen saturation and nausea were assessed. Mean time to onset of satisfactory analgesia (VAS ≤ 3, out of 10) was 18.9 (15.8-21.9 95% CI) min at a mean target remifentanil concentration of 2.02 ng/ml (1.87-2.16 95% CI). There were no episodes of hypoxaemia (oxygen saturation <95%) and the lowest respiration rate was 9 breaths per min. Nausea occurred in 26.6% of patients and 10% vomited. The majority of patients were only slightly sedated (mean sedation score: 2.1 out of 6).

We did not measure remifentanil blood concentrations and so we could not estimate the performance of the remifentanil TCI on the patients studied. However, the pharmacokinetic data used to program the TCI controller have been shown to be sufficiently reliable. Pharmacokinetic bias and precision, expressed as relative and absolute percent performance error, are reported to be 26% and 19%, respectively[20], which are comparable to data obtained for TCI-PCA alfentanil and sufentanil[23]. Even if we knew the actual remifentanil blood concentrations, this would only be a minor contribution since the pharmacodynamic variability of the required target concentrations between the individual patients (about 200%) exceeds the expected pharmacokinetic error.

Another possible source of inaccuracy could be the physical performance of the infusion pump and the dilution of the drug. A remifentanil concentration of 50 µg/ml has been reported to be associated with a high incidence of opioid-induced adverse effects when used as a manual infusion[9]. The choice of intravenous tubing, dead space of taps or three-way valves and changes in flow rates of additional fluids may substantially influence moment-to-moment delivery, resulting in varying drug concentrations. Therefore we used a low concentrated remifentanil of 20 µg/ml, which was connected to the proximal port of the intravenous line, flushed by a constant rate of Ringer's lactate. Even taking these precautions into account, our preliminary experience does not yet support the use of this system without adequate supervision and monitoring.

These preliminary results of a patient-maintained TCI of remifentanil imply a safe and effective tool in the early postoperative period after anaesthesia using remifentanil as the analgesic component. Currently this technique is evaluated

Table 2
Therapeutical suggestions for the transition to postoperative analgesia following remifentanil-based anaesthesia

Type of surgery	Intraoperative management	Postoperative management
Minor surgery	Morphine 0.15-0.2 mg/kg	Non-steroidal analgesics
	Local block (bupivacaine)	Non-steroidal analgesics
Major surgery	Morphine/Piritramide 0.2 mg/kg (15 min before surgery ends)	PCA Morphine/Piritramide
	Start of epidural analgesia	Epidural analgesia
	Remifentanil TCI *	Patient-maintained remifentanil TCI*

* not yet approved for official use

double-blind, double-dummy against standard morphine PCA after major abdominal surgery.

Conclusion

Over the past years a significant body of knowledge on the transition from anaesthesia to adequate postoperative analgesia following remifentanil-based anaesthesia has been gathered. However, regarding this issue specific recommendations based on unbiased studies that guarantee a high degree of effectiveness and safety are still lacking. A summary of suggested therapeutic options is given in table 2.

Without a feasible and clinically attractive solution for the transition of anaesthesia to postoperative analgesia, remifentanil will only be of limited additional value to the anaesthetist in daily practice. Combined analgesic strategies and target-controlled infusion of remifentanil together with the application of a patient controlled device could help to achieve a smooth transition from remifentanil anaesthesia to a satisfactory postoperative analgesia.

References

1. Kapila A, Glass PS, Jacobs JR, Muir KT, Hermann DJ, Shiraishi M, Howell S, Smitz RL. Measured context-sensitive half-times of remifentanil and alfentanil. Anaesthesiology 1995; 83:968-75.

2. Fleisher LA, Glass PSA, Roizen MA, Twersky R, Tuman K, Warner DS, Colopy M, Jamerson BD, and the SOURCE Investigators. Remifentanil provides superior hemodynamics and faster time to extubation than a fentanyl based anesthetic in a large scale trial of effectiveness. Anesthesiology 1998; 89:A33.
3. Dershwitz M, Randel GI, Rosow CE, Fragen RJ, Connors PM, Librojo ES, Shaw DL, Peng AW, Jamerson BD. Initial clinical experience with remifentanil, a new opioid metabolised by esterases. Anesth Analg 1995; 81:619-23.
4. Roizen M, Lampe G, Benefiel D. Is increased operative stress associated with worse outcome? Anesthesiology 1987; 67:A1.
5. Mangano DT, Siciliano D, Hollenberg M, Leung JM, Browner WS, Goehner P, Merrick S, Verrier E, SPI Research Group. Postoperative myocardial ischemia: Therapeutic trials using intensive analgesia following surgery. Anesthesiology 1992; 76:342-53.
6. Philip BK, Scuderi PE, Chung F, Conahan TJ, Maurer W, Angel JJ, Kallar SK, Skinner EP, Jamerson BD, and the remifentanil/alfentanil outpatient TIVA group. Remifentanil compared with alfentanil for ambulatory surgery using total intravenous anaesthesia. Anesth Analg 1997; 84:515-21.
7. Minkowitz H, Yarmush J, Rung G, Melson T, Weiss J, Wentz A. Postoperative analgesia with morphine sulfate following remifentanil-based anesthesia. Anesth Analg 1998; 86:S484.
8. Albrecht S, Schüttler J, Fechner J, Moecke HP, Maass AB, Upadhyaya B, Haigh CG. Postoperative pain management following remifentanil-based anesthesia for major abdominal surgery. Anesth Analg 1998; 86:S253.
9. Bowdle TA, Camporesi EM, Maysick L, Hogue CW, Miguel RV, Pitts M, Streisand JB. A multicenter evaluation of remifentanil for early postoperative analgesia. Anesth Analg 1996; 83:1292-7.
10. Bowdle TA, ReadyLB, Kharash ED, Nichols WW, Cox K. Transition to postoperative epidural or patient-controlled intravenous analgesia following total intravenous anaesthesia with remifentanil and propofol for abdominal surgery. Eur J Anaesth 1997; 14:374-9.
11. Schüttler J, Albrecht S, Breivik H, Osnes S, Prys-Roberts C, Holder K, Chauvin M, Viby-Mogensen J, Gustafson I, Lof L, Noronha D, Kirkham AJT. A comparison of remifentanil and alfentanil in patients undergoing major abdominal surgery. Anaesthesia 1997; 52:307-17.
12. Smith MA, Morgan M. Remifentanil (editorial). Anaesthesia 1997; 52:291-93.
13. Yarmush JM, D´Angelo RD, Kirkhart BS, et al. A comparison of remifentanil and morphine sulphate for acute postoperative analgesia after total intravenous anesthesia with remifentanil and propofol. Anesthesiology 1997; 87:235-43
14. Sá Rêgu MM, Inagaki Y, White PF: Remifentanil administration during monitored anesthesia care: Are intermittent boluses an effective alternative to a continuous infusion? Anesth Analg 1999; 88:518-22.
15. Babenco HD, Conard PF, Gross JB. The pharmacodynamic effect of a remifentanil bolus on ventilatory control. Anesthesiology 1998;89:A502.
16. Peacock JE, Luntley JB, O´Connor B, Reilly CS, Ogg TW, Watson BJ, Shaikh S. Remifentanil in combination with propofol for spontaneous ventilation anaesthesia. Br J Anaesth 1998; 80:509-11.
17. Murdoch JAC, Hyde RA, Kenny GNC. Target-controlled remifentanil in combination with propofol for spontaneously breathing day case patients: effects on respiration. Br J Anaesth 1998; 80(Supp1):A.42.
18. Kenny NC, White M: A portable target controlled propofol infusion system. Int J Clin Monit Comp 1992; 9:179-82.

19. Irwin MG, Jones DM, Visram AR, Kenny GN. Patient-controlled alfentanil. Target-controlled infusion for postoperative analgesia. Anaesthesia 1996; 51:427-30.
20. Minto CF, Schnider TW, Egan TD, Youngs E, Lemmens HJ, Gambus PL, Billard V, Hoke JF, Moore KH, Hermann DJ, Muir KT, Mandema JF, Shafer SL. Influence of age and gender on the pharmacokinetics and pharmacodynamics of remifentanil. I. Model development. Anesthesiology 1997; 86:10-23.
21. Rosow C: Remifentanil - A unique opioid analgesic [editorial]. Anesthesiology 1993; 79:875-6.
22. Schraag S, Kenny GNC, Mohl U, Georgieff M. Patient-maintained remifentanil target-controlled infusion for the transition to early postoperative analgesia. Br J Anaesth 1998; 81:365-8.
23. Van den Nieuwenhuyzen MC, Engbers FH, Burm AG, Vletter AA, van Kleef JW, Bovill JG. Target-controlled infusion of alfentanil for postoperative analgesia: a feasibility study and pharmacodynamic evaluation in the early postoperative period. Br J Anaesth 1997; 78:17-23.

TARGET CONTROLLED INFUSION FOR POSTOPERATIVE ANALGESIA

Marjolein C.O. van den Nieuwenhuyzen

Leiden, The Netherlands

Introduction

The vast majority of patients after surgery require administration of opioids to treat postoperative pain. However, opioids are associated with serious and sometimes life-threatening side effects. Therefore, the search for an optimal postoperative analgesic regimen continues. To optimize postoperative pain management a variety of opioids have been explored. In addition, various modes and routes of administration have been examined, in order to improve the quality of analgesia and to minimise the incidence of side effects.

The degree of postoperative pain varies widely between individuals and also fluctuates in time. A technique for administering analgesics that is tailored to the needs of the individual patient should, therefore, provide optimal pain relief. At present Patient-Controlled Analgesia (PCA) is the only individually tailored technique to provide postoperative analgesia that is widely accepted in clinical practice. Since the patients are able to self-administer small doses of opioid when they experience pain, the PCA technique offers the psychological advantage of being in control over one's own pain. The current PCA devices rely on the administration of bolus doses. Consequently, the plasma concentration, the concentration in the central nervous system, and the analgesic effect will vary considerably during the intervals between doses. From a pharmacokinetic point of view the optimal lockout time and the optimal background infusion rate vary in time during the postoperative period. Theoretically, a low or absent back-

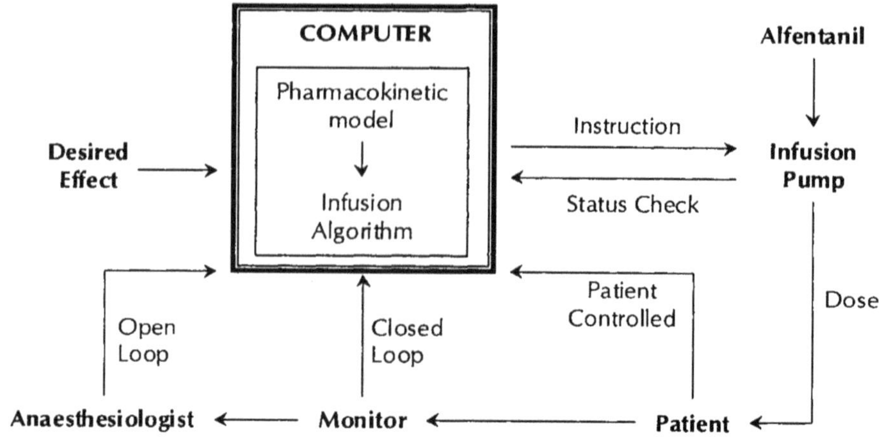

Figure 1
Schematic diagram of target controlled drug delivery. For intra-operative use the open-loop system is generally used. Feed back of information from monitors to the computer changes the system in a closed-loop system. For use as a postoperative analgesic delivery system the system can be made patient-controlled. (Modified from: Reves JG, Jacobs JR Glass PSA. Automated drug delivery in anesthesia. ASA refresher course in anesthesiology. Philadelphia, JB Lippincott, 1991;19.)

ground infusion and a long lockout time can lead to ineffective analgesic concentrations at the start of therapy. On the contrary, a short lockout time or a high background infusion may result in overdosing the patient at a later stage.

The administration of an infusion at a continuously changing rate can only be managed reliably using a computer controlled infusion pump. The main advantage of drug administration by target controlled infusion (TCI) is that it allows rapid adjustments of blood concentrations to individual patient's requirements. In the postoperative period there is a considerable variability in both inter- and intra-individual requirements, even after standardised operations. At the same time, the therapeutic window for most opioids is narrow in the postoperative period. It is therefore difficult for the anaesthetist in the operating room to predict and to anticipate on the requirements of the individual patient in the postoperative phase. Consequently, the availability of a technique that allows rapid titration to the individual patient's requirements would be advantageous. In this respect TCI could be the technique of choice for intravenous administration of opioids. Especially in the era where new

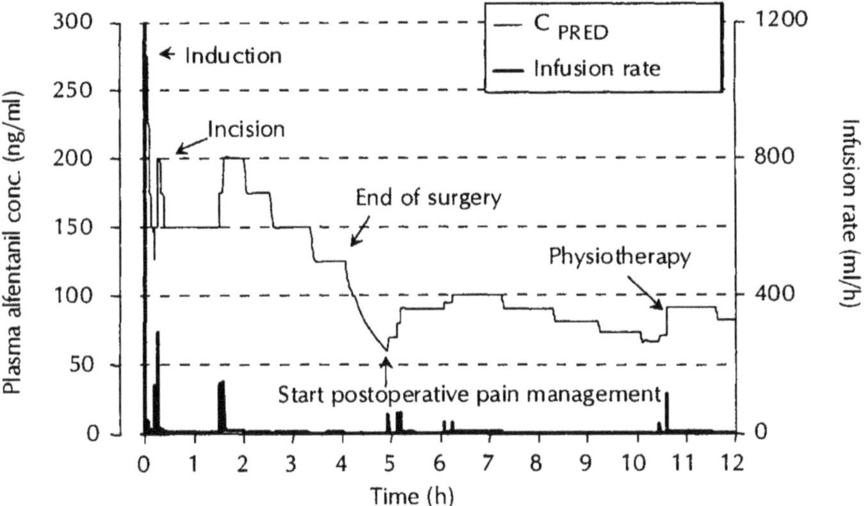

Figure 2
Hypothetical case with predicted plasma (C_{PRED}) concentrations of alfentanil that could be achieved by TCI during general anaesthesia and in the postoperative period. The infusion rates are automatically adjusted by the computer to achieve and maintain the desired target. (For the simulation the population pharmacokinetics of alfentanil as described by Maitre et al.[1] were used).

short-acting anaesthetics and analgesics are introduced, a reliable and effective postoperative analgesic technique associated with few side effects, will optimize patient's recovery and satisfaction and permit early discharge from the postanaesthesia care unit.

TCI settings in postoperative analgesia

TCI systems are maintaining desired target concentrations of a drug by automatically changing the infusion rate. A schematic presentation of a TCI device is shown in figure 1. The computer is programmed with a pharmacokinetic model as well as pharmacokinetic data. The computer translates predictions from the model into instructions to control the infusion device. The program calculates at frequent intervals, every 5-10 s the infusion rate needed to achieve and maintain the desired target plasma concentration. The infusion pump then delivers the required infusion rate. Intraoperatively, the target concentration is selected directly by the anaesthetist. Likewise, in the immediate postoperative period the anaesthetist has to select the target concentration that provides an adequate and acceptable level of analgesia, before the patient can take over the control of the system.

As shown in figure 2 for alfentanil this target concentration does not have to be kept constant over time, but may be increased or automatically decreased, according to the clinical need of the patient.

Several studies from different investigators have explored the efficacy of TCI for postoperative analgesia.[2-10] The pharmacologic properties of alfentanil make it a suitable drug for use in this setting. Alfentanil has a rapid onset of action, a favourable characteristic for the patient in pain. Its pharmacokinetics allow rapid changes in target concentrations even after prolonged infusions. Its rapid blood-brain equilibration results in corresponding rapid changes of effect, which may be advantageous when alterations in analgesic effect are required or when side effects occur. Remifentanil has a comparable rapid blood-brain equilibration as alfentanil and its unique metabolism results in rapid offset of drug effect regardless of the duration of the infusion. The experience with TCI remifentanil in the postoperative period is still limited.[9]

Pharmacokinetic data used in TCI systems are subject to interindividual pharmacokinetic variability. In general, individually predetermined data are not available. Therefore, the application of a relevant and valid pharmacokinetic parameter set in a TCI system, especially, when the TCI system is to be used in the postoperative period, is important. None of the published pharmacokinetic data sets of opioids has been shown to be valid during prolonged (up to several days) infusion for postoperative pain relief. Pharmacokinetic research on the postoperative period is scarce. Since pharmacokinetic parameters are often derived from a small, relatively homogeneous population it is not easy to select an appropriate data set for TCI. As demonstrated in figure 3, the measured blood or plasma concentrations in patients may differ considerably from the concentrations predicted by the TCI system's computer. A median performance error of less than 15% and an absolute median performance error of less than 30% are generally considered acceptable for drugs used for intra-operative and postoperative patient care. Pharmacodynamic variability between patients and the variation in responses (e.g. changes in heart rate, blood pressure) to stimuli

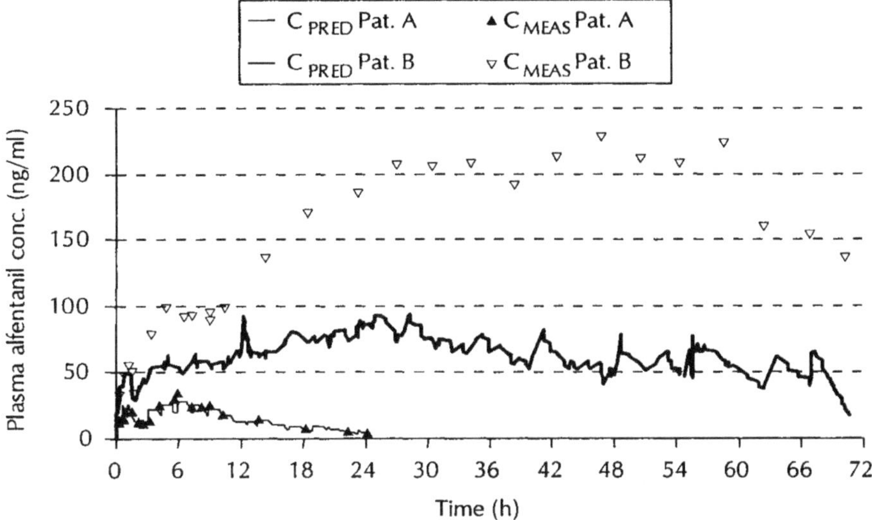

Figure 3
The best (pat. A) and the worst (pat. B) patient's performance of a patient-controlled TCI system when used to administer alfentanil in the postoperative period. The lines represent the predicted concentration by the computer and the wedges (▽) and triangles (▲) the measured concentrations of alfentanil.

during and after a procedure, force the anaesthetist to adjust the target concentration during and after anaesthesia.

Rational administration of opioids in the postoperative period requires not only reliable pharmacokinetic data but also reliable pharmacodynamic data. Therefore, concentration-effect relationships have to be established in order to identify not only the target concentration of the drug that provides satisfactory postoperative analgesia but also a rational step size to increase the target concentration and to automatically decrease the target concentration of the opioid.

Clinical experience of TCI in postoperative analgesia

Hill et al.[11,12] were the first to document the use of a computer controlled infusion pump with an algorithm that utilised predetermined individual pharmacokinetic parameters and showed that pharmaco-kinetically tailored opioid infusions produced stable plasma concentrations of alfentanil and morphine within 10 min after its start. These investigators used the TCI system to obtain stable drug concentrations to investigate concentration-effect relationships and intensities of side-effects produced by equianalgesic plasma concentrations of opioids.[13] The same group documented the analgesic efficacy of TCI-morphine for the treatment of persistent pain in cancer patients undergoing bone marrow transplantation and also used predetermined individual pharmacokinetic parameters for their patients who used the TCI system for up to 2 weeks to relief pain from oral mucositis and found the TCI system to be a safe and effective alternative to conventional Patient-Controlled Analgesia (PCA).[14-16]

Davies et al.[2] described a nurse-controlled TCI system of alfentanil to provide postoperative analgesia following aortic bifurcation graft surgery in 14 patients. The anaesthetist initially selected the optimum target concentration of alfentanil in the immediate postoperative period in order to achieve satisfactory analgesia. For the rest of the postoperative period the target concentration was altered by the nursing staff in response to the patient's request. These alterations could increase or decrease the target concentration by only 5 ng/ml. The control software also slowly reduced the target concentration over a period of time if no activation of the system was detected. As an added safety feature, the system could be linked to a pulse oximeter, so that, if the oxygen saturation would fall below a predefined limit the infusion rate would rapidly be reduced by the computer until the saturation level again rises above the preset limit. Later on, the nurse-controlled system has been modified, so that the target concentration is increased in response to activation of the system by the patient.[4,6] Irwin et al. described the use of such a patient-controlled, pharmacokinetic-based infusion of alfentanil in a single patient crossover comparison with PCA-morphine.[4] By double pressing the demand button within 1 s, the patient was now enabled to increase the target concentration of alfentanil by 5 ng/ml, with a lockout time of 2 min. If analgesia was not demanded, the target concentration declined every 15 min during the first 4 h of use, every 30 min during the next 4 h period and every 60 min thereafter, until the target concentration reached the baseline value of 15 ng/ml. When compared to PCA-morphine bolus administration (bolus 1 mg, lockout 5 min), the time to achieve satisfactory analgesia was delayed in the initial postoperative period, while using the TCI regimen. The patient experienced difficulties manipulating the handset, which required double activation of the button to permit successful drug delivery. Once the patient became proficient in the use of the system and a predicted alfentanil target concentration in the range of 54-64 ng/ml had been achieved, pain relief, respiratory rates and sedation scores were comparable to those achieved with morphine. In a following study Irwin et al. studied 20 patients scheduled to undergo major thoracolumbar spinal surgery.[6] Patients either received PCA-morphine or TCI-alfentanil with the same settings as described in the earlier report.[4] The initial postoperative target concentration of alfentanil in this study was 30 ng/ml. The TCI alfentanil system was demonstrated to be equally effective as a postoperative analgesic technique in comparison with conventional PCA-morphine. However, equianalgesia to morphine was not achieved until after about 6 h of infusion. There were no hypoxaemic episodes (oxygen saturation < 94%), no differences in sedation scores, and the incidence of nausea (30%) was the same in both groups. The TCI system had a significant tendency to underestimate actual drug concentrations. This inaccuracy was particularly pronounced at concentrations less than 40 ng/ml.

In a series of studies we also demonstrated the efficacy of TCI alfentanil in the postoperative period.[3,5,7,10] In contrast to the experimental system developed in Glasgow, our initial step-size to increase the target concentration was 10 ng/ml with a lockout interval of 10 min in a trial where 20 patients after orthopaedic surgery were studied.[3] After a loading period, where the target concentration was increased by the investigator, the step-size was reduced to 5 ng/ml when the patient was controlling the system and the target concentration was maintained for 2 h after the last rewarded demand, before it was automatically decreased by 5 ng/ml every 15 min until the next demand was made. In contrast to the earlier reported studies by Irwin et al.[4,6] and despite the longer lockout interval, the onset of satisfactory analgesia (visual analogue score # 3.0 on a scale from 0 to 10 and no request for additional analgesia) was faster in the TCI-alfentanil group (median 20 min, range 10-80 min) than in the PCA-morphine group (median 50 min, range 20-163 min). The validity of the pharmacokinetic data set described by Maitre et al.[1] was affirmed with a median performance error of 8% and a median absolute performance error of 22%, this in contrast to the underprediction of the system of the actual plasma concentration of alfentanil in Chinese patients as reported by Irwin et al.[6](median performance error of 58% and an absolute median performance error of 75%).

In a more recent study, including 120 patients recovering from cardiac surgery, TCI-alfentanil was again compared with conventional PCA-morphine.[8] After bypass patients in the TCI-alfentanil group continued to receive alfentanil and returned to the intensive care unit with an initial target concentration set at an appropriate level. When the patients in the TCI-alfentanil group were able to use a PCA handset, when they opened their eyes and obeyed simple commands, the handset was plugged into the TCI system. With a successful demand the target concentration of alfentanil was increased by 5 ng/ml with a lockout time of 2 min. If analgesia was not requested for 30 min, the target concentration was automatically reduced in steps of 5 ng/ml every 30 min for the first 4 h of use, every 45 min for the next 4 h and every 60 min thereafter. The system was programmed to deliver a minimum plasma concentration of 15 ng/ml and a maximum concentration of 150 ng/ml. The overall median pain scores were lower in the TCI alfentanil group compared to the PCA morphine group, but they were both in the zone of analgesic success defined by Mantha et al.[17] Both systems did not differ with respect to overall sedation scores, the frequency of postoperative nausea and vomiting, haemodynamic instability, myocardial ischaemia or hypoxaemia.

To overcome the disadvantage of immediate painful conditions after stopping infusions of remifentanil, Schraag et al.[9] studied 30 male patients in the early postoperative period after orthopaedic surgery to assess the efficacy, safety and feasibility of a patient-maintained target controlled infusion of remifentanil. Approximately 10 min before the anticipated end of surgery, the infusion of propofol was stopped and the target concentration of remifentanil was reduced progressively in decrements of 0.1 ng/ml until patients were breathing spontaneously at a ventilatory frequency ∃ 10 bpm. The target concentration of remifentanil at which each individual patient regained consciousness and tracheal extubation occurred was maintained until they were transferred to the post-anaesthesia care unit. A handset was connected to the TCI controller and the patient was given control. By pushing the demand button twice within 1 s when pain relief was required, the patient was able to increase the target concentration of remifentanil. The target concentration of remifentanil was increased by 0.2 ng/ml after every successful demand. The double push for every demand was chosen to ensure a minimum of alertness of the patient. There was a lockout time of 2 min after each increase in target concentration. In the absence of a demand within a 30-min period, the target concentration was automatically reduced by 0.2 ng/ml during the first 4 h and further reductions of 0.2 ng/ml were made every 45 min during the following 4 h. The mean target remifentanil concentration at which spontaneous ventilation was first noted after the end of surgery was 1.05 (95% confidence interval: 0.97-1.14) ng/ml, significantly less than that required for adequate analgesia after operation, which was 2.02 (1.87-2.16) ng/ml. Mean time to adequate analgesia was 18.9 (15.9-21.9) min. The frequency of nausea and vomiting was 26.6% and 10%, respectively, and occurred predominantly in patients with relatively high and rapid increases in target concentrations of remifentanil. Patient-demand target controlled infusion of remifentanil was found to be an effective tool for the transition to sufficient analgesia in the early postoperative period.

The potential advantage of improving the onset time of adequate analgesia using a TCI technique may be particularly useful, when pain is most intense, i.e. soon after waking up. The static settings of the lockout period and the maximum dosage in time with conventional PCA are actually a compromise between the shortest onset time for pain relief and a possible overdosing later on, once the drug is distributed to all the compartments in the body. By combining TCI systems with PCA and using short-acting drugs with a relative short blood-brain equilibration half-time such as alfentanil and remifentanil, a fast onset can be combined with a maintenance of analgesia for prolonged periods, when the plasma concentration of the analgesic drug is sustained within the therapeutic window. In consequence, superimposed on the TCI algorithms, extra algorithms are necessary that decide on the step-size in target concentration, the lockout interval, and at what point in time the predicted concentration is to be reduced, as well as on the step-size of the reduction of the target concentration needed to avoid unnecessary high delivery of opioids, once the intensity of the pain stimulus has decreased. These algorithms will influence the performance and efficacy of the system and might in part explain the differences in onset of satisfactory analgesia when TCI alfentanil is used. These algorithms should be well described as they will differ between experimental systems. In figure 4, an example of such an algorithm is demonstrated.

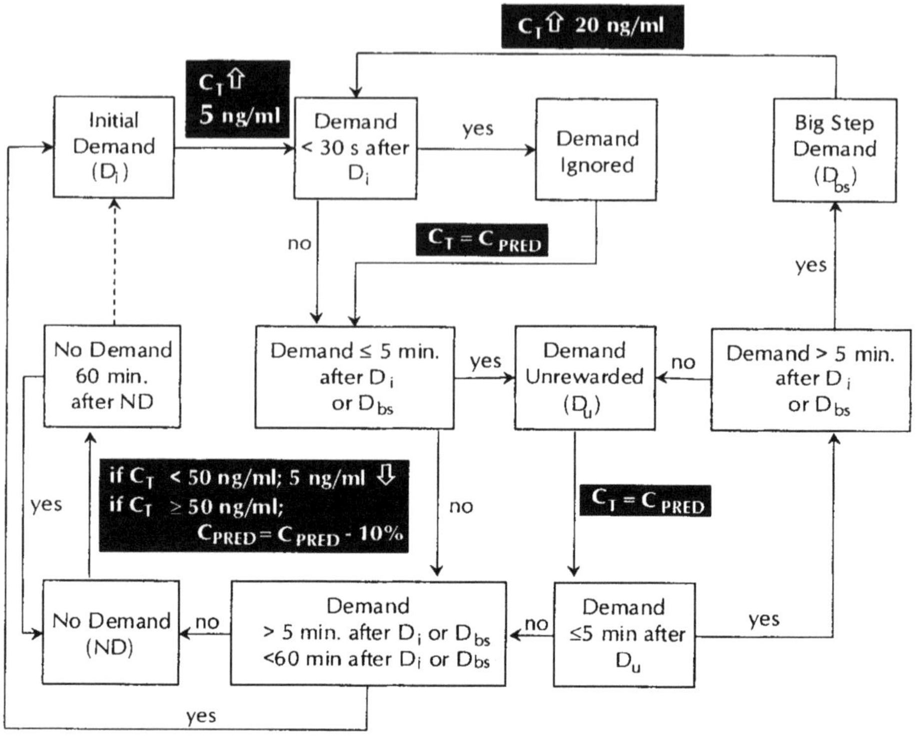

Figure 4
Flow diagram of the changes in target plasma concentration (C_T) of alfentanil using a Target Controlled Infusion of alfentanil for patient-controlled postoperative analgesia.

Conclusion

The use of TCI systems outside the operating room offers potential benefits to patient care. Several investigations describe that target controlled infusion devices of alfentanil and remifentanil can provide satisfactory analgesia. However, data from double-blind randomised controlled trials are scarce. The rapid onset of action, together with the flexibility of TCI, in particular when it is used in the patient-controlled mode, can be of benefit to future patients in pain. Overall, the bias and inaccuracy associated with the pharmacokinetic data, implemented in the TCI system used in the studies, are acceptable. However, occasionally, deviations between predicted and actually achieved plasma concentrations in individual patients may be considerable (see figure 3).

Further investigations are necessary to determine whether there are any advantages of the use of TCI administration of a specific opioid for postoperative analgesia. The optimal pharmacokinetic data sets for administration of prolonged infusions in specific patient populations, the optimum target concentrations and steering algorithms are yet to be determined. Target controlled infusions for postoperative pain relief are not necessarily restricted to opioids like alfentanil and remifentanil, with a rapid blood-brain equilibration. However, when for example morphine would be used by target controlled infusion, the rapid onset of action cannot be achieved, unless plasma concentrations are allowed to exceed the effect site concentrations. This potentially dangerous situation can theoretically be avoided if the effect site concentration, rather than the plasma concentration, is chosen as the target. However, current effect-site controlled infusion systems are still experimental.

When TCI is used in the patient-controlled mode, steering algorithms are necessary to adapt the target (the output of the TCI algorithm) to the varying pain stimuli in the postoperative period. One has to be aware of the fact that with the varying intensity of pain the effective analgesic concentration is constantly changing in the postoperative period. The target concentration is therefore fluctuating. TCI settings enable rapid titration to desired analgesic levels whenever the intensity of pain increases, but may require further optimization with respect to the downward titration (a larger step down and/or shorter interval between subsequent decreases) when pain diminishes. Therefore, when used in the postoperative period these algorithms are more important than the algorithms of the TCI system itself and need to be fully described in order to be able to compare experimental systems.

Improvements are also possible with respect to the safety of the TCI system. Coupling a respiration monitor to the TCI system could result in early detection of respiratory slowing. However, currently available respiration monitors appear to be insufficient and result in an unacceptably high incidence of false alarms and artefacts.

Further investigations of the TCI analgesic delivery systems in the patient-controlled mode compared to well-established existing analgesic techniques have to evaluate whether or not patient-controlled TCI delivery of analgesics will become a worthwhile addition to the existing armamentarium. Preliminary experience does not yet support the use of the patient-controlled TCI systems for postoperative analgesia without adequate supervision and monitoring.

References

1. Maitre PO, Vozeh S, Heykants J, Thomson DA, Stanski DR. Population pharmacokinetics of alfentanil: The average dose-plasma concentration relationship and interindividual variability in patients. Anesthesiology 1987;66:3-12.
2. Davies FW, White M, Kenny GNC. Postoperative analgesia using a computerised infusion of alfentanil following aortic bifurcation graft surgery. Int J Clin Monit Comput 1992;9: 207-12.
3. van den Nieuwenhuyzen MCO, Engbers FHM, Burm AGL, Lemmens HJM, Vletter AA, van Kleef JW, Bovill JG. Computer-controlled infusion of alfentanil for postoperative analgesia. Anesthesiology 1993;79:481-92.
4. Irwin MG, Jones RDM, Visram AR, Kornberg JP. A patient's experience of a new post-operative patient-controlled analgesic technique. Eur J Anaesthesiol 1994;11: 413-5.
5. van den Nieuwenhuyzen MCO, Engbers FHM, Burm AGL, Vletter AA, van Kleef JW, Bovill JG. Computer-controlled infusion of alfentanil versus patient-controlled administration of morphine for postoperative analgesia: A double-blind randomized trial. Anesth Analg 1995;81:671-9.
6. Irwin MG, Jones RDM, Visram AR, Kenny GNC. Patient-controlled alfentanil. Target-controlled infusion for postoperative analgesia. Anaesthesia 1996;51:427-30.
7. van den Nieuwenhuyzen MCO, Engbers FHM, Burm AGL, Vletter AA, van Kleef JW, Bovill JG: Target-controlled infusion of alfentanil for postoperative analgesia: a feasibility study and pharmacodynamic evaluation in the early postoperative period. Br J Anaesth 1997;78:17-23.
8. Checketts MR, Gilhooly CJ, Kenny GNC. Patient-maintained analgesia with target-controlled alfentanil infusion after cardiac surgery: a comparison with morphine PCA. Br J Anaesth 1998;80:748-51.
9. Schraag S, Kenny GN, Mohl U, Georgieff M Patient-maintained remifentanil target-controlled infusion for the transition to earley postoperative analgesia. Br J Anaesth 1998;81:365-8.
10. van den Nieuwenhuyzen MCO, Engbers FHM, Burm AGL, Vletter AA, van Kleef JW, Bovill JG: Target-controlled infusion of alfentanil for postoperative analgesia: contribution of plasma protein binding to intrapatient and interpatient variability. Br J Anaesth 1999;82:580-5.
11. Hill HF, Mackie AM, Jacobsen RC. Infusion-based Patient-Controlled Analgesia systems, In: Ferrante FM, Ostheimer GW, Covino BG, eds. Patient-Controlled Analgesia. Boston, Blackwell Scientific, 1990; pp 214-22.
12. Hill HF, Saeger L, Bjurstrom R, Donaldson G, Chapman CR, Jacobson R. Steady-state infusions of opioids in human volunteers. I. Pharmacokinetic tailoring. Pain 1990;43:57-67
13. Hill HF, Chapman CR, Saeger LS, Bjurstrom R, Walter MH, Schoene RB, Kippes M. Steady-state infusions of opioids in human volunteers. II. Concentration-effect relationships and therapeutic margins. Pain 1990;43:69-79.

14. Hill HF, Mackie AM, Coda BA, Iverson K, Chapman CR. Patient-controlled analgesic administration. A comparison of steady-state morphine infusions with bolus doses. Cancer 1991;67:873-82.
15. Hill HF, Jacobson RC, Coda BA, Mackie AM. A computer-based system for controlling plasma opioid concentration according to patient need for analgesia. Clin Pharmacokinet 1991;20:319-30.
16. Hill H, Mackie A, Coda B, Schaffer R, Jacobson R, Benedetti C. Evaluation of the accuracy of a pharmacokinetically-based patient-controlled analgesia system. Eur J Pharmacol 1992;43:67-75.
17. Mantha S, Thisted R, Foss J, Ellis JE, Roizen MF. A proposal to use confidence intervals for visual analogue scale data for pain management to determine clinical significance. Anesth Analg 1993;77:1041-7.

SEROTONIN: ITS IMPLICATIONS IN POST-OPERATIVE NAUSEA AND VOMITING

Alain Borgeat

Zürich, Switzerland

Introduction

Postoperative nausea and vomiting (PONV) still remain the most frequent and feared side effects for patients observed in the recovery room. One of the most recent advances in this clinical context is the introduction of the specific 5-HT3 antagonists for the prevention and/or treatment of PONV. The introduction of the 5-HT3 antagonists in anaesthetic practice was empirical for the relationship between serotonin concentrations and the effect of surgery and anaesthesiology are still unknown.

Physiology and pharmacology of serotonin (5-hydroxytryptamine)

An unidentified agent with vasoconstrictor activity was observed more than a century ago in coagulated blood. This substance was noted to be released from platelets which were known to be degraded in the clotting process. This unknown agent was isolated in a pure form in 1948 and in the following year was named 5-Hydroxytryptamine (5-HT). Five-hydroxytryptamine is found in the intestine, blood and in the central nervous system. About 80% (4-8 mg) is located in the enterochromaffin cells of the intestinal tract, 10% of the remaining

Table 1
Metabolism of serotonin (5-Hydroxytryptamine)

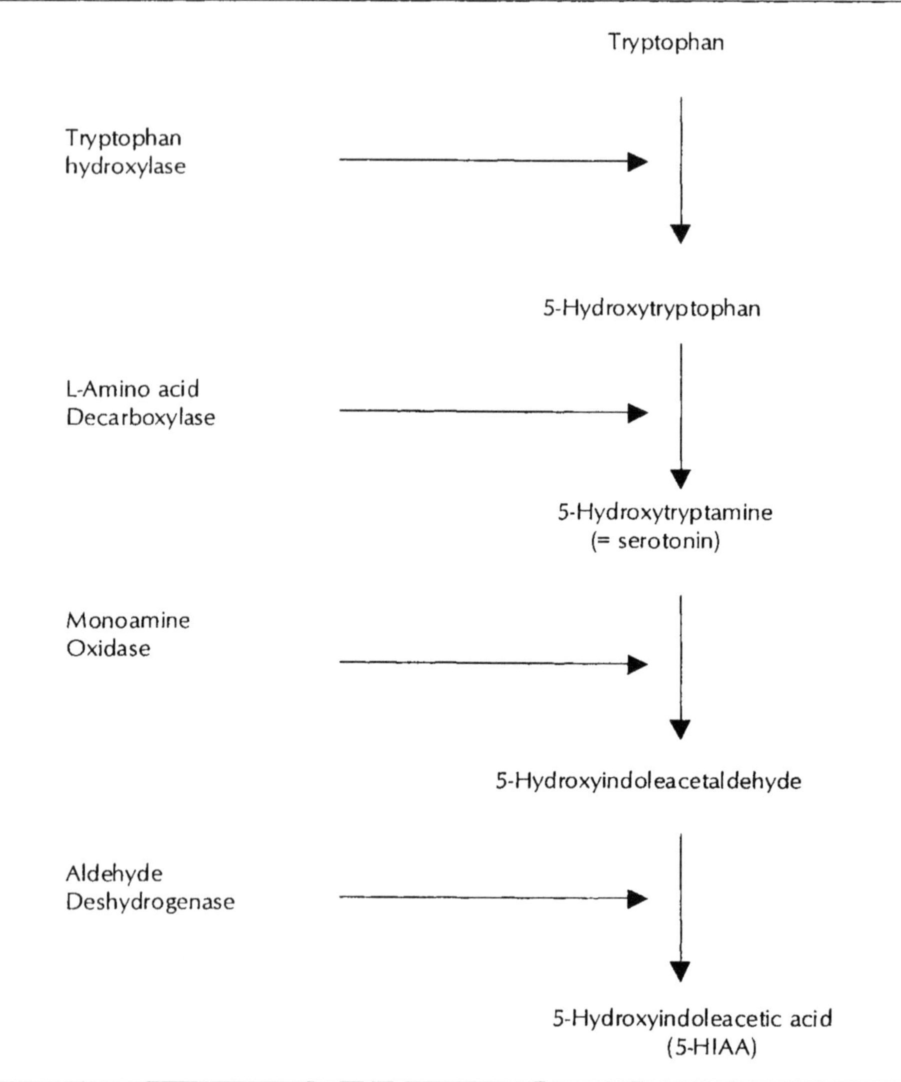

5-HT is also found in the myenteric plexus of the intestine, where it is believed to function as an excitatory neurotransmitter. Furthermore, 5-HT is present in high concentrations in platelets. Platelets release 5-HT during aggregation at a site of vessel wall injury (platelet release reaction). Lastly, 5-HT is also present in

Table 2
The modern classification of 5-HT receptors

5-HT receptor	Agonist ligands	Tissue activity
5-HT_1	Flesinoxan	Anxiolytic
5-HT_{1A}	Urapidil	Hypotension
5-HT_{1B}	5-HT	Autoreceptor (↓ acetylcholine and noradrenaline release)
5-HT_{1C}	5-HT	Vasodilatation
5-HT_{1D}	Sumatriptan, 5-HT	Migraine
5-HT_2	Ketanserine	Anxiety, depression, pain signals, platelet aggregation
5-HT_3	2-methyl-5-HT Phenybiguanide	Anxiety, nausea, pain signals, neural transmission
5-HT_4	Metoclopramide	EEG activity, gastric mobility, cardiac inotropy

the brain, particularly in the midbrain areas and the spinal cord. 5-HT is synthesised from tryptophan; approximately 1% from dietary tryptophan is converted to 5-HT. Degradation of 5-HT occurs by oxidative deamination mechanisms in the liver, brain, lung and numerous other tissues (table 1). The principal metabolite, 5-hydroxyindoleacetic acid (5-HIAA), is excreted in urine (2-10 mg/24 h in an average adult). Measurement of this product in urine may be used clinically as an indicator of the level of endogenous 5-HT metabolism in the body.

Eleven receptors now exist and the majority of these have been cloned and purified[1-3] (table 2). In contrast with the G protein 5-HT receptors, 5-HT3 receptors are ligand-gated, cation-selective ion channels, mediating membrane depolarisation and neuronal excitation.

Serotonin and emesis

The discovery and use of 5-HT3 receptor antagonists in the management of cisplatin-induced vomiting[4] has led to considerable interest in the role of serotonin in emesis and the neuronal pathways involved in the emetic reflex. Several experimental studies have shown that serotonin mediates its emetic sequelae by acting on 5-HT3 receptors situated both centrally, in the area postrema[5] and peripherally on nerve plexuses (vagal and splanchnic) within the wall

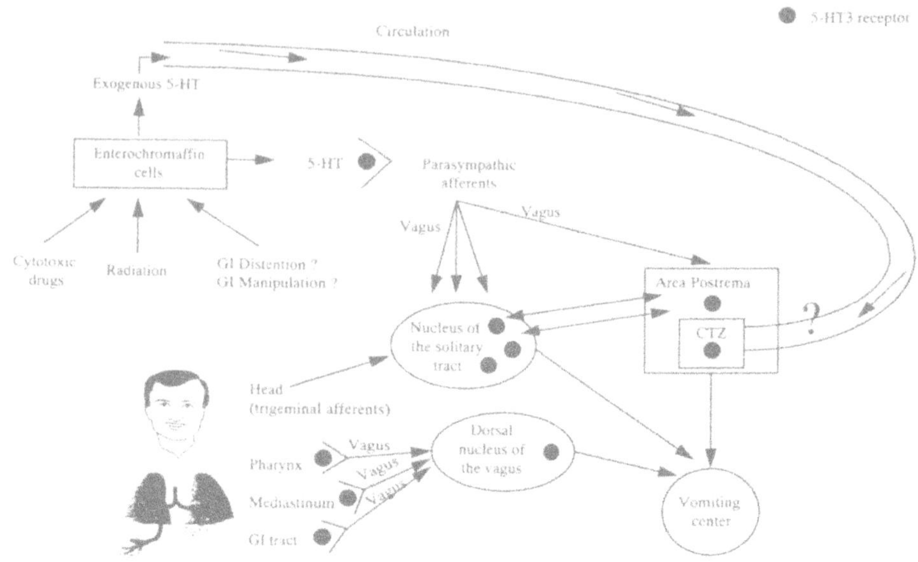

Figure 1
Links between 5-HT and emesis.

of the small intestine.[6] It was demonstrated that cisplatin caused damage to intestinal mucosa[7], resulting in the release of serotonin. The released serotonin acts on 5-HT3 receptors located on parasympathic nerve afferents in the myenteric plexus of the intestinal wall to initiate the emetic reflex.[5] Some studies in the cat revealed that the major part of the antiemetic effect of 5-HT3 antagonists after cisplatin administration was targeted on the peripheral myenteric intestinal part of the reflex rather than on the 5-HT3 receptors located in the area postrema.

The different possible links between serotonin and emesis are summarized in figure 1. The vomiting reflex itself is believed to have evolved as a protective mechanism for the removal of ingested toxins. It comprises a complex sequence of events involving different systems and is co-ordinated via nuclei situated in the medulla oblongata of the brain. The concept of a discrete vomiting center within the reticular formation was proposed by Borison and Wang.[8] The vomiting center itself does not respond to chemical application, although an area anatomically close to it, the chemoreceptor trigger zone, does respond and is closely linked to the initiation of the vomiting reflex. The chemoreceptor trigger zone is located within the area postrema, a structure that is more permeable than other nuclei within the brain to blood borne substances because of the lack of a blood-brain-barrier. This would then facilitate the diffusion of circulating emetogenic stimuli to stimulate the emetic reflex. However, it should be noted that an additional nucleus, the nucleus tractus solitarius, which lies immediately below the area postrema, is also likely to be involved in emesis. These two nuclei have rich neuronal connections[9] and, indeed, many of the functions of the nucleus tractus solitarius are encompassed in the vomiting process. Researchers have identified a relatively large density of 5-HT3 receptors within the area postrema and nucleus tractus solitarius.[10,11] The highest density of receptors was within the dorso-medial nucleus tractus solitarius, which may be of importance, since this region receives the highest density of vagal afferents which originate from the gut.[12] The vagal afferents posses 5-HT3 receptors. This is relevant, since the vagal nerve has actions in the mediation of the vomiting reflex and may provide a second and peripheral site of drug action.[13-15]

Serotonin and cancer chemotherapy

Chemotherapy regimens for the treatment of cancer are better known for their toxicity than for their efficacy. Among the side effects, nausea and vomiting are for patients the most feared complications. The comprehension of the role of serotonin as well as of the development and use of the 5-HT3 antagonists in this context come from studies performed during cancer chemotherapy. In 1990 Cubeddu et al.[16] measured the urinary excretion of 5-hydroxyindoleacetic acid (5-HIAA) in 24 patients receiving cisplatin therapy. An increase of 5-HIAA peaked between 6 and 8 h later and returned to baseline 24 h afterwards. In a second study,[17] the same authors included a control group which was hydrated and received mannitol just as the patients undergoing cisplatin treatment. In contrast to the treated group, no change in 5-HIAA excretion was observed in the control group. In the same study, no changes in the content of serotonin per platelet were found. These studies support the serotonin hypothesis and confirm results from the following trials. First, cisplatin was found to increase the turnover of ileal serotonin in the ferret.[18] Second, the depletion of tissue serotonin with p-chloro-phylalanine inhibited cisplatin-induced emesis in the ferret.[19] Third, administration of cisplatin in the isolated mesenteric beds induced the release of serotonin in guinea pigs.[20] Fourth, the presence of 5-HT3 receptors in vagal afferent fibers, when activated by serotonin, increased the firing rate of these fibers.[21] Lastly, increases in serotonin release, that occur in close relationship in time with the development of nausea and vomiting, have been reported following cisplatin-based chemotherapies in cancer patients.[10, 22] Thus, the association between nausea and vomiting and serotonin release during the first 24 h following cancer chemotherapy has clearly been established. In contrast, the relationship between nausea and vomiting and serotonin release during the delayed phase, the period during which consistent antiemetic control remains elusive, has not been extensively investigated. This issue was challenged by Wilder-Smith et al.[22], who studied the urinary excretion of 5-HIAA during the first 24 h after cisplatin treatment. The authors found a significant peak of 5-HIAA excretion 6 h after induction of chemotherapy, a return to baseline 16 h later and no 5-HIAA concentration peaks thereafter. The authors concluded that the absence of an increase of serotonin secretion during the delayed phase may question the use of the 5-HT3 antagonists during this period and explain the relative inefficacy of this class of drugs in the treatment of nausea and vomiting after the first 24 h following cancer treatment. From the results of these studies it is concluded that the 5-HT3 antagonists are very efficient in treating nausea and vomiting associated with an increased serotonin secretion, but that their efficacy may be less or absent when other mechanisms are involved.

Serotonin and anaesthesia

The introduction of the 5-HT3 antagonists in anaesthetic practice was purely empirical. At that time, no study had been done on the interactions of surgery, anaesthesiology and the metabolism and/or secretion of endogenous serotonin. Indeed, in contrast to the emetic responses to cytotoxic chemotherapy and radiotherapy, relatively little is know on the mechanisms involved in the control of postoperative nausea and vomiting (PONV). The first results dealing with this issue were promising. Leeser and Lip[23] administered 16 mg of ondansetron or a placebo, orally, in a double-blind study. The doses were given 1 h before operation and 8 h later in 84 ASA I-III patients undergoing major intraabdominal gynaecological surgery under general anaesthesia induced with thiopentone and maintained with 67% nitrous oxide and isoflurane in oxygen. Muscular relaxation was provided by vecuronium and analgesia was assured with alfentanil. Neuromuscular blockade was antagonised with neostigmine and atropine, when needed. Postoperative analgesia was provided with morphine and assessments of PONV were made at 1 and 24 h after operation. One hour after operation the incidence of nausea and vomiting was 52% and 40% in the placebo group, versus 17% and 12% in the ondansetron group, respectively. During the first 24 h after the surgical procedure 67% and 60% of the patients that received a placebo complained of nausea and vomiting, compared to 29% and 26% in the patients that received ondansetron. The efficacy of intravenous 5-HT3 antagonists in the treatment and prophylaxis of PONV was confirmed in several studies. Larijani et al.[24] studied 36 patients suffering from PONV after orthopaedic and gynaecological surgery. The patients were allocated randomly to receive either ondansetron 8 mg, i.v., or a placebo, in a double-blind study over 2-5 min. Ondansetron was statistically more effective than the placebo and control of nausea was achieved in 78% and 28% in the patients receiving ondansetron or the placebo, respectively. Although the majority of studies have shown the superiority of 5-HT3 antagonists over placebo or other often used antiemetics, some investigations were not able to demonstrate any advantages of the 5-HT3 antagonists in the prevention or treatment of PONV. Koivuranta et al.[25] investigated in a prospective, randomised, double blind, placebo-controlled trial the antiemetic efficacy of ondansetron, 4 mg, given prophylactically in 63 patients undergoing cholecystectomy. The general anaesthesia procedure was standardised for all patients. During the first 24 h postoperative, nausea was experienced by 64% of the patients in the ondansetron group and 56% in the placebo group, and emetic episodes occurred in 45% and 50% of the patients in the two groups, respectively. Sniadach and Alberts[26] compared ondansetron to droperidol in a randomised, prospective, double blind study in women undergoing gynaecologic laparoscopies. No difference in the number of women experiencing PONV was found during the first 24 postoperative hours. In children undergoing strabismus repair, Litman et al.[27] compared in a prospective, double-blinded, randomised trial droperidol with ondansetron. The children received either 0.15 mg/kg ondansetron, iv, or 0.075 mg/kg droperidol, iv, shortly after induction of anaesthesia. The anaesthetic technique was standardised. The incidence of nausea and vomiting was recorded during the first 24 postoperative hours. In the ondansetron group 94% were emesis free as compared to 81% in the droperidol group on the day of surgery. There were no significant differences in the number of episodes of emesis on the day after surgery or in the time of discharge. The contradictory results observed with the 5-HT3 antagonists in cancer chemotherapy during the delayed phase and in anaesthetic practice for the prevention and/or the treatment of PONV require a better understanding of the relationship that may exist between serotonin metabolism, surgical procedures and anaesthetic agents and techniques. The basic knowledge of the mechanisms involved in PONV is still limited and therefore, the beneficial effects of 5-HT3 antagonists in this context poorly understood. Various surgical procedures may excite 5-HT3 receptors on mucosal vagal afferents, thereby activating the afferent arm of the vomiting reflex, a mechanism similar to the one observed with cancer chemotherapy or radiation. The anaesthetic itself could disrupt mucosal enterochromaffin cells and induce release of paracrine transmitters, including serotonin, resulting in afferent vagal firing and initiation of the vomiting reflex. A similar mechanism of cell disruption may be induced as well by gastrointestinal distention caused by diffusion of nitrous oxide into the lumen of the gastrointestinal tract[28]. In addition, a laparotomy, involving manipulation and irritation of the gastrointestinal tract, could activate vagal afferents via mucosal serotonin release. Although these peripheral mechanisms are speculative, they may provide an explanation for the anti-emetic effects of the 5-HT3 antagonists in PONV. Outside the gastrointestinal tract, vagal peripheral afferents coming from the abdominal and the thoracic systems terminate in distinct, adjacent regions of the nucleus tractus solitarius.[29] It is also possible that stimulation of these afferent nerves may involve the 5-HT3 receptors and/or the serotonin of central origin to initiate the emetic reflex. It is known that patients undergoing surgery in the head and neck region are high-risk groups to PONV.[28] In this context, it was demonstrated that sensory afferent fibers of the trigeminal nerve terminate in the nucleus tractus solitarius.[30] Thus, surgery involving the head and neck may sensitise the nucleus tractus solitarius to induce emesis via stimulation of trigeminal afferents. Borgeat et al.[31] have investigated in a prospective study the consequences of the pneumoperitoneum during gynaecological or digestive procedures, both procedures being associated with a very high incidence of PONV, on the secretion of serotonin. The authors compared the excretion of the serotonin metabolite 5-hydroxyindoleacetic acid in 40 women undergoing either gynaecologic laparoscopic surgery or a traditional open laparotomy. Premedication, anaesthetic technique and postoperative pain treatment were standardised. The excretion of 5-HIAA corrected to creatinin was measured in all patients immediately after the induction of anaesthesia and this was repeated regularly until 9 h after induction. There was no difference in the excretion of 5-HIAA between the two groups and no increase was observed in either group. The incidence of nausea and vomiting was 50% and 35%, respectively, in the laparoscopy group versus 60% and 15%, in the laparotomy group (not significantly different). The excretion of 5-HIAA/creatinine was comparable in patients of both groups among those who vomited and those who did not. The authors conclude that an increase of serotonin secretion from the gut may not explain PONV associated with this type of surgery. The same group[32] investigated the relationship between the excretion of 5-HIAA corrected to creatinin excretion between 23 gravid women with hyperemesis gravidarum, 10 gravid women without nausea and vomiting, both groups within the first 3 months of pregnancy, and 10 non-gravid women of similar age not taking oral contraceptives. No significant difference in the urinary excretion of 5-HIAA/creatinine was found between the groups.

Conclusion

The role of serotonin in PONV still is unclear. The relationship between the different types of surgery, the anaesthetic drugs and techniques has not yet been investigated. A peripheral mechanism associated with an increase of serotonin release may not explain the PONV associated with laparoscopic surgery. The beneficial effect of the 5-HT3 antagonists after gynaecological laparoscopic surgery is most likely explained by an interaction within the central nervous system on the 5-HT3 receptor and/or the serotonin release, possibly within the nucleus tractus solitarius. Further studies on the complex interaction between peripheral and/or central serotonin release, peripheral or central 5-HT3 receptor stimulation or blockade, are needed to improve our understanding of the mechanisms associated with PONV and to better define the indications of 5-HT3 antagonists in PONV.

References

1. Hoyer D, Schoeffer P: 5-HT receptors. Subtypes and second messengers. J Receptor Res 1991; 11: 197-244
2. Peroutka SJ. 5-Hydroxytryptamine subtypes. Pharmacol Toxicol 1990; 67: 373-83
3. Zifa E, Fillion G. 5HT receptors. Pharmacol Rev 1992; 44: 401-58
4. Miller AD, Monaka S. Mechanisms of vomiting induced by serotonin 3 receptor agonists in the cat. Effect of splenectomay, vagotomy on area postrema lesions. J Pharmacol Exp Ther 1992; 260: 509-17
5. Tyers MG, Freeman AJ. Mechanisms of antiemetic activity of 5HT3 antagonists. Oncology 1991; 49: 263-8
6. Andrews PLR, Davis CJ, Bingham S, Davidson HIM, Hawthorn J, Maskell L. The abdominal visceral innervation and the emetic reflex: pathways, pharmacology and plasticity. Can J Physiol Pharmacol 1990; 68: 325-45
7. Milano S, Simon C, Grelot L. In vitro release and tissue release of ileal serotonin after cisplatin induced emesis in the cat. Clin Autonomic Research 1991; 1: 275-80
8. Borison HL, Wang SC. Physiology and pharmacology of vomiting. Pharmacol Rev 1953; 5: 193-230
9. Leslie RA, Gwyn DG. Neuronal connections of the area postrema. Fed Proc 1984; 43: 2941-3
10. Barnes NM, Costall B, Naylor RJ, Tattersall FD. Identification of 5-HT3 recognition sites in the ferret area postrema. J Pharm Pharmacol 1988; 40: 586-8
11. Kilpatrick GJ, Jones BJ, Tyers MB. The distribution of specific binding of the 5-HT3 receptor ligand (^{3}H)GR65630 in rat brain using quantitative receptor autoradiography. Neurosci Lett 1988; 94: 156-60
12. Leslie RA. Neuroactive substances in the dorsal vagal complex of the medulla oblongata; nucleus of the tractus solitarius, area postrema and dorsal motor nucleus of the vagus. Neurochem Int 1985; 7: 191-5
13. Andrews PLR, Bingham S, Davis CJ. Retching evoked by stimulation of abdominal vagal afferents in the anaesthetised ferret. J Physiol 1984; 358: 103P
14. Hawthorn J, Ostler KJ, Andrew PLR. The role of the abdominal visceral innervation and 5-hydroxytryptamine M-receptors in vomiting induced by the cytotoxic drugs cyclophosphamide and cisplatin in the ferret. Quart J Exp Physiol 1988; 73: 7-21
15. Andrews PLR, Hawthorn J. Evidence for an extra-abdominal site of action for the 5-HT3 receptor antagonist BRL43694 in inhibition of radiation-evoked emesis in the ferret. Neuropharmacology 1987; 26: 1367-70
16. Cubeddu LX, Hoffman IS, Fuenmayor NT et al. Efficacy of ondansetron (GR 38032F) and the role of serotonin in cisplatin induced nausea en emesis. N Engl J Med 1990; 322: 810-6
17. Cubeddu LX, Hoffmann IS, Fuenmayor NT et al. Changes in serotonin metabolism in cancer patients: Its relationship to nausea and vomiting induced by chemotherapeutic drugs. Br J Cancer 1992; 66: 198-203
18. Stables P, Andrews PLR, Bailey HE et al: Antiemetic properties of the 5-HT3-receptor antagonist, GR38032F. Cancer Treat Rev 1987; 14: 333-6
19. Barnes NM, Barry JM, Costal B et al: Antagonism by para-chlorophenylalanine of cisplatin-induced emesis. Br J Pharmacol 1987; 92: 649P
20. Schworer H, Racke K, Kilbinger H: Cisplatin increases the release of 5-hydroxytryptamine (5-HT) from the isolated vascularly perfused small intestine of the guinea-pig: Involvement of the 5-HT3 receptors. Naunyn Schmiedebergs Arch Pharmacol 1991; 344: 143-9

21. Andrews PRL. Neuropharmacology of emesis induced by cytotoxic drugs and radiation, in Diaz Rubio E, Martin M (eds); Antiemetic therapy: Current Status and Future Prospects. Madrid, Spain, Creaciones Elba, SA, 1992, pp 18-39
22. Wilder-Smith OHG, Borgeat A, Chappuis P, Fathi M, Forni M. Urinary serotonin metabolite excretion during cisplatin chemotherapy. Cancer 1993; 72: 2239-41
23. Leeser J, Lip H. Prevention of postoperative nausea and vomiting using ondansetron, a new, selective, 5-HT3 receptor antagonist. Anesth Analg 1991; 72: 751-5
24. Larijani GE, Gratz I Afshar M, Minassian S. Treatment of postoperative nausea and vomiting with ondansetron: a randomised, double blind comparison with placebo. Anesth Analg 1991; 73: 246-9
25. Koivuranta MK, Läärä E, Rhyänen PT. Anitemetic efficacy of prophylactic ondansetron in laparoscopic cholecystectomy. Anesthesia 1996; 51: 52-5
26. Sniadach MS, Alberts MS. A comparison of the prophylactic antiemetic effect of ondansetron and droperidol on patients undergoing gynecologic laparoscopy. Anesth Analg 1997; 85: 797-800
27. Litman RS, Wu CL, Lee A, Griswold JD, Voisine R, Marshall C. Prevention of emesis after strabismus repair in children: a prospective, double-blinded, randomized comparison of droperidol versus ondansetron. J Clin Anesth 1995; 7: 58-62
28. Cookson RF. Mechanisms and treatment of postoperative nausea and vomiting. In: Davies CJ, Lake-Bakaar GV, Grahame-Smith DG, eds Nausea and Vomiting: Mechanisms and Treatment. Berlin: Springer-Verlag, 1986; 130-50
29. Kalia M, Mesulam MM. Brain stem projections of sensory and motor components of the vagus complex in the cat: II. Laryngeal, tracheobronchial, pulmonary, cardiac and gastroinetstinal branches. J Comp Neurol 1980; 193: 467-508
30. Arbab MAR, Delagdo T, Wiklund L, Svendgaard NA. Brain stem terminations of the trigeminal and upper spinal ganglia innervation of the cerebrovascular system: WGA-HRP transganglionic study. J Cerebr Blood F Met 1988; 8: 54-63
31. Borgeat A, Hasler P, Fahti M. Gynecologic laparoscopic surgery is not associated with an increase of serotonin metabolites excretion. Anesth Analg 1998; 87: 1104-8
32. Borgeat A, Fathi M, Valiton A. Hyperemesis gravidarum: Is serotonin implicated ? Am J Obstet Gynecol 1997; 176: 476-7

www.ingramcontent.com/pod-product-compliance
Ingram Content Group UK Ltd.
Pitfield, Milton Keynes, MK11 3LW, UK
UKHW021833190726
13853UKWH00003B/1287

* 9 7 8 9 4 0 1 5 9 6 0 5 3 *